Disability in Africa

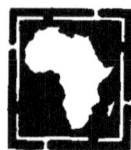

Rochester Studies in African History and the Diaspora

Toyin Falola, Series Editor
The Jacob and Frances Sanger Mossiker Chair in the Humanities
and University Distinguished Teaching Professor
University of Texas at Austin

Recent Titles

Plantation Slavery in the Sokoto Caliphate: A Historical and Comparative Study
Mohammed Bashir Salau

African Migration Narratives: Politics, Race, and Space
Edited by Cajetan Iheka and Jack Taylor

Ethics and Society in Nigeria: Identity, History, Political Theory
Nimi Wariboko

African Islands: Leading Edges of Empire and Globalization
Edited by Toyin Falola, R. Joseph Parrott, and Danielle Porter-Sanchez

Catholicism and the Making of Politics in Central Mozambique, 1940–1986
Eric Morier-Genoud

Liberated Africans and the Abolition of the Slave Trade, 1807–1896
Edited by Richard Anderson and Henry B. Lovejoy

The Other Abyssinians: The Northern Oromo and the Creation of Modern Ethiopia, 1855–1913
Brian J. Yates

Nigeria's Digital Diaspora: Citizen Media, Democracy, and Participation
Farooq A. Kperogi

West African Masking Traditions: History, Memory, and Transnationalism
Raphael Chijioke Njoku

Cultivating Their Own: Agriculture in Western Kenya during the "Development" Era
Muey C. Saeteurn

A complete list of titles in the Rochester Studies in African History and the Diaspora series may be found on our website, www.urpress.com.

Disability in Africa

Inclusion, Care, and the Ethics of Humanity

Edited by
Toyin Falola and Nic Hamel

UNIVERSITY OF ROCHESTER PRESS

Copyright © 2021 by the Editors and Contributors

All rights reserved. Except as permitted under current legislation, no part of this work may be photocopied, stored in a retrieval system, published, performed in public, adapted, broadcast, transmitted, recorded, or reproduced in any form or by any means, without the prior permission of the copyright owner.

First published 2021

University of Rochester Press
668 Mt. Hope Avenue, Rochester, NY 14620, USA
www.urpress.com
and Boydell & Brewer Limited
PO Box 9, Woodbridge, Suffolk IP12 3DF, UK
www.boydellandbrewer.com

ISBN-13: 978-1-58046-971-5
ISSN: 1092-5228; v. 91

Library of Congress Cataloging-in-Publication Data

Names: Falola, Toyin, editor, author. | Hamel, Nic, editor, author.
Title: Disability in Africa : inclusion, care, and the ethics of humanity / edited by Toyin Falola and Nic Hamel.
Description: Rochester : University of Rochester Press, 2021. | Series: Rochester studies in African history and the diaspora, 1092-5228 ; 91 | Includes bibliographical references and index.
Identifiers: LCCN 2020056460 (print) | LCCN 2020056461 (ebook) | ISBN 9781580469715 (hardback) | ISBN 9781787446717 (ebook) | ISBN 9781787449909 (epub)
Subjects: LCSH: Sociology of disability--Africa. | People with disabilities—Africa—Social conditions.
Classification: LCC HV1559.A35 D57 2021 (print) | LCC HV1559.A35 (ebook) | DDC 362.4096—dc23
LC record available at https://lccn.loc.gov/2020056460
LC ebook record available at https://lccn.loc.gov/2020056461

This publication is printed on acid-free paper.

Printed and bound in Great Britain by
TJ Books Ltd, Padstow, Cornwall

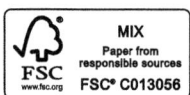

For our students, the University of Texas at Austin:
Anna Lee Carothers, Abikal Borah, Devon Hiaso, Simi Hassan,
and Shannon Doyle

Contents

Part One. Introducing the Field

1. Africanizing Disability: Toward an Articulation of African Disability Studies   1
   Toyin Falola and Nic Hamel

2. Disability Studies: A Disciplinary Overview   47
   Toyin Falola, Anna Lee Carothers, and Nic Hamel

Part Two. Theorizing Disability in Africa

3. An African Ethics of Social Well-Being: Understanding Disability and Public Health   75
   Maria Berghs

4. Rethinking African Disability Studies: From the Cultural-Deficit Model to a Socioeconomic Perspective   91
   Fikru Negash Gebrekidan

5. Disability in Africa: A Cultural/Religious Perspective   115
   Mary Nyangweso

6. Disability and Cultural Meaning Making in Africa   137
   Kathryn Linn Geurts

Part Three. Representation and Cultural Expressions

7. Disfiguration, Trauma, and Disability: Reclaiming the Body and the Case against Prosthetics   161
   Ernest Cole

8. Paradoxical Dramaturgies: Disability, Ritual, and Resistance in the Plays of Wole Soyinka   185
   Nic Hamel

9. Demonizing Madness: Mental Disorders as *Deus Ex Machina* in Nollywood Movies 209
Kolawole Olaiya

10. Masculinity, Disability, and Empire in J.M. Coetzee's *Waiting for the Barbarians* 228
Saloua Ben Zahra

Part Four. Education, Community, and Caregiving

11. Addressing Poverty and Inequality in Sub-Saharan Africa: Fostering Inclusive Education of Children with Disabilities 241
Serges Djoyou Kamga

12. Inclusive Education and Cultural Relevance in East Africa 255
Angi Stone-MacDonald and Ozden H. Pinar-Irmak Tanzania

13. Youth, Women, and Disability in Africa: Economic Empowerment and Community Strategies to Leave No One Behind 286
Ntombekhaya Tshabalala, Elizabeth Ladjer Bibi Agbettor, and Theresa Lorenzo Ghana + S. Africa

14. Caregiving and Support in African Context: A Personal Perspective 306
Frances Emily Owusu-Ansah — Ghana

Part Five. Activism and Barriers to Inclusion

15. So That the Stew Reaches Everybody: Women's Negotiations of Leadership and Power in Ghana's DPO's 319
Denise M. Nepveux — Ghana

16. Disability Policy, Movement Activism, and the Nonenforcement of a Disability Act: The Case of Ghana 343
Emmanuel Sackey — Ghana

17. Students with Disabilities' Lack of Opportunity for Sport and Recreational Activities: The Case of South African Universities 361
Desire Chiwandire

18. Rehabilitation and the Realization of Disability Rights 389
Serges Djoyou Kamga

Conclusion: A Research Agenda for African Disability Studies   405
Anna Lee Carothers and Toyin Falola

Selected Bibliography   423

Notes on Contributors   425

Index   431

Part One
Introducing the Field

Chapter One

Africanizing Disability

Toward an Articulation of African Disability Studies

Nic Hamel and Toyin Falola

That impairment is an actual or potential condition of all living bodies in all places is indisputable. The way that societies treat people with impairments certainly varies, but as disability studies scholars have repeatedly illustrated, the overwhelming tendency is to treat those with impairments poorly. And social mistreatment can be as disabling, if not more so, than physical or mental impairments themselves. To address the forms of disablement that Africans face requires confronting a variety of challenges to social acceptance that arise from specific conditions of history, geography, and economic factors. Among the most prominent challenges to disabled Africans are indigenous, colonial, and postcolonial stigmas, legacies of armed conflict, dense urban zones, vast rural areas, epidemiological risks, misplaced governmental and humanitarian priorities, as well as financial exploitation and underdevelopment. However, Africa has also seen prominent social mobilizations of disabled people who have secured substantial, if still incomplete, gains across the continent. Most African nations now formally acknowledge the special status of disabled people. Aid organizations operating in Africa are beginning to incorporate more socially conscious approaches to disability. Africans' own communalist traditions and practices are enabling more social inclusion for people with disabilities. An African approach to disability combines the insights of disability studies with the actual contexts of African experiences and acknowledges both how Africa creates problems for traditional disability studies approaches, even as it also offers exciting new potentialities.

Disability studies as an academic discipline emerged in the late twentieth century as an arm of the Anglo and European political movements for disability empowerment. However, tools developed in the minority world left disability scholars unequipped to fully address lived experiences of disability in low- and middle-income countries where "exclusion and inaccessibility are by no means unique to people with disabilities."[1] Recent attention has been paid to the process of "globalizing" disability studies by recognizing the particular challenges of disability in the Global South. From this process, a field is emerging that combines issues of debilitation, development, and humanitarian policy with traditional disability studies critiques of stigma, ostracization, and disempowerment. As disability studies comes to terms with its inherently problematic universalisms, care should be taken to also adequately describe the particular conditions in individual Global South contexts. We argue here that Africa specifically, beyond generalizations of the Global South, presents a range of challenges and opportunities for the discipline of disability studies that warrants consideration as an identifiably important field.

As recently as 2007, Benedicte Ingstad, a Norwegian medical anthropologist researching disability in Botswana, reportedly was asked by a reviewer, "Is being blind in Africa really so fundamentally different from being blind in Norway?"[2] This question relies on two dubious assumptions: first, that disability is predominantly or primarily a biomedical condition of an individual body, and second, that lived experiences of people in Africa and Europe are fundamentally similar. The first assumption has been endlessly critiqued by swaths of disability scholars,[3] while the second has consistently

---

1   Clare Barker and Stuart Murray, "Disabling Postcolonialism: Global Disability Cultures and Democratic Criticism," in *The Disability Studies Reader*, Lennard J. Davis, 4th ed.(New York and London: Routledge, 2013), 70.

2   Benedicte Ingstad, "Seeing Disability and Human Rights in the Local Context: Botswana Revisited," in *Disability in Local and Global Works*, eds. Benedicte Ingstad and Susan Reynolds Whyte (Berkeley: University of California Press, 2007), 250.

3   This volume includes an introductory chapter that summarizes key developments and issues in traditional disability studies, intended primarily for readers who may have limited experiences of the concerns of disability studies as a discipline.

been disproved by Africanists and other postcolonial theorists.[4] While the social critique developed by Northern disability studies is a necessary component for addressing disability in African contexts, as Ingstad illustrates, other hotly debated problems in the field are entirely irrelevant: "Thus for a poor hearing-impaired woman in a village in the Kalahari it is presently of little interest whether she is called 'deaf,' 'disabled,' or a 'person with a disability.' (She does not have equivalent words in her language anyway.) Her agenda would be more realistically be summarized as access to food and firewood, and care from her children tomorrow."[5] This volume argues that fundamental theoretical questions about disability and Africa, as well as the myriad practical consequences that emerge from them, require a methodology that combines the postcolonial, subaltern, and indigenous approaches of African studies with a disability studies focus on access, embodiment, and rehabilitation. We suggest that a reactivation of an African communalist ethos is necessary to improve the lives of Africans with disabilities. This can be accomplished through (1) a critical evaluation of African cultures and belief systems with regard to disability; (2) an investment in local communities of families, caregivers, and disabled peoples' organizations; and (3) productive cooperation among national governments, NGOs, and the international humanitarian community to recognize and respond the unique situations of disabled people in Africa.

Outside of disability studies, the concept of disability is often used as a metaphor for African colonial and postcolonial conditions. A prominent example is Nelson Mandela's apartheid-era pronouncement that "Africans want a just share in the whole of South Africa; they want security and a stake in society. Above all, we want equal political rights, because without them our disabilities will be permanent."[6] Such statements serve to emphasize the similar sorts of oppression experienced both by Africans and by people with disabilities worldwide. Indeed, such rhetoric was instrumental for early disability movements in the global North. Vic Finkelstein, a disabled white

---

4   See V. Y. Mudimbe, *The Invention of Africa: Gnosis, Philosophy and the Order of Knowledge* (Bloomington: Indiana University Press, 1988); Mahmood Mamdani, *Citizen and Subject: Contemporary Africa and the Legacy of Late Colonialism* (Princeton, NJ: Princeton University Press, 1996); Achille Mbembe, *On the Postcolony* (Berkeley: University of California Press, 2001); and Boaventura de Sousa Santos, *Epistemologies of the South* (New York and London: Routledge, 2015).

5   Ingstad, "Seeing Disability and Human Rights in the Local Context," 250.

6   Nelson Mandela, *The Struggle is My Life* (New York: Pathfinder, 2013), 306.

South African exiled for his political activities, used apartheid as an analogy for the treatment of disabled people in Britain.[7] The rhetorical link from Africans to disabled people generally emphasizes the experiences of marginalization and exploitation shared by persons inhabiting each category.[8]

Similarly, Frantz Fanon often scathingly described colonial debilitation in terms related to disability, both directly and indirectly. Direct references to colonial disablement include Fanon's 1952 polemic "North African Syndrome," where he describes a malady in colonized North Africans that European physicians refused to adequately recognize "pain without lesion, this illness distributed in and over the whole body, this continuous suffering."[9] Similarly, Fanon explicitly argued in 1963, after the Algerian revolution, that "the truth is that colonization, in its very essence, already appeared to be a great purveyor of psychiatric hospitals"[10] In a more explicitly metaphorical vein, Fanon also criticized the colonial endeavor in Algeria as an "attempt to decerebralize a people"[11] and claimed that "apart from the pathology of torture, the pathology of the tortured and that of the perpetrator, there is a pathology of the entire atmosphere in Algeria."[12] Prominent disability studies scholars in the Global North often deploy Fanon's theoretical heft to emphasize the magnitude of oppression that disabled people experience.[13] Again, the language of postcolonial resistance is intricately

---

7   Mark Priestley, "Disability Studies: The International Context," *Disability and Social Change: A South African Agenda* (2006): 23.
8   For an analogous argument concerning the disability inflected Pan-African rhetoric of Kwame Nkrumah, see Evelyn Kissi, "Sankofa: The Critical Nkrumahist Theory," *Africology: The Journal of Pan African Studies* 12, no. 7 (2018): 154–174.
9   Frantz Fanon, *Toward the African Revolution*, trans. Haakon Chevalier (New York: Grove Press, 1967), 7.
10 Fanon, *Wretched of the Earth*, trans. Richard Philcox (New York: Grove Press, 2004), 181.
11 Fanon, *Toward the African Revolution*, 53.
12 Fanon, *Wretched of the Earth*, 216.
13 See James L. Charlton, *Nothing About Us Without Us: Disability Oppression and Empowerment* (Berkeley: University of California Press, 2000); Tom Shakespeare, *Help* (Birmingham: Venture Press, 2000); Lennard J. Davis, *Bending Over Backwards: Disability, Dismodernism, and Other Difficult Positions* (New York: New York University Press, 2002); Rosemarie Garland-Thomson, *Staring: How We Look* (Oxford: Oxford University Press, 2009); David T. Mitchell and Sharon L. Snyder, "Disability as Multitude:

intermingled with the language of disability in a manner that operates in both directions simultaneously.

However, metaphorical uses of disability also often make disability scholars uncomfortable. As media theorist Vivian Sobchack asserts, disability metaphors are often reductive and reduce the complexity of disabled bodies.[14] By treating disability as a metaphor rather than a social and material fact, Mandela and Fanon's language dismisses the lived experiences of the substantial number of Africans who have disabilities. This dismissal is particularly galling since, as Nirmala Erevelles argues, disabled people in the Global South "run the risk of almost complete erasure, and, subsequently, face the most extreme dehumanization on account of this non-recognition."[15] The fundamental activist claim of disability studies is the argument that disabilities are most insidious in their manifestations of social barriers, stigma, and dehumanization. Social and material conditions for disabled people in Africa exacerbate many of these challenges even as they present a number of others; thus, they require urgent and unique approaches that both acknowledge and radically revise the methods of traditional disability studies.

Our project in this volume is not merely to extend disability studies to incorporate the insights of African studies. Rather, we wish to stage a productive encounter at the intersection of these disciplines: an encounter that can develop new approaches to African disability based on the realities faced by disabled Africans. Within disability studies, scholars increasingly recognize that the discipline overwhelmingly relies on "a one-way transfer of ideas and knowledge from the North to the South"[16] (Finkelstein and Fanon notwithstanding) and that the field thus requires a process of decolonization. A growing number of researchers have recently begun to suggest approaches to

---

Re-Working Non-Productive Labor," *Journal of Literary and Cultural Disability* 4, no. 2 (2010): 179–193; Dan Goodley, *Dis/Ability Studies: Theorising Disablism and Ableism* (New York and London: Routledge, 2014); Robert McRuer, *Crip Times: Disability, Globalization and Resistance* (New York: New York University Press, 2018).

14 Vivian Sobchack, "A Leg to Stand On: Prosthetics, Metaphor, and Materiality," in *Carnal Thoughts: Embodiment and Moving Image Culture* (Berkeley: University of California Press, 2004), 209.

15 Nirmala Erevelles, *Disability and Difference in Global Contexts: Enabling a Transformative Body Public* (London: Palgrave Macmillan, 2011), 122.

16 Helen Meekosha, "Decolonising Disability: Thinking and Acting Globally," *Disability & Society* 26, no. 6 (2011): 668.

disability based on "a critical postcolonial disability research agenda,"[17] or are explicitly framed by African worldviews. Many of these scholars proceed from the assumption that "African knowledge, and its method of acquisition, has a practical, collective and social or interpersonal slant"[18] and that this has significant implications for the way that Africans can and should approach issues around disability.[19] Historian Jenifer L. Barclay pushes this encounter in an expressly censorious direction when she claims that "Africanizing knowledge about impairment and disability, then, demands greater attention to African cosmologies, ontologies, and epistemologies, but it also requires a more critical assessment of scholarship about disability across the continent today and in the past."[20] The authors in this volume utilize a multiplicity of critical disciplinary methodologies to reflect and advance an African disability studies that is keenly attentive to the possibilities offered by the uniqueness and diversity of African contexts.

This chapter will attempt to address the breadth of issues central to African disability studies: African conceptions of disability, African disability rhetoric, structural barriers, and opportunities, as well as challenges to African disability activists and policymakers. We begin with an overview of indigenously African definitions and conceptual understandings of disability, impairment, and debility, as well as the influences and legacies of colonialism on these concepts. We then consider the various ways in which African disability is framed, especially in terms of human rights, intersectionality, caregiving, and communalism. We outline the uniquely African circumstances that complicate and aggravate the experiences of people with disabilities across the continent, including challenges related to poverty, geography, and globalized biopolitics. We then conclude with a consideration of the

---

17 Tsitsi Chataika, "Disability, Development and Postcolonialism," in *Disability and Social Theory: New Developments and Directions*, eds. Dan Goodley, Bill Hughes, and Lennard Davis (London: Palgrave Macmillan, 2012), 253.

18 Frances E. Owusu-Ansah and Gubela Mji, "African Indigenous Knowledge and Research," *African Journal of Disability* 2 (2013): 2.

19 Theresa Lorenzo, Mzolisi ka Toni, and Mark Priestley, "Developing a Disability Studies *Programme*: Engaging Activism and Academia," in *Disability and Social Change: A South African Agenda*, ed. Brian Watermeyer et al. (Cape Town, South Africa: Human Sciences Research Council, 2006), 180.

20 Jennifer L. Barclay, "Differently Abled: Africanisms, Disability, and Power in the Age of Transatlantic Slavery," in *Bioarchaeology of Impairment and Disability*, ed. Jennifer F. Byrnes and Jennifer L. Muller (New York: Springer, 2017), 82.

successes and difficulties in implementing disability policy in Africa, as well as descriptions of the successful approaches taken by local, national, and international organizations.

African Concepts of Disability: Meaning Making, Indigeneity, and Colonialism

The terms "Africa" and "disability" share a variety of features. Both terms are widely used and understood, even as each contains multiple and actively contested meanings. Both terms have historically tended to carry negative connotations, even as many argue for their positive value. Both terms may be said to have existed for all of human history, even as their boundaries were arbitrarily formalized in the minority world of the nineteenth century. Kenyan Africanist Ali A. Mazrui stressed that "Africa is a *concept*, pregnant with the dreams of millions of people. It is one of the great ironies of modern African history that it took European colonialism to inform Africans that they were Africans. . . . Europe's supreme gift was the gift of African identity, bequeathed without grace of design—but a reality all the same."[21] Meanwhile, Cameroonian philosopher Achille Mbembe offers a somewhat less optimistic framing: "To a great degree, what is called *Africa* is first and foremost a geographical accident. Moving from the sphere of geography to the sphere of representation, this accident is subsequently invested with a multitude of significations, diverse imaginary contents, or even fantasies, which by force of repetition, end up becoming authoritative narratives."[22] Both definitions emphasize how "Africa" is a term both historically contingent and externally enforced but nevertheless also a term that has profound real-world implications for a significant percentage of the world's population. With merely a few alterations, the same claims may be made about "disability."

Just as the ancient landmass contributes only a fraction of meaning to the word "Africa," so does the continuous existence of impairments fail to adequately define "disability." With particular reference to Nigeria and the Mali empire, Barclay interrogates how "the notions of 'impairment' and

---

21 Ali A. Mazrui, "The Re-Invention of Africa: Edward Said, V. Y. Mudimbe, and Beyond," *Research in African Literatures* 36, no. 3 (2005): 74.

22 Achille Mbembe, "On the Power of the False," trans. Judith Inggs, *Public Culture* 14, no. 3 (2002): 631–632.

'disability' appear to be precisely the kind of concepts that do not hold up as universal, transhistorical categories of analysis. These terms convey a sense of lack, limitation, disempowerment, and negativity that fails to adequately capture perceptions of some people with embodied differences as empowered in precolonial West African societies."[23] By combining both overdetermined signifiers into a consideration of African disability, the conventional associations become particularly insidious. Nepveux and Smith Beitiks examine cultural representations of African disability and find that disability in Africa represents "inertia, interpersonal violence and indifference, and fatalism . . . the message is clear that Africa is the home of disability, yet it is *no* place to be disabled."[24]

It seems that disability, another colonial import, continues to function in a way that extracts value from African bodies in order to satisfy the desires of the minority world. According to historian Matthew Heaton the connection of impaired Africans to European self-consciousness has in fact always been a part of the colonial project in Africa, portraying Africans as "naturally diseased, unsanitary people ignorant of basic hygiene and medical practices. This became the unifying narrative of colonialism regarding African "salvation" and "civilization."[25]

If the predominant connotations of African disability have evolved from a colonial superiority to a patronizingly humanitarian one, the important task becomes to locate and examine Afrocentric definitions to evaluate how Africans actually experience disability.

Indigenous Conceptions of Disability

Even as the most widespread assumptions of disabled Africans are overwhelmingly figures of pity or pathos, the actual attitudes on the continent are far more varied. Indigenous African concepts of disability are as diverse as Africa itself and contain a range of both positive and negative representations

---

23 Barclay, "Differently Abled," 81.
24 Denise Nepveux and Emily Smith Beitiks, "Producing African Disability through Documentary Film: Emmanuel's Gift and Moja Moja," *Journal of Literary and Cultural Disability Studies* 4, no. 3 (2010): 244.
25 Matthew Heaton, "Health and Medicine in Colonial Society," in *The Palgrave Handbook of African Colonial and Postcolonial History*, ed. Martin Shanguhyia and Toyin Falola (London: Palgrave Macmillan, 2018), 307.

of disabled people. There is substantial evidence that in ancient Egypt, people with physical impairments, especially dwarves, were well treated and often included in the mainstream of social life.[26] Sunjata, the founder of the Mali empire, is said to have been born unattractive and unable to walk but became a great military and political leader.[27] In contemporary East Africa, "integration into community life" and "fit within the social norms" are more important to social acceptance than impairment.[28] The Chagga of Tanzania consider people with physical impairments to be "pacifiers of the evil spirits."[29] In Somalia, "the Hubeer do not discriminate firmly between disability and disease . . . the same values and indicators of health are used for both categories."[30]

With particular reference to the Côte d'Ivoire, anthropologist Patrick J. Devlieger claims that "the category of the extraordinary in West-African societies is clearly conceptually marked as 'not belonging.' Such a conceptual distinction need not necessarily result in social exclusion. Instead, the

---

26   See Chahira Kozma, "Dwarfs in Ancient Egypt," *American Journal of Medical Genetics* 140, no. 4 (2006): 303–311; David Jeffreys and John Tate, "Disability, Madness, and Social Exclusion in Dynastic Egypt," *Madness, Disability and Social Exclusion: The Archaeology and Anthropology of "Difference,"* ed. Jane Hubert (New York and London: Routledge, 2001), 87–95.

27   Barclay describes how the story of Sunjata could be criticized through a traditional disability studies approach "as yet another version of an 'overcoming narrative' of disability. This interpretation, however, rests on the belief that able-bodiedness is always appreciated as "normal" and "superior." Read through a different lens, this moment in the epic instead dramatizes the ways in which assumptions about embodied forms of difference lead some to underestimate those with differently abled bodyminds, denying them strength and power. That Sunjata, the powerful Lion, ultimately arose by leaning on his aged, deformed mother lends further support to this interpretation." See Barclay, "Differently Abled," 85.

28   Angi Stone-MacDonald and Gretchen Butera, "Cultural Beliefs and Attitudes about Disability in East Africa," *Review of Disability Studies: An International Journal* 8, no. 1 (2012): 69.

29   Chomba Wa-Munyi, "Past and Present Perceptions towards Disability: A Historical Perspective," *Disability Studies Quarterly* 32, no. 2 (2012).

30   Bernhard Helander, "Disability as Incurable Illness: Health, Process, and Personhood in Southern Somalia," in *Disability and Culture*, eds. Benedicte Ingstad and Susan Reynolds Whyte (Berkeley: University of California Press, 1995), 89.

presence and care of persons with visible differences is characterized by social tolerance."[31] Among the Anlo of Ghana, the emphasis is on interdependence and "relations of being" that are not affected by impairment.[32] In northern Nigeria, "A spirit may have crippled you, but stigma is not attached to 'you', though the spirit who wounded you or is possessing you (and causing you to behave oddly) may be stigmatized. . . . If, as with a disability, there is no recovery, so be it: your 'housing' is defective, but 'you' are not."[33] Also of particular note in Nigeria:

> In Igbo- and Yorubaland, children born with certain physical marks who developed seizures or forms of madness in which they heard voices were (and sometimes still are) thought of as *àbikú* or *ògbánge* children . . . *Àbikú* or *ògbánge* children often receive special treatment from their mothers who coax them to stay in the material world where, because of their perceived spiritual power, they have license to create special songs and dances that they perform in festivals. If they survive to adulthood, *àbikú* or *ògbánge* simply become ordinary members of society because it is believed that their parents' kindness convinced them to stay in the material world.[34]

In Cameroon, Bantu farmers with physical impairments are incorporated into farm work, while disabled people in Baka are fed and taken care of by their extended families.[35] A similar communal investment is evident in Botswana, where "Batswana understand impaired relationships to generate body misfortune, which in turn is managed as disability. . . . While people are very interested in opportunities to do for themselves, they also rightly understand themselves to be living in a web of dependencies, and they strive

---

31 Patrick J. Devlieger, "At the Interstices of Classification: Notes on the Category of Disability in Sub-Saharan Africa," *Research in Social Science and Disability* 5 (2010): 92.
32 Kathryn Geurts, *Culture and the Senses: Bodily Ways of Knowing in an African Community* (Berkeley: University of California Press, 2002), 215.
33 Murray Last, "Social Exclusion in Northern Nigeria," in *Madness, Disability and Social Exclusion: The Archaeology and Anthropology of "Difference,"* ed. by Jane Hubert (New York and London: Routledge, 2001), 221.
34 Barclay, "Differently Abled," 86–87.
35 Mikako Toda, "Disability and Charity Among Hunter-Gatherers and Farmers in Cameroon," *Senri Ethnological Reports* 143 (2017): 79.

to manage and foster the nurturing side of these dependencies."[36] Proverbs across sub-Saharan Africa caution against laughing at people with disabilities: "The proverb *Tosepanga lemene, Efile kiakupanga* ('Don't laugh at the disabled person, God keeps on creating you') is widely used among the Songye ... Among the Shona of Zimbabwe, the proverb *Seka hurema wafa* ('Laugh at disability after you are dead') is widely used and in Swahili (Tanzania and parts of Kenya) many similar proverbs exist."[37]

While such encouraging and nuanced characterizations of disability are prevalent across Africa, stigmatization of people with disabilities is also certainly present, not unlike the situation in the Global North. Just as many proverbs dictate civil treatment of disabled people, so do many advocate avoidance, "as in the Wolof proverb *Ku bëgë dundël 9 walaakaana 10 kel len* ("If you want to feed nine disabled persons, you will end up being the 10th") or the Zambian proverb *Simweenda aumineme ayebo ulaminama* ("You who walk with a deformed person, will also be deformed")."[38] In Morocco, the cultural tendencies are even less generous, since "disability is often associated with some hereditary weakness and most often perceived as a curse from God, a punishment that is afflicted on those who deserve it." [39] McKenzie and Chataika document how disabled people in Africa are often associated with malign spirits and/or family transgression, including "witchcraft, a curse or punishment from God, anger of ancestral spirits, bad omens, reincarnation, heredity, incestuous relationships and the misdemeanours of the mother."[40]

Children stigmatized for these reasons may be beaten, neglected, or even killed to cleanse them of evil spirits. While the prevalence of spiritual

---

36   Julie Livingston, *Debility and the Moral Imagination in Botswana* (Bloomington: Indiana University Press, 2005), 10.

37   Patrick J. Devlieger, "Frames of Reference in African Proverbs on Disability," *International Journal of Disability, Development and Education* 46, no. 4 (1999): 441–442.

38   Devlieger, "Frames of Reference in African Proverbs on Disability," 446.

39   Gulnara Z. Karimova, Daniel A Sauers, and Firdaousse Dakka, "The Portrayal of People with Disabilities in Moroccan Proverbs and Jokes," *Journal of Arab & Muslim Media Research* 8, no. 3 (2015): 245.

40   Judith McKenzie and Tsitsi Chataika. "Supporting Families in Raising Disabled Children to Enhance Childhood Development," in *The Palgrave Handbook of Disabled Children's Childhood Studies*, ed. Katherine Runswick-Cole, Tillie Curran, and Kirsty Liddiard (London: Palgrave Macmillan, 2018), 318.

accounts of disability in Africa undoubtedly affects the way that individuals with disabilities are treated, a danger for disability scholars would be to dwell in a perceived exoticism of these beliefs rather than their practical and material consequences.[41]

Perhaps the most disturbing aspect of indigenous African approaches to disability has to do with the practice of infanticide, a practice in which many cultures across the world have engaged throughout history. In Maasiland, there have been reports of children with disabilities murdered by their parents, "with the excuse that such children cannot endure long treks in search of pastures especially in the dry season."[42] Among the Beng of the Côte d'Ivoire, "having a developmental disability or having been identified as a *snake* in childhood may have three possible outcomes: being killed, being left to die, or being allowed to live in the community as the 'other', non-human."[43]

Even the Songye, whose admonition against ridiculing the disabled was earlier cited, "a deformed child can be 'returned' to God by throwing it into a river or burying it in an anthill."[44] While such practices still occur, they are perhaps unsurprisingly sensationalized, particularly by media and humanitarian organizations seeking donations.

Islamic and Christian Conceptions of Disability

As we have seen, indigenous spiritual and religious approaches to disability are prevalent throughout Africa. The influences of Islamic and Christian conceptions of disability are also substantial, even as they also vary widely depending on local context. The Qur'an specifically addresses the treatment of people with impairments: "There is not upon the blind any guilt or upon the lame any guilt or upon the ill any guilt. And whoever obeys Allah and His messenger—He will admit him to gardens beneath which rivers flow:

---

41 Susan Reynolds Whyte, "Constructing Epilepsy: Images and Contexts in East Africa," in *Disability and Culture*, ed. Benedicte Ingstad and Susan Reynolds Whyte (Berkeley: University of California Press, 1995), 237.

42 Kaganzi Rutachwamagyo, "A Profile of Tanzanians with Disabilities," *Disability, Society, and Theology: Voices from Africa*, ed. Samuel Kabue et al. (Limuru, Kenya: Zapf Chancery, 2011), 365.

43 Mojdeh Bayat, "The Stories of Snake Children," *Journal of Intellectual Disability Research* 59 (2015): 7–8.

44 Devlieger, "Frames of Reference in African Proverbs on Disability," 75.

but whoever turns away He will punish him with a painful punishment."[45] According to historian Sara Scalenghe in her work on disability in the medieval Arab cultural context, "The foundational texts of Islam generally reject a causal relationship between guilt, disease, illness, and infirmity, and the rejection of the Christian notion of the original sin. . . . People believed that impairments were rooted in the physical body and rarely attributed them to supernatural forces or to the moral, spiritual, or intellectual qualities of the impaired."[46]

However, it is something of a misnomer to assume that early Arabic cultures conceptualized disability in the contemporary sense. Rather, "The equivalent classical Arabic term *aha* literally means 'blight' or 'damage,' and it can refer to objects both inanimate (crops, trees) and animate (human and non-human animals). The category of blightedness certainly encompasses 'disability,' but it incorporates aesthetics and character."[47] In pre-modern Egypt, the Islamic influence may be seen in the treatment of people with leprosy, where "no connection was posited between pollution, corruption, and leprosy, and there is little evidence that leprosy was deemed a product of divine punishment, or that moral or spiritual stigma was attached to it."[48]

The contemporary influence of Islam on disability in Africa can be observed in the attitudes of people with disabilities in Guinea-Bissau, where a recent study found that "individuals with a disability that had a Muslim background to be more positive about their disability. Muslims believe that everything is 'written', and so, whatever it is that one wishes to do will only occur if it is within God's plan."[49] Treatment of people with disabilities by African Muslims also often retains Qur'anic injunctions toward charity and care. However, the charity extended does often not ensure disabled people's well-being, as in northern Nigeria where:

---

45 Quoted in Hiam Al-Aoufi, Nawaf Al-Zyoud, and Norbayah Shahminan, "Islam and the Cultural Conception of Disability," *International Journal of Adolescence and Youth* 17, no. 4 (2012): 207.

46 Sara Scalenghe, "Disability in the Premodern Arab World," in *The Oxford Handbook of Disability History*, ed. Michael Rembis, Catherine Kudlick, and Kim E. Nielsen (Oxford: Oxford University Press, 2018), 79.

47 Kristina L. Richardson, *Difference and Disability in the Medieval Islamic World: Blighted Bodies* (Edinburgh: Edinburgh University Press, 2012), 36.

48 Scalenghe, "Disability in the Premodern Arab World," 78.

49 Willem M. Otte et al., "Cultural Beliefs Among People with Epilepsy or Physical Impairment in Guinea-Bissau: Differences and Similarities," *Epilepsy and Behavior* 29 (2013): 506.

> Giving alms *(sadaka)* to the unfortunate is not so much for their relief as a 'sacrifice', a gift to earn protection for the donor from the powers that cause the misfortune. . . . People who are mad or impaired are fed and given shelter anyway; they (especially their real selves) are part of the household and provided for, house by house, personally. They are not a special category. The general disinterest suggests not stigma so much as neglect; victims are unfortunate rather than dangerous or evil.[50]

More distressingly, some Muslims in Africa appear to have either forgotten, mislearned, or simply ignored traditional Islamic treatments of disability. Literary scholar Saloua Ali Ben Zahra suggests that spurious Qur'anic quotes may even be intentionally repurposed by some contemporary Muslims to justify ableist and misogynist behavior. In Tunisia, Ben Zahra contends that "in a context of westernizing efforts, certain native and positive ways of saying, knowing and naming have become obsolete in the eyes of a large number of Tunisian sons and daughters. The nearly forgotten ways seem to have been a compassionate, endearing, and polite way of speaking about the disabled."[51]

Christian missionaries to Africa brought with them both medical assistance and European ideologies, along with their concomitant contradictions about disability bound up in both. Some contemporary Africans speak highly of missionary work and how it affected the treatment of disability. Rosallie B. Bukumunhe, a disabled Ugandan woman, describes how,

> The European missionaries began to visit individual homes. . . . The missionaries showed them love and gave them material help, too. . . . The Europeans told people that they did not have disabled children because the Creator hated them, nor had they offended Him in any way.[52]

Missionaries were often the first outsiders in African communities that gave any sort of positive attention to people with disabilities. For instance, in Madagascar, "missionaries provided social amenities to win locals," including

---

50   Last, "Social Exclusion in Northern Nigeria," 223.
51   Saloua Ali Ben Zahra, *Arab Islamic Voices, Agencies, and Abilities: Disability Portrayals in Muslim World Literature and Culture* (Lanham, MD: Lexington, 2018), 37.
52   Rosallie B. Bukumunhe, "'I Will Definitely Go,'" in *Imprinting Our Image: An International Anthology by Women with Disabilities*, ed. Diane Driedger and Susan Gray (Ottawa: Gynergy, 1992), 76.

"schools for the blind and for the deaf."[53] The work of missionaries was not solely to promote the social well-being of Africans, but rather to save their souls. So, even as they were often the only source of advanced medical care in their communities, "Christian missionaries tended to see the health problems of Africans in terms of their lack of Christian morals, in which physical illness was a representation of African moral failing, very much in keeping with images of Africa as a 'Dark Continent' of 'backward' and child-like people in need of education and salvation."[54] Some Africans rejected such European approaches to both medicine and religion, though many adapted the missionaries' assistance to more practical uses, combining European medicine with community traditions.[55] Contemporary manifestations of missionary Christianity abound and have a tendency to maintain a retrograde conception of disability. For instance, Nigerian Christians tend to express that "the concept of disease and disability is usually interpreted as a punishment for sin or wrongdoing. This belief is widespread in the Nigerian Christian community of all denominations." Because the evangelical impulse so often coincides with conservative forms of Christianity, it is a small wonder that many African Christians have a retrograde view of disability.

Colonial Impositions of Disability

The late nineteenth-century scramble for Africa and subsequent colonization left indelible marks across the entire continent, many on the bodies of Africans. The scale of trade and production imposed upon Africa was instrumental in the spread of disease, as well as physical and mental strains that often resulted in impairment and disability. Colonizers brought medical models of disability to Africa, even as they brought little medicine (at least for the colonized). The perpetual racism and frequent brutality of African colonization have been frequently explored,[56] but comparatively little has

---

53 Ralphine Razaka, "Persons with Disabilities in Madagascar," in *Disability, Society, and Theology: Voices from Africa*, ed. Samuel Kabue et al. (Limuru, Kenya: Zapf Chancery, 2013), 20.
54 Heaton, "Health and Medicine in Colonial Society," 309.
55 Mario J. Azevedo, *Historical Perspectives on the State of Health and Health Systems in Africa, vol. 1, The Pre-Colonial and Colonial Eras* (London: Palgrave Macmillan, 2017), 361.
56 See Walter Rodney, *How Europe Underdeveloped Africa* (Washington, DC: Howard University Press, 1981); A. Adu Boahen, *African Perspectives on*

been written about the role of disability in colonial Africa. This appears to be an unfortunate omission, especially given not only how colonialism contributed so much to increased debilitation and disablement across the African continent but also to the medicalization of disability understanding. Undoubtedly, contemporary African culture, politics, and policy toward disability cannot be sufficiently understood without a consideration of the colonial era and its residue.

The hallmark of British colonial administration in Africa was a policy of indirect rule, which is to say a reliance on local district governments comprising indigenous leaders. This method allowed the British to retain control because it encouraged factionalization and removed much of the impetus of effective governance from the colonial power. This was a convenient excuse for abdicating much of the responsibility for the well-being of colonized Africans and justified the lack of investment in major public provisions, "including state-funded education, social welfare, and health care."[57] Since missionaries had set up medical centers to serve the indigenous population, the British prioritized care facilities in areas adjacent to white colonizer populations, and "where large numbers of Africans were employed, so that the process of production would go on." The resulting policy was one where "government concentrated on cities, plantations, mines, and railroads, the missions established hospitals in isolated rural areas. However, total facilities (of both government and missions) rarely reached more than 20 percent of the population."[58] That British health resources were anemic at best was particularly egregious considering that colonialism was a significant contributor to ill health in Africa during the period. For instance, "In British Somaliland . . . it was likely the combination of natural calamities such as drought and the social conditions brought about by colonialism, that constituted the major factor in the escalation of the frequency of diseases and epidemics, some of which were either endemic or latent and never seen before."[59] That such diseases as malaria, yellow fever, and smallpox caused mass fatalities is well documented, but they

---

Colonization (Baltimore: Johns Hopkins University Press, 1989); and Thomas Pakhenham, *The Scramble for Africa: White Man's Conquest of the Dark Continent from 1876 to 1912* (New York: Avon, 1992).

57 Heaton, "Health and Medicine in Colonial Society," 209.

58 Steven Feierman, "Struggles for Control: The Social Roots of Health and Healing in Modern Africa," *African Studies Review* 28, no. 2/3 (June–September 1985):122–123.

59 Azevedo, *Historical Perspectives*, 218.

also almost certainly would have produced debilitating short- and long-term conditions as well. Further, British colonials pathologized a variety of conditions that were inconvenient to their rule. Sloan Mahone describes circumstances in Kenya where prophets and their followers were labeled as psychiatrically abnormal, and "a wealth of research on the increasing impact of 'acculturation', saw the 'semi-educated' and the 'semi-converted' as straddling conflicting worlds leaving them virtually on the brink of madness."[60]

Thus, the British colonial governments only provided medical care for a small percentage of colonized Africans, engaged in industry and trade that increased exposure and incidence of infectious diseases, and also regarded acts of resistance as psychiatric disorders rather than legitimate reactions to colonial rule.

Despite the shortcomings of British colonials in Africa, it would be inaccurate to suggest that their influence was exclusively negative. For instance, British doctors in Nigeria made a concerted effort to improve the lot of mothers and children to the extent that "at the end of World War II, Nigeria was ahead of most other colonies in the provision of maternal and child care, accompanied by a campaign waged against antenatal and postnatal obstetrical and gynecologic diseases through the provision of health services that targeted mothers and children at the time."[61] Given the prevalence of impairments acquired in gestation and childbirth, this effort likely reduced rates of congenital disability. Further, there is evidence that the British government would also provide prosthetics to disabled children, particularly those with polio, at a reduced price for their families.[62] The British colonial government also was the first to train African doctors in Sierra Leone,[63] who likely had a firmer grasp on indigenous African cultural conceptions of impairment and disability than their European counterparts.

The French colonial governments in Africa, with their contrasting direct rule models, were substantially more proactive when it came to the health and welfare of colonized Africans. This is certainly not to say that French provisions were sufficient for ensuring the well-being of Africans, but rather that they were far more consistent in their token efforts at good governance

---

60   Sloan Mahone, "The Psychology of Rebellion: Colonial Medical Responses to Dissent in British East Africa," *Journal of African History* 47 (2006): 256–257.
61   Azevedo, *Historical Perspectives*, 225.
62   Azevedo, *Historical Perspectives*, 230.
63   Azevedo, *Historical Perspectives*, 239.

among their African colonies. Neither should the existence of marginally better health and disability policies necessarily impute more righteous motives to the French, since the intention of such policies was seemingly to pacify regions that were increasingly opposed to foreign control. The French pursued a *mission civilisatrice*, which "assumed a cultural superiority that was paradoxically understood to be normative, therefore any 'other' (lower) culture could be labeled pathological. The colonized subject—uncivilized, unclothed, 'uncultured'—was characterized by inherent cultural and intellectual deficiencies."[64] The French thus presumed that Africans were implicitly disabled by their inferior culture, which appears to imbue their comparatively generous welfare projects with the condescension of noblesse oblige. Also, similar to Britain and other colonizing powers, French colonial avarice appears to have contributed to the spread of disease in the colonies. The rapid spread of sleeping sickness in colonial Chad was likely due to European interference: "At the end of the nineteenth century, the increased contact between people unknown to each other before helped spread it, transforming it into a recurrent epidemic."[65]

Hygiene became a particular preoccupation for French colonizers in Africa, not least because "since the French National Assembly had rejected race as a policy in Africa, racist colonialists invoked acceptance of French living standards and hygienic practices by Africans as a sine qua non for integrated living."[66] Rather than the explicitly racialized segregation imposed by the British, the French opted for de facto segregation enforced through the ideology of "hygiene," of which Africans were considered incapable. The hygienic discourse remained through the postcolonial period, as evidenced by Senegal where

> during the Senghorian regime, for example, disabled people were aligned not only with ideas of politico-economic dependence and stagnancy, but with more generalized notions of contamination and ordure. Due in part to the economic potential of French tourism, Senegal embraced an ideal of hygiaesthetic (hygenic and aestheticized) public spaces and public bodies, making visible for itself and for outsiders an able, ordered, orderly, contained, and 'healthful' urban body politic—one worthy of courting, one worthy of *living*. Those citizens seen to counter this national fiction—the physically and

---

64 Julie Nack Ngue, *Critical Conditions: Illness and Disability in Francophone African Women's Writing* (Lanham, MD: Lexington, 2012), 145.
65 Azevedo, *Historical Perspectives*, 254–255.
66 Azevedo, *Historical Perspectives*, 237.

mentally disabled, lepers, albinos, prostitutes, and beggars alike—came to be identified as 'social plagues' or 'human obstructions,' terms directly inherited from the colonial era.[67]

Similarly, the French ideological modes of thought concerning disability inundated both colonial and postcolonial North Africa. Ben Zahra contends that societies in North Africa display an "assimilation of European norms" where "able-bodied Arab/Muslims see their disabled fellow citizens as deviant" and thus "are unable to accept them and by extension, reject, and oppress them."[68] Liberal French notions are also substantially at odds with disabled bodies and so have ramifications in their colonies and postcolonies. In particular, "the principle of French universalism and *laïcité* (secularism)—principles that insist on a body politic stripped of its possible religious cultural, or personal affiliations and resulting in a 'model' that is visibly Franco-French (white), male, able-bodied, and in all other ways 'fit.'"[69] Such ideals of normalcy render both the disabled body and the nonwhite body as profoundly outside the bounds of citizenship. A disabled African body was thus anathema to French liberal principles.

French colonial welfare provisions, even if they originated from spuriously racist and ableist motives, provided material supports for disabled Africans in their colonies. Notably, "the French created the Medical Assistance Program in French West Africa as early as 1905, which provided Africans free medical care, free consultation, free immunization, and emergency care for children under-five as well as free health insurance for them, and free maternal and child services for all Africans."[70] The French government also instituted pensions following both world wars, specifically for disabled veterans. In North Africa, "The indigenous war-disabled, as ex-soldiers, were among the few categories of people who could apply for French naturalization."[71] This process, however, was often arbitrary and personalized to the whims of

---

67 Julie Van Dam (Nack Ngue), "Re-Viewing Disability in Postcolonial West Africa: Ousmane Sembène's Early Resistant Bodies in *Xala*," *Journal of Literary & Cultural Disability Studies* 10, no. 2 (2016): 212.
68 Ben Zahra, *Arab Islamic Voices, Agencies, and Abilities*, 125.
69 Van Dam, "Re-Viewing Disability in Postcolonial West Africa," 211.
70 Azevedo, *Historical Perspectives*, 249.
71 Gildas Brégain, "Reintegrating Without Changing Colonial Hierarchies? Ethnic and Territorial Inequalities in the Policies to Assist War-Disabled Men from the French Colonial Empire (1916–1939)," *Alter: European Journal of Disability Research* 13, no. 4 (2019): 261.

colonial officials. The pensions provided for war-disabled Africans following World War I were also tiered by colony, so that where North Africans and Senegalese received pensions comparable to the war-disabled French citizens, the amounts were progressively less for Africans in French West Africa, French East Africa, Côte des Somalis, and Madagascar—where they sometimes received only 25 percent of the sum accorded to war-disabled French citizens.[72] The war-disabled policy, though unevenly distributed across the colonies, was nevertheless a rare concession to civilized Africans by a colonial power. According to historian Gildas Brégain, "This social policy, which was costly for France, was a priority because of the political imperative of showing gratitude for those who sacrificed themselves for the country, but also and above all to maintain the backing of the colonized populations and the political support of the disabled and former combatants in a context of growing anti-colonial nationalism."[73]

Other European colonizers in Africa also prefaced their own brutality in disingenuously humanitarian terms. The Belgian colonization of Central Africa was justified specifically by the promise of fewer impairments under Belgian rule:

> Leopold stated at that time that his actions were necessary and legitimate because Belgian colonization would put an end to the widespread reign of Arabic slavery and the related practices of forced mutilation. . . . Interestingly, while Leopold II used the threat of Arabic slavery and mutilation as a principle for Belgian involvement in Central Africa, it was not long before Belgian atrocities toward the Congolese people replaced the atrocities of others.[74]

The Germans in 1910, proposed that the Cameroonian city of Duala be segregated, with white colonists occupying the harbor and black Africans at least a kilometer away due to supposed health concerns: "The segregated housing and the unequal water and sewerage services that accompanied it remained as a legacy for the French to uphold."[75] The Italian colonizers in Libya set

---

72 Brégain, "Reintegrating Without Changing Colonial Hierarchies?," 258.
73 Brégain, "Reintegrating Without Changing Colonial Hierarchies?," 261.
74 Pieter Verstraete, Evelyne Verhaegen, and Marc Depaepe, "One Difference is Enough: towards a History of Disability in the Belgian-Congo, 1908–1960," in *The Routledge History of Disability*, ed. Roy Hanes, Ivan Brown, and Nancy E. Hasan (New York and London: Routledge, 2017), 232.
75 Daniel R. Headrick, "*The Tentacles of Progress: Technology Transfer in the Age of Imperialism, 1850–1940* (Oxford: Oxford University Press, 1988), 164.

up concentration camps for Bedouin where "Italian medical provision was minimal and even in areas that avoided mass starvation, many Bedouin suffered from malnutrition and its connected diseases. Exacerbating this, basic hygiene provision was poor and typhus and other diseases were endemic."[76]

Despite Lusotropicalist pretensions of a kinder and gentler colonialism, conscription and forced labor in the Portuguese colony of Mozambique became increasingly debilitating. Eric Allina documents how "physical assaults by employers, their supervisors, and company police, combined with a near unending work regime, left laborers with little sense that even control of their own bodies was allowed or possible."[77] Colonialism in Africa certainly resulted in not only physical and mental disablement but also in an ideological legacy that continues to be a significant barrier to the well-being of disabled Africans. Geographer Marcus Power suggests, following Mamdani, that

> in both Angola and Mozambique, there is a sense in which the institutional segregation of 'citizens' and 'subjects' has not been completely overhauled, and neither have the state machineries inherited from colonialism been fully transformed. There continues to be a sense, therefore, in which post-colonial state power in both countries remains bifurcated and Janus-faced, an inherited impediment, centered upon urban spaces and a notion of citizens as bearers of state-protected rights rather than as a focus of moves to build equality and widen access to participation.[78]

However, there is substantial evidence that postcolonial Africa is not completely trapped within unhelpful Eurocentric modes of thought. Rather, African indigenous conceptions of kinship and community offer an attractive way forward for dismantling disability oppression in Africa. It is to these considerations that we now turn.

---

76 David Atkinson, "Encountering Bare Life in Italian Libya and Colonial Amnesia in Agamben," in *Agamben and Colonialism*, ed. Marcelo Svirsky and Simone Bignall (Edinburgh: Edinburgh University Press, 2012), 164.

77 Eric Allina, *Slavery by Any Other Name: African Life Under Company Rule in Colonial Mozambique* (Charlottesville: University of Virginia Press, 2012), 54.

78 Marcus Power, "War Veterans, Disability, and Postcolonial Citizenship in Angola and Mozambique," in *War, Citizenship, Territory*, ed. Deborah Cowen and Emily Gilbert (New York and London: Routledge, 2008), 191.

Rhetoric, Community, and Humanity

While colonial underdevelopment, postcolonial shortsightedness, and neoliberal exploitation may undermine traditional African values, indigenous ways of knowing are still evident across the continent. Spiritual dimensions of disability in African cultures are often closely bound up with the community dimensions. In the case of disability, then, many Africans take impairments to be a result of damaged relationships within personal and spiritual communities.[79] Julie Livingston discusses how cultural understandings of the Tswana in southern Africa directly link disability and bodily impairment to a larger sense of community impairment, the result being that the Tswana "rightly understand themselves to be living in a web of dependencies, and they strive to manage and foster the nurturing side of these dependencies."[80] In West Africa, Geurts and Komabu-Pomeyie draw attention to "an important indigenous phenomenon encapsulated in the term *seseleme* (literally 'perceive-perceive-at-flesh-inside', or 'feeling in the body')." [81] In the east African country of Rwanda, Wallace et al. suggested that "there is evidence that traditional forms of social assistance, or community solidarity, known in Rwanda as '*ubumwe*', are still strong features of everyday life."[82] Traditional African attitudes and behavior emphasize interdependent and communitarian webs of support, which afford a conceptualization of disabled people as central to (and supported through) ties of nonbiological kinship.

Even in African communities that may still mark people with disabilities as inhuman others, a cultural model built around collective meaning making and the embrace of otherness already has deep roots. The concept of *ubuntu* has come to signify a Pan-African communalism, where "one is not considered a human being unless one is concerned about the well-being of other

---

79   Owusu-Ansah and Mji, "African Indigenous Knowledge and Research," 2.
80   Julie Livingston, *Debility and the Moral Imagination in Botswana* (Bloomington: Indiana University Press, 2005), 10.
81   Kathryn Linn Geurts and Sefakor G. M. A. Komabu-Pomeyie, "From 'Sensing Disability' to Seselame: Non-Dualistic Activist Orientations in Twenty-First-Century-Accra," in *Disability in the Global South*, ed. Shaun Grech and Karen Soldatic (New York: Springer, 2016), 88.
82   Derron Wallace, Evariste Karangwa, and Jeannette Bayisenge, "'Boys Don't Rule Us': Exploring Rwandan Girls with Disabilities' Resistance to Masculine Dominance at School," *International Journal of Inclusive Education* 23, no. 3 (2019): 268.

people.... This principle is based on the Nguni saying: *Umuntu ngumuntu ngabantu* (A person is a person through other people)."[83] Theresa Lorenzo advocates an *ubuntu* approach to disability that "seeks to cultivate a spirit of interdependence in meeting physical, emotional, and spiritual needs as a means of human development."[84] Medical anthropologist, Maria Berghs, suggests that *ubuntu* allows for considerations of disability at multiple levels simultaneously:

> Using *ubuntu* we can ask why the social responsibilities of ethical actions are enabled or disabled individually, socially, by the state or structurally ... *Ubuntu* does not place individual blame on a child, nor mother, but asks why a community, institution or state is failing in its compassionate responsibilities towards upholding respect for human diversity, who is filling the gap and why and what can be done to change such discourses and practices.[85]

An *ubuntu* approach to disability thus can incorporate the social construction claims of traditional disability studies but also goes farther to activate African communities toward creating and sustaining collective well-being. As a matter of practical disability activism and social policy, Mji et al. emphasize the deployment of *ubuntu* rhetorics as particularly effective strategies for social change in Africa: "In keeping with a community-based, *ubuntu* approach, persons with disabilities ... have tried to show how persons with disabilities have been marginalized by society at different levels."[86] *Ubuntu* rhetoric has an established use in reference to economic and racial issues, particularly in South Africa, where "the morality of *Ubuntu* has created a common understanding of discrimination and poverty, explained as a result of the past

---

83 Sindile A. Ngubane-Mokiwa, "Ubuntu Considered in Light of Exclusion of People with Disabilities," *African Journal of Disability* 7 (2018): 1.

84 Theresa Lorenzo, "No African Renaissance Without Disabled Women: A Communal Approach to Human Development in Cape Town, South Africa," *Disability & Society* 18, no. 6 (2003): 774.

85 Maria Berghs, "Practices and Discourses of Ubuntu: Implications for an African Model of Disability?," *African Journal of Disability* 6 (2017): 6.

86 Gubela Mji et al., "Networking in Disability for Development: Introducing the African Network for Evidence-to-Action on Disability (AfriNEAD)," *Disability & International Development: Towards Inclusive Global Health*, ed. Malcolm MacLachlan and Leslie Swartz (New York: Springer, 2009), 70.

segregation practice of apartheid."[87] Framing disability in terms of *ubuntu*, then, is a logical extension of recent successful practices.

However, even as it offers intriguing opportunities for a specifically African disability studies, an *ubuntu* approach is not without its limits and its detractors. Disability theorists Dan Goodley and Leslie Swartz note that as a community-based ethics, *ubuntu* relies on definitions of precisely who is inside and outside a given community. Goodley and Swartz claim that in practice, "the extent to which *ubuntu* grants equal rights may be seriously constrained by ideas of gender and lineage."[88] Further, global development scholar David A. McDonald regards *ubuntu* to be a "tired and tainted . . . political idea"[89] that has been co-opted by decades of neoliberal capitalism and might no longer have purchase in creating contemporary social change. McDonald is largely dismissive of utilizations of *ubuntu* to influence public policy, claiming that "they are, at best, a naive appeal by liberal academics for rapid changes in governance culture . . . and at worst a distraction from the deeper structural impediments to the inequities in health, education and jurisprudence."[90] These critics of an *ubuntu* approach to disability in Africa focus on the practical implementation of *ubuntu* rhetorics more than on the concept itself, and while their concerns are certainly cautionary, they do not take issue with the communitarian form of ethics central to the concept.

At first glance, it might appear that an *ubuntu* approach would be incompatible with the rhetoric of human rights, which often focuses on individuals instead of communities. Indeed, several disability scholars are skeptical about using human rights concepts in African and other Global South contexts. Meekosha and Soldatic forcefully challenge the discourse of human rights, which they interpret as couched in the "language of universalism," which "assumes developing countries will evolve to the 'higher' standards of Western

---

87   Camilla Hansen and Washeila Sait, "'We Too Are Disabled': Disability Grants and Poverty Politics in Rural South Africa," in *Disability and Poverty: A Global Challenge*, ed. Arne H. Eide and Benedicte Ingstad (Bristol, UK: Bristol University Press, 2011), 111.

88   Dan Goodley and Leslie Swartz, "The Place of Disability," in *Disability in the Global South*, ed. Shaun Grech and Karen Soldatic (New York: Springer, 2016), 78.

89   David A. McDonald, "Ubuntu Bashing: The Marketisation of 'African Values' in South Africa," *Review of African Political Economy* 37, no. 124 (2010): 140.

90   McDonald, "Ubuntu Bashing," 145.

human rights, such as the recognition of individual rights."[91] Kenyan legal scholar Makau Mutua cites postapartheid South Africa to demonstrate the shortcomings of human rights discourse, which he calls "traditional and conservative. Except for largely cosmetic effects, there is little possibility that the particular conceptualization of rights in the new South Africa will alter the patterns of power, wealth, and privilege established under apartheid."[92] While Mutua grants that human rights has been an effective organizing principle for activists, he rejects how it typically incorporates "the liberal conception of the individual as the state's primary antagonist."[93]

Human rights may yet be vindicated for the purpose of reducing disability oppression in Africa if it can be synthesized with the communitarian ethos of *ubuntu*. Philosopher Polycarp Ikuenobe argues that in fact, rights are unthinkable without the underlying assumption of a functioning community: "Without a community, rights cannot provide the substantive basis for individuals' well-being and flourishing."[94] Ikuenobe maintains that *ubuntu* already contains a conception of individual human rights, if not exactly in the same terms as those traditionally imagined by those in the Global North.[95] Legal scholar Serges Djoyou Kamga suggests that "the trademark feature of disability in Africa is 'voicelessness' and institutional neglect of disabled people, who are often forced to take positions on the outermost margins of their societies."[96] A rhetoric and practice of human rights that incorporates the principles of *ubuntu* is keenly positioned to help bring disabled Africans back from the margins.

If we are to take seriously the rights of every disabled African, attention must be paid to the range of intersectional identities that disability affects. Of course, African disability is already fundamentally located at an intersection,

---

91 Helen Meekosha and Karen Soldatic, "Human Rights and the Global South: The Case of Disability," *Third World Quarterly* 32, no. 8 (2011): 1388.

92 Makua Mutua, *Human Rights: A Political and Cultural Critique* (Philadelphia: University of Pennsylvania Press, 2013), 128–129.

93 Mutua, *Human Rights*, 84.

94 Polycarp Ikuenobe, "Human Rights, Personhood, Dignity, and African Communalism," *Journal of Human Rights* 17, no. 5 (2018): 599.

95 Ikuenobe, "Human Rights ," 598.

96 Serges Alain Djoyou Kamga, "A Call for a Protocol to the African Charter on Human and Peoples' Rights on the Rights of Persons with Disabilities in Africa," *African Journal of International and Comparative Law* 21, no. 2 (2013): 222.

but it would be an oversimplification to presume that a variety of factors, including gender, sexuality, age, and religion, do not also play prominent roles in the lives of disabled Africans. Women with disabilities often have markedly different life circumstances in Africa than men do. Sexuality for disabled people of all genders is rife with stereotypes and misconceptions, but women are often perceived as unable to marry, bear children, or raise a family.[97] In North Africa, Ben Zahra highlights how disability and gender combine with religion and culture in particularly debilitating ways: "Women with disabilities living in Arab and Muslim society have traditionally been isolated, silenced, and buried alive in the house institution."[98] Joanne Neille and Claire Penn indicate how isolating environments for disabled women in South Africa can put them at increased risk for sexual exploitation, since the place of women is traditionally relegated to the home.[99] Tsitsi Chataika further emphasizes the particularly distressing vulnerability of disabled women in Africa:

> Disabled women are more exposed to violence and rape than women without disabilities, and less likely to ask the police to intervene, or at least seek legal protection . . . The popular belief that people with sexually transmitted diseases can be cured if they have sexual relations with a virgin creates a particular risk for girls with disabilities due to the misconception that disabled people are sexually inactive, and therefore virgins.[100]

Opportunities to avoid violence and isolation can be limited by barriers to education, as in Malawi where "some parents do not send girls with disabilities to school in order to protect them from the stigma associated with

---

97   Ngubane-Mokiwa, "Ubuntu Considered," 6.
98   Ben Zahra, *Arab Islamic Voices*, 58.
99   Joanne Neille and Claire Penn, "The Interface Between Violence, Disability, and Poverty: Stories from a Developing Country," *Journal of Interpersonal Violence* 32, no. 18 (2017): 2853.
100 Tsitsi Chataika, "Disabled Women, Urbanization, and Sustainable Development in Africa," in *Women, Urbanization and Sustainability: Practices of Survival, Adaptation, and Resistance*, ed. Anita Lacey (London: Palgrave Macmillan, 2017), 183.

education."[101] In Zimbabwe, "children are discriminated by family members, paternal relatives, neighbors and church members."[102]

Notably, disabled African women find ways to exert their own authority, even in multiply disabling conditions. Wallace et al. found that disabled girls in Rwanda can often effectively resist disabling environments by elevating their social standing through academic or athletic achievements.[103] In Ethiopia, Katsui and Majtahedi observe that despite having their options limited only to domestic labor, "being good at household chores becomes an important way to defend their space in their respective households."[104] Also in rural Ethiopia, "disabled women are not considered for marriage, and this creates an opportunity for them to go to school . . . Disabled women move to metropolitan areas of the country for education, and paradoxically, this separation seems to inspire disabled women to succeed."[105]

The responsibilities of care for disabled relatives fall predominantly on women in Africa and are made even more difficult by the typical lack of external support. Judith McKenzie argues that despite the prevalence of home family care for disabled Africans, disability policy often fails to recognize the importance (or even existence of) the caretakers themselves: "The family caregiver becomes invisible when only the rights of the disabled person are taken into account in the distribution of social goods."[106] Caretakers for disabled people in Africa reportedly experience stigmas themselves, in

---

101 Jim Nyanda, "Confronting the Double Marginalisation of Girls with Disabilities: Practical Challenges for the Realisation of the Right to Education for Girls with Disabilities Under the Disability Act of Malawi," *African Disability Rights Yearbook* 3 (2015): 112.

102 Elise Jantine Van der Mark and Hebe Verrest, "Fighting the Odds: Strategies for Female Caregivers of Disabled Children in Zimbabwe," *Disability & Society* 29, no. 9 (2014): 1420.

103 Wallace et al., "'Boys Don't Rule Us,'" 306.

104 Hisayo Katsui and Mina C. Mojtahedi, "Intersection of Disability and Gender: Multi-Layered Experiences of Ethiopian Women with Disabilities," *Development in Practice* 25, no. 4 (2015): 571.

105 Belaynesh Tefera, "The Disability Paradox: Better Opportunities Versus the Hardships of High-Achieving Disabled Women of Ethiopia," *Canadian Journal of Disability Studies* 5, no. 1 (2016): 120–121.

106 Judith Ann McKenzie, "An Exploration of an Ethics of Care in Relation to People with Intellectual Disability and Their Family Caregivers in the Cape Town Metropole in South Africa," *Alter* 10, no. 1 (2016): 70.

addition to the stigmas of their disabled child or family member.[107] A study conducted in Tanzania by Heather Aldersey found that families of people with intellectual disabilities expressed common thought patterns: "This process often fell into subcategories of learning that 'something is wrong', seeking a cure for disability, and finally, acceptance."[108] Van der Maark and Verrest identify the responses to caregiving displayed by women in Zimbabwe:

> As formal state and non-governmental organization facilities have deteriorated and social support networks are limited, women deploy three strategies to provide care and comfort for their child: *reducing the effects of poverty* by deploying basic household activities and providing health/hygiene to their child; *learning skills* to provide the necessary medical care; and *training* the child for independence. The lack of external support causes stress, pain, and feelings of neglect among women. A fourth developed strategy, *acceptance*, addresses this and supports women in finding peace with their situation.[109]

Faith, spirituality, and reflection are indicated as major coping mechanisms for many caregivers in Africa. Speaking from her personal experiences and her work as a therapist in Ghana, Frances Owusu-Ansah emphasizes how "the experience of caregiving *does* change the caregiver in many ways. Among other things, it provides occasions for deep and personal introspection, reappraisal of own values, and opportunities for self-transcendence."[110]

Debility, Geography, and Biopolitics

The impairment/disability distinction that resides at the center of the traditional social model of disability has received criticism among disability scholars for reasons independent of African or Global South concerns. In African contexts, the social model takes on a variety of particular challenges that are related to these criticisms but have significant nuances at levels both ideological and material. Shaun Grech, arguing from a postcolonial perspective,

---

107 Heather M. Aldersey, "Family Perceptions of Intellectual Disability: Understanding and Support in Dar es Salaam," *African Journal of Disability* 1, no. 1 (2012): 10.
108 Aldersey, "Family Perceptions of Intellectual Disability," 9.
109 Van der Mark and Verrest, "Fighting the Odds," 1423.
110 Frances E. Owusu-Ansah, "Sharing in the Life of the Person with Disability: A Ghanaian Perspective," *Africa Journal of Disability* 4, no. 1 (2015): 2.

suggests that disability studies' disdain for medical frameworks does not map easily onto the Global South, where "it is not surprising that disabled people may look for the abhorred medical 'fixing' because they are hardly subjected to the medical gaze; their disabled bodies are often rendered docile by extraordinary, unmedicated pain, and the desperate need to work to ensure survival means the priority is refocused on achieving previous body functioning"[111] Western and northern models of disability studies can, in some ways, afford to make vituperative antimedical arguments because medical care of disabled bodies is largely the hegemonic norm. In the Global South, such treatment is often not available or easily accessible, and consequently the role of medical care in an African disability studies needs to be substantially different from hegemonic social models.

Another distinction that takes on greater importance in Africa—and elsewhere in the Global South—is how an impairment was acquired, or the sense that a culture has about how and why it was acquired. In her study of Botswana, Julie Livingston suggests that it is more than just a distinction between impairment and disability: what is required to effectively theorize in some parts of Africa is a distinction between disability and debility. Livingston uses the term "debility" to indicate "both the frailties associated with chronic illness and aging and as the impairments underlying the word disability . . . it highlights the overlaps between impairment, chronic illness, and senescence. I discuss debility in terms of physical misfortune."[112] This distinction is important in the particular case of Botswana because of the set of cultural attitudes toward impairment and disability that are substantially different than those typically found in the Global North: "Batswana understand impaired relationships to generate body misfortune, which in turn is managed as disability."[113] Further, Livingston asserts that in Botswana, debility is tied to a colonial history both in material fact and in its cultural understanding, so that "the crisis of debility (as remembered and experienced) stretches back in time for people in Botswana and is intertwined with the story of 'modernization'—the influx of a particular web of western

---

111 Shaun Grech, "Disability and the Majority World: A Neocolonial Approach," in *Disability and Social Theory: New Developments and Directions*, ed. Dan Goodley, Bill Hughes, and Lennard Davis (London: Palgrave Macmillan, 2012), 63.
112 Livingston, *Debility and the Moral Imagination in Botswana*, 6.
113 Livingston, *Debility and the Moral Imagination in Botswana*, 10.

institutions, ideas, and capital"[114] Global structures of neocolonialism, racism, economic injustice, and ecological catastrophe produce and maintain disability throughout the Global South through processes of debilitation that often go unnoticed. Ironically, even "economic booms have negative consequences by engendering impairment through social upheaval and increases in pollution affecting chronic, neurological or mental health conditions limiting the ability to work."[115] By emphasizing debilitation in the African context, an African disability studies would specifically engage with relationships not only between disabled and nondisabled bodies but also between and among intersecting global systems of biopolitical control.

In postconflict zones, which are unfortunately rife in Africa, disability can be particularly debilitating. Landmines create disabilities, both during wartime and long after, particularly for civilians. And even though much of Africa has made great strides in landmine removal, their legacy often remains in the lived experiences of people disabled by them. Interestingly, in areas where such impairments are common, there are indications that disability stigma has been significantly lessened. In Somaliland, "There is a hierarchy of recognition of disability—war and mine injuries being acknowledged, and some provision made, children and adults with other disabilities (including blindness and deafness) and learning difficulties (still termed mental handicap) often being unacknowledged and stigmatized."[116] Ulrich Tietze reports from Angola (where many landmines still remain) that "the woman on crutches with a baby on her back, carrying a basket of dried fish on her head to the marketplace, hardly evokes any extra sympathy in Luena. The customers haggle over her prices just as vigorously as over those of the other fish sellers at the market."[117] People who received punitive amputations during wartime, as in the civil war in Sierra Leone, appear to be less well integrated. Ernest Cole suggests that the case of punitive amputation is fundamentally

---

114 Livingston, *Debility and the Moral Imagination in Botswana*, 4.

115 Berghs, "The New Humanitarianism: Neoliberalism, Poverty, and the Creation of Disability," in *Disability, Human Rights and the Limits of Humanitarianism*, ed. Michael Gill and Cathy J. Schlund-Vials (Farnham, UK: Ashgate, 2014), 29.

116 Sally Tomlinson and Osman Ahmed Abdi, "Disability in Somaliland," *Disability & Society* 18, no. 7 (2003): 914.

117 Ulrich Tietze, "Possibilities for Working with Cultural Knowledge in the Rehabilitation of Mine Victims in Luena, Angola," in *Disability in Different Cultures: Reflections on Local Concepts*, ed. Brigitte Holzer, Arthur Vreede, and Gabriele Weigt (Bielefeld, Germany: Transcript Verlag, 1999), 182–183.

different than other disabilities because it "is anchored in feelings of resentment to the victimizer and pain at the loss of the limb."[118] This is exacerbated by the cultural context of Sierra Leone, where "in a country that is predominantly Muslim, in strict interpretations of Islamic or *Sharia* law, a relationship exists between the loss of a hand and theft. . . . Rebels understood that both locally and globally amputation would be treated with condemnation, sympathy, and pity, but also voyeurism and interest."[119]

Poverty, as a result of African underdevelopment and neoliberal debilitation, is inextricable from disability. Chalklen et al. contended that "severe poverty disempowers people and severely limits the extent to which people can organize themselves into successful DPOs (disabled people's organizations)."[120] The often causal relationships between disability and poverty have been well documented by disability scholars, even in the Global North. Specifically in Africa, the combination of disability and poverty can lead to situations such as those documented in Kenya by Grut et al., where "poor families seem to have lost what we may call a 'fighting spirits' and have given up. Faced with the many losses and obstacles that poverty creates, the care for a disabled family member is one burden too many and just becomes too much."[121] Particularly in places where governmental or NGO resources for disability care are scarce or nonexistent, the family becomes the primary caregiver; so when the family is burdened by poverty, there are often direct effects on the care received by disabled family members. Alternately, there are indications that the opposite may also be the case. Wallace et al. report that in Rwanda

> increased affluence, especially in urban areas, can mean that family members are likely to be fully occupied away from home most of the day, leaving children

---

118 Ernest Cole, *Theorizing the Disfigured Body: Mutilation, Amputation, and Disability Culture in Post-Conflict Sierra Leone* (Trenton, NJ: Africa World, 2014), 54–55.

119 Maria Berghs, *War and Embodied Memory: Becoming Disabled in Sierra Leone* (Farnham, UK: Ashgate, 2012), 75–76.

120 Shuaib Chalklin, Leslie Swartz, and Brian Watermeyer, "Establishing the Secretariat for the African Decade of Persons with Disabilities," in *Disability and Social Change: A South African Agenda*, ed. Brian Watermeyer et al. (Cape Town, South Africa: Human Sciences Research Council, 2006), 96.

121 Lisbet Grut, Joyce Olenja and Benedicte Ingstad, "Disability and barriers in Kenya," in *Disability and Poverty: A Global Challenge*, ed. Arne H. Eide and Benedicte Ingstad (Bristol, UK: Bristol University Press, 2011), 163.

with disabilities in the care of paid workers or family members. Children with disabilities in these families seem to be socially isolated and sometimes "hidden." By contrast, children with disabilities growing up in income-poor households, especially in rural communities, were found to be active participants in the wide circle of the extended family and community.[122]

The complex relationship between disability and poverty may be further exacerbated by inadequate definitions not only of "disability" but also of "poverty." In reference to Morocco and Tunisia, Trani et al. follow the capability approach of economist Amartya Sen to emphasize the importance of a "multidimensional" definition of poverty to determine overall well-being. For instance, health-care facilities are comparatively easy to access in Morocco and Tunisia, yet the study still found "long waiting times, high costs for drugs and tests, unavailability of needed devices, uncertain diagnoses, and a lack of respect and courtesy from medical staff during interactions with patients"[123]

The compounding challenges for disabled people living in poverty becomes even more complex in Africa's many rural communities, and even when such areas are targeted by antipoverty initiatives, such measures "exclude disabled individuals—by default, if not by intent."[124] As a consequence, many people with disabilities leave rural communities for cities, where they are in closer proximity to caregiving bodies and DPOs.[125] In Uganda, Muyinda and Whyte document how opportunities to relocate to urban communities are unequally distributed: "Most women were tied to their life in the rural areas mainly because of family obligations of looking after children and/or protecting their marriages . . . Most men, on the other hand, had no fear of losing their spouses if they left them in the rural areas; instead, many used this as an opportunity to get some source of income in

---

122 Wallace et al., "'Boys Don't Rule Us,'" 275. See also Rutachwamagyo, "A Profile of Tanzanians with Disabilities," 367.

123 Jean-Francois Trani et al., "Disability and Poverty in Morocco and Tunisia: A Multidimensional Approach," *Journal of Human Development and Capabilities* 16, no. 4 (2015): 523.

124 Margaret Booyens, Ermien van Pletzen, and Theresa Lorenzo, "The Complexity of Rural Contexts Experienced by Community Disability Workers in Three Southern African Countries," *African Journal of Disability* 4, no. 1 (2015): 8.

125 Eide and Ingstad, *Disability and Poverty*, 8.

town to support their families in the rural camps."[126] Migration from rural to urban areas, also tends to debilitate rural zones, since the people who are left behind are often those who lack either the resources or the capacity to move to the cities.[127] However, as is the case with poverty, there are reports from rural areas, particularly in Ghana[128] and northern Nigeria[129], where people with disabilities are treated significantly better than in the cities.

For Africans with disabilities who migrate to cities, begging becomes a possible avenue for income due to increased opportunities for social interaction: "Begging is a source of income that is practiced in urban, not rural, social space. . . . Wheelchairs are an asset here [in Accra], because they put the beggars at a convenient height for interacting with car passengers and allow rapid, efficient coverage of several cars in the space of a red light."[130]

The *documentaires* in Kinshasa engage in a particularly innovative approach to begging by utilizing printed documents to solicit donations.[131] According to anthropologist, Clara Devlieger, "The *documentaires* have created a remarkable system that reflects the tensions of social judgment in the city. Rather than using references to religious charity, they speak the language of NGO work and state responsibility for deserving citizens, while also evoking civic obligations of contractual dependency between individuals."[132] An urban location may also put disabled people in

---

126 Herbert Muyinda and Susan Reynolds Whyte, "Displacement, Mobility, and Poverty in Northern Uganda," in *Disability and Poverty: A Global Challenge*, ed. Arne H. Eide and Benedicte Ingstad (Bristol: Bristol University Press, 2011), 131.
127 Fikru Negash Gebrekidan, "Disability Rights Activism in Kenya, 1959-1964: History from Below," *African Studies Review* 55, no. 3 (2012): 107.
128 Juliana Abena Owusu, "Struggle of Disabled Women in Ghana," in *Imprinting Our Image: An International Anthology by Women with Disabilities*, ed. Diane Driedger and Susan Gray (Ottawa: Gynergy, 1992), 58.
129 Last, "Social Exclusion in Northern Nigeria," 235.
130 Susan Reynolds Whyte and Herbert Muyinda, "Wheels and New Legs: Mobilization in Uganda," in *Disability in Local and Global Worlds*, ed. Benedicte Ingstad and Susan Reynolds Whyte (Berkeley: University of California Press, 2007), 289.
131 Clara Devlieger, "Contractual Dependencies: Disability and the Bureaucracy of Begging in Kinshasa, Democratic Republic of Congo," *American Ethnologist* 45, no. 4 (2018): 455.
132 Devlieger, "Contractual Dependencies," 466.

proximity to DPOs, who tend to focus their advocacy on the issues directly confronting disabled people in the cities.[133]

However, increased proximity to people and resources may create its own problems for urban Africans with disabilities. A study by Maart, et al. indicated that disabled South Africans in the urban Western Cape reported more physical barriers than those in the rural Eastern Cape.[134] The authors suggest that this is because "living in an urban, built up environment poses more barriers with regard to mobility and accessibility."[135] Jori De Coster argues that contemporary ideological factors also further debilitate some disabled urban people: "Within the megalopolis that Kinshasa has become, this capacity 'to belong', to socially posit oneself within as many different collectives as possible, and thereby to obliterate anonymity (in itself an almost unthinkable concept), is crucial to survive and to exist beyond the raw reality of mere survival and bare life."[136] Indeed, many rural people return to their homes (or attempt to) because they perceive that there is more social support despite fewer resources.[137] Chataika also identifies the "clear relationship between patterns of urbanization in African states and issues of environmental degradation and climate change."[138] The increasing frequency of drought draws food-insecure migrants to the cities, where they are often relegated to the debilitating environment of the slums.

---

133 David R. Penna, "Empowering Rural Deaf Citizens through Organizations and Social Movements," in *Citizenship, Politics, Difference: Perspectives from Sub-Saharan Signed Language Communities*, ed. Audrey C. Cooper and Khadijat K. Rashid (Washington, DC: Gallaudet University Press, 2015), 186.

134 Soraya Maart et al., "Environmental Barriers Experienced by Urban and Rural Disabled People in South Africa," *Disability & Society* 22, no. 4 (2007): 364.

135 Maart et al., "Environmental Barriers Experienced by Urban and Rural Disabled People in South Africa," 365.

136 Jori De Coster, "A Dialogue with Society: Disability, Theatre, and Being Human in Kinshasa, DR Congo," in *Rethinking Disability: World Perspectives in Culture and Society*, ed. Patrick Devlieger et al. (Antwerp: Garant, 2016), 183.

137 Collins Airhihenbuwa, "Framing an African-Centred Discourse on Global Health: Centralising Identity and Culture in Theorising Health Behavior," *The Study of Africa, vol. 1, Disciplinary and Interdisciplinary Encounters*, ed. Paul Tiyambe Zeleza (Dakar: Council for the Development of Social Science Research in Africa, 2006), 381.

138 Chataika, "Disabled Women, Urbanization, and Sustainable Development in Africa," 183.

The debilitating effects of Africa's HIV/AIDS pandemic are intimately bound up with issues of disability, both because of the impairments and stigmatizations caused by the disease and because of the increased risk among people with disabilities for acquiring HIV. Women with disabilities are often at a higher risk of acquiring HIV because of inadequate health provisions: "A generalised assumption among healthcare service providers is that women with disabilities will not be sexually active, and thus do not require reproductive healthcare. This leads to increased vulnerability to sexually transmitted infections."[139] More distressing still are circumstances such as those reported by Peta and McKenzie in Zimbabwe, where "traditional healers prescribe sex with disabled women not only as a cure for HIV but also for curing epilepsy and getting rich."[140] Yet even as HIV infection risk is higher for women with disabilities, and even while many of the concerns of Africans with HIV are similar or identical to those with other impairments, this does not necessarily translate into disability solidarity. As Evans, Adjei-Amoako, and Atim report, "People living with HIV in Africa and others with chronic illness . . . may identify with others on the basis of their biomedical diagnosis rather than according to strategic notions of 'disability.'"[141] Indeed the treatment of HIV/AIDS as a biomedical condition rather than a socioeconomic one, even for the purposes of social activism, is an approach foreign to traditional disability studies: it appears to exchange a medical approach for the field's foundational distinctions between impairment and disability.

Albinism, while not considered a disability in many parts of the world, is certainly a disability issue in Africa, as well as a humanitarian one. Indeed, albinism in Africa may well be a disability without any actual impairment, since "deficiency in melanin, the chemical responsible for producing pigments that determine human colours, can lead to the absence of pigment from the skin, hair and eyes. In some cases, it leads to poor vision. But albinism is not a chronic medical condition; a person with albinism is generally

---

139 Lisbet Grut, Joyce Olenja, and Benedicte Ingstad, "Disability and Barriers in Kenya," *Disability and Poverty: A Global Challenge*, ed. Arne H. Eide and Benedicte Ingstad (Bristol, UK: Bristol University Press, 2011), 157.

140 Christine Peta and Judith McKenzie, "Bodies (Im)politic: The Experiences of Sexuality of Disabled Women in Zimbabwe," in *The Palgrave Handbook of Disability and Citizenship in the Global South*, ed. Brian Watermeyer, Judith McKenzie, and Leslie Swartz (London: Palgrave Macmillan, 2019), 257.

141 Ruth Evans, Yaw Adjei-Amoako, and Agnes Atim, "Disability and HIV: Critical Intersections," *Disability in the Global South*, ed. Shaun Grech and Karen Soldatic (New York: Springer, 2016), 354.

as healthy as the rest of the population."[142] Nevertheless, albinism is treated as an impairment by many in Africa, and the stigma that results can be especially dangerous to people with the condition. In Malawi and Tanzania, people with albinism are frequently murdered or mutilated because common beliefs in these countries assume albinos have supernatural powers, including the power to heal through the use of body parts.[143] Although Tanzania has been labeled "ground zero," similar beliefs and victimizations are documented in Zimbabwe, Kenya, and Burundi, as well as Cameroon, Ghana, and Benin, and trafficking in the body parts of people with albinism is reported across the continent.[144] In Zimbabwe, the mistaken belief that people with albinism cannot die has led to ritual rapes, particularly by people with HIV/AIDS.[145] As Bright Nkrumah argues, "The ongoing persecution not only violates the right to life of albinos but also constitutes discrimination and persecution, which has triggered mass fear in their lives."[146]

As with albinism, the practice of female genital mutilation (FGM) may also be considered a disability in parts of Africa without necessarily involving an impairment, though serious impairments certainly can and do result. Owojuyigbe et al. argue forcefully for the treatment of FGM as a disability, since:

> the victims of FGM are often thought to be portrayed in a negative light when they are unable to cope with the negative and disabling effects of the practice . . . The psychological trauma and issues of painful intercourse which are attendant problems when mention to others may paint the disabled as helpless and suffering and create a situation where the disabled may be shamed into silence.[147]

---

142 Kolawole Olaiya, "Commodifying the 'Sacred,' Beatifying the 'Abnormal': Nollywood and the Representation of Disability," *Global South* 7, no. 1 (2013): 149.

143 Ken Junior Lipenga and Emmanuel Ngwira, "'Black on the Inside': Albino Subjectivity in the African Novel," *Disability and the Global South* 5, no. 2 (2018): 1473.

144 Mark P. Mostert and Martha M. Weich, "Ablinism in Africa: A Proposed Conceptual Framework to Understand and Effectively Address a Continental Crisis," *African Disability Rights Yearbook* 5 (2017): 103.

145 Collis Garikai Machoko, "Albinism: A Life of Ambiguity—A Zimbabwean Experience," *African Identities* 11, no. 3 (2013): 330.

146 Bright Nkrumah, "The Hunted: UDHR and Africans with Albinism," *International Migration* 57, no. 1 (2019): 193.

147 Michael Owojuyigbe, Miracle-Eunice Bolorunduro, and Dauda Busari, "Female Genital Mutilation as Sexual Disability: Perceptions of Women and

Unlike most other disabilities, however, FGM is not a de facto source of stigma or social marginalization. Discussing the prevalence in Kenya, Mary Nyangweso explains that "in indigenous communities, female circumcision was perceived as a practice that assures female fertility, that provides a source of identity, and that prescribes social status whereas the lack of circumcision can lead to social exclusion and shunning."[148] Whether or not FGM necessarily qualifies as a disability by itself, it certainly has frequent consequences that are undeniably disabling. Ntiense Ben Edemikpong argues that the surgery involved in FGM "constitutes a serious threat to the child, and that the painful operation is a source of major psychological, as well as physical, trauma."[149] Further, FGM presents a variety of risks to physical health, including increased risk of infection, excessive bleeding, urinary retention, and/or sterility, each of which are likely disabling conditions for African women.[150]

Disability Policy, Activism, and Humanitarianism

The United Nations' 2006 Convention on the Rights of People with Disabilities (CRPD) frames disability as a fundamental human rights concern and has had a substantial impact on public policy initiatives in nations across Africa. As Hansen and Sait describe it, "The Convention requires a specific disability focus with a strong focus on discrimination and the responsibility to create a society that incorporated and makes reasonable accommodations for people with disabilities."[151] African countries like South Africa, Ghana, and Uganda have implemented substantial disability policies, and most others have become signatories to the CRPD.[152] Uganda even implements quotas in their parliament, with five seats reserved specifically for people with

---

   Their Spouses in Akure, Ondo State, Nigeria," *Reproductive Health Matters* 25, no. 50 (2017): 87.
148 Mary Nyangweso Wangila, "Beyond Facts to Reality: Women in 'Female Circumcising' Communities," *Journal of Human Rights* 6 (2007): 405.
149 Ntiense Ben Edemikpong, "'We Shall Not Fold Our Arms and Wait': Female Genital Mutilation," in *Imprinting Our Image: An International Anthology by Women with Disabilities*, ed. Diane Driedger and Susan Gray (Ottawa: Gynergy, 1992), 130.
150 Wangila, "Beyond Facts to Reality," 399.
151 Hansen and Sait, "'We Too Are Disabled,'" 98.
152 Evans, Adjei-Amoako, and Atim, "Disability and HIV," 361.

disabilities.[153] Further, Meekosha and Soldatic indicate how the Convention adds legitimacy to the arguments of disabled activists:

> Local activists have also seized upon the UNCRPD as a central instrument of dissent against neoliberal social policy restructuring. A central component of their strategic orientation has involved harnessing the international moral authority for the UNCRPD as a means to contest, and resist, the radical implantation of neoliberal nation-state policy regimes that seek to privatise and individualise disabled people's structural location of disadvantage.[154]

However, despite the excitement and quick adoption of policies, the CRPD may have provided false hope to many African nations. Eide et al. caution that "optimism surrounding the CRPD in particular may have a bleak flipside, that is, the celebration of good policies with no effect on the lives of persons with disabilities, in particular in poor contexts where the gap between policy and reality is most pronounced."[155] The convention was crafted to be global but in some ways is incompatible with the values and challenges faced by Africans "notwithstanding the broad and meaningful participation of African states and non-state actors in the adoption of the CRPD, the convention failed to cover some concerns of the African disability discourse including albinism, HIV/AIDS, and the effects of harmful traditional practices and beliefs on the rights of PWDs."[156]

The CRPD's incompatibility with local practices was put into striking relief when "South Africa—in seeking to realise the rights incorporated into the CRPD including the right to care in the community—began a process of de-institutionalising over two thousand mental health patients to under-resourced community-based organisations with inadequately trained staff, resulting in the deaths of at least 94 people."[157] Nevertheless, on balance the

---

153 Emmanuel Sackey, "Disability and Political Participation in Ghana: An Alternative Perspective," *Scandinavian Journal of Disability Research* 17, no. 4 (2015): 376.

154 Meekosha and Soldatic, "Decolonising Disability," 1386.

155 Arne H. Eide, Watson Khupe, and Hasheem Mannan, "Development Process in Africa: Poverty, Politics, and Indigenous Knowledge," *African Journal of Disability* 3 (2014): 4.

156 Kamga, "A Call for a Protocol," 228.

157 Faraaz Mohomed, Janet E. Lord, and Michael Ashley Stein, "Transposing the Convention on the Rights of Persons with Disabilities in Africa: The

convention remains a positive development for Africa since it commits its nations to acknowledging the importance of disabled Africans, even if its full and effective implementation is far from complete.

One of the largest barriers to effective disability policies is the unevenness of reliable and actionable statistical data on the prevalence and concentration of disability. Berghs contends that "the absence of usable information reflects an imbalance of power in terms of data-collection, which remains top-down and occurs without the participation of disabled people advocating their needs."[158] A lack of statistical data has made effective policy responses difficult, since activists cannot present governments with the actual rates of disability.[159] Where data is collected, it is often insufficiently engaged with local knowledge and customs. For instance, in Zambia: "Most assessment instruments that are currently in use for the diagnosis of learning disabilities are standardized using Western norms. This raises ethical issues as a lack of sensitivity to cultural differences can result in misdiagnosis or mislabelling."[160]

Even when disability policies are in place in African nations, there are often major gaps and/or barriers to effective implementation. In South Africa, despite some of the most promising policies on the continent, "The majority of persons with disabilities are not yet experiencing meaningful change in their quality of life, in access to equal rights and in levels of community integration."[161] In Nigeria, policies often purport to assist people with disabilities, but "these efforts have yielded few dividends, leading to declining quality of life for millions of people who have disabilities."[162] While in Zimbabwe, one of the earliest African nations to officially address

---

Role of Disabled Peoples' Organizations," *African Journal of International and Comparative Law* 27, no. 3 (2019): 343.
158 Berghs, "New Humanitarianism," 32.
159 Arne H. Eide and Mitch E. Loeb, "Data and Statistics on Disability in Developing Countries," *Disability Knowledge and Research Programme Executive Summary* (London: 2005), 6.
160 Mika Paananen et al., "Learning Disability Assessment," in *Assessment of Learning Disabilities: Cooperation Between Teachers, Psychologists and Parents—African Edition*, ed. Tuija Aro and Timo Ahonen (Jyvaskyla, Finland: Uniprint, 2011), 32.
161 Mji et al., "Networking in Disability for Development," 77.
162 Paul M. Ajuwon, "Disabilities and Disability Services in Nigera: Past, Present and Future," *The Routledge History of Disability*, ed. Roy Hanes, Ivan Brown, and Nancy E. Hasan (New York and London: Routledge, 2017), 141.

disability policy and establish disability rights, "The enjoyment of such rights is limited by the insufficient resources provided by the State toward disability issues."[163]

Concerns about the cost of disability programs often led to insufficient (or even nonexistent) implementation. Privilege Haang'andu asserts that "it is not irrational for host governments to accept legislative proposals accompanied by economic benefits and other political incentives with no intention to implement them."[164] Educational spending is prone to disability cuts, since "special education often has a much higher cost per pupil than educating a non-disabled student. Moreover, regardless of the time and funds invested, there is no guarantee that the cost-benefit ratio will ever equal that for the non-disabled child."[165] Even when inclusive educational requirements are in place, as in South Africa, "we see a pattern of HEIs [higher education institutions] falling back to a position of minimal accommodation for SWDs [students with disabilities] and an approach of minimum legal compliance."[166]

Gaps in disability policy are common throughout Africa, particularly with regard to privileging certain disabled populations over others: "Extreme cases include countries such as Cape Verde, Eritrea, Madagascar, Morocco, Mozambique, and Swaziland, which do not even make the pretense of recognizing deaf people as equal citizens."[167] South African disability grants are

---

163 Tafadzwa Rugohu and France Maphosa, "Socio-Economic Barriers Faced by Women with Disabilities in Zimbabwe," in *The Routledge Handbook of Disability in Southern Africa*, ed. Tsitsi Chataika (New York and London: Routledge, 2018), 238.

164 Privilege Haang'andu, "Transnationalizing Disability Policy in Embedded Cultural-Cognitive Worldviews: The Case of Sub-Saharan Africa," *Disability in the Global South* 5, no. 1 (2018): 1302.

165 Karen L. Biraimah, "Moving Beyond a Destructive Past to a Decolonised and Inclusive Future: The Role of Ubuntu-Style Education in Providing Culturally Relevant Pedagogy for Namibia," *International Review of Education* 62, no. 1 (2016): 58.

166 Desire Chiwandire and Louise Vincent, "Funding and Inclusion in Higher Education Institutions for Students with Disabilities," *African Journal of Disability* 8 (2019): 8.

167 Alem Hailu, "Adopting Human Development as the Universal Goal: Inclusive Strategies for Sociopolitical Transformation in Africa," in *Citizenship, Politics, Difference: Perspectives from Sub-Saharan Signed Language Communities*, ed. Audrey C. Cooper and Khadijat K. Rashid (Washington, DC: Gallaudet University Press, 2015), 151.

only available for people with physical disabilities,[168] while "in the Sudan, those with mental disabilities are kept together with the mentally sick in hospitals, as their case is not properly understood."[169] After the fall of the Gaddafi government in Libya, "any war-wounded casualty could have international care paid for by the government regardless of personal wealth. But people who acquired disability outside a revolutionary context and did not have personal wealth to draw on were dependent on a post-revolutionary public rehabilitation system that was barely functioning."[170]

Much of the pressure for effective disability policy across Africa has come from the activist work of DPOs. In South Africa, "The disability movement (DPOs) . . . has made self-experiences and self-representations a political agenda, emerging with the transformational process of creating access for all."[171] DPOs present opportunities for disabled people to coordinate with one another for both political and social purposes. As Lara Bezzina illustrates, "In Burkina Faso, where there are people with disabilities who did not know that there are other people with disabilities like them before they joined a DPO, the sense of identity emerging from belonging to a group of people with disabilities takes on an accentuated significance."[172] During and after North Africa's Arab Spring, DPOs were able to secure substantial gains, particularly in Egypt and Tunisia.[173] Prodemocracy movements in Egypt employed human rights rhetoric that was then picked up by disability protesters in the country, resulting in significant gains for each movement.[174]

The priorities, organizational vision, and sustainability of DPOs present unique challenges. DPO leadership is often restricted to a small segment of the disability community: "DPO leaders are those who possess a certain level of education but are not necessarily the ones who have the DPO's and

---

168 Hansen and Sait, "'We Too Are Disabled,'" 94.
169 Michael Karanja, "Disability in Contexts of Displacement," *Disability Studies Quarterly* 28, no. 4 (2009): 3.
170 Anne Cusick and Rania M. Hamed El Sahly, "People with Disability in Libya Are a Medicalised Minority: Findings of a Scoping Review," *Scandinavian Journal of Disability Research* 20, no. 1 (2018): 151.
171 Hansen and Sait, "'We Too Are Disabled,'" 99.
172 Lara Bezzina, "Disabled People's Organizations and the Disability Movement: Perspectives from Burkina Faso," *African Journal of Disability* 8 (2019): 4.
173 Mohomed, Lord, and Stein, "Transposing the Convention," 338.
174 Sharon N. Barnartt, "The Arab Spring Protests and Concurrent Disability Protests: Social Movement Spillover or Spurious Relationship," *Studies in Social Justice* 8, no. 1 (2014): 75.

its members interests at heart. Unfortunately, these leaders tend to form an 'elite' group whose members are re-elected in consecutive elections, simply rotating roles from election to election"[175] As Muyinda and Whyte note, "Even disabled people's organisations (DPOs) at both grass-roots and national level tended to downplay or even be unaware of the diversities that existed among people with disabilities."[176] Governments can be unresponsive to DPO claims or assume that the activity of DPOs makes government interventions unnecessary.[177] Further complicating the work of DPOs is the lack of resources and continual disappointments, which can sometimes lead to despair: "Numerous DPOs comment on the fact that meetings are no longer held because of the fact that the members feel that they are not getting anything."[178] While the challenges facing local DPOs, as well as many national and international bodies, are substantial, recent decades have seen a variety of disability policy success stories that can be learned from and built upon.

With typically better resources than DPOs, community-based rehabilitation (CBR) programs are frequently employed to assist people with disabilities in Africa. As summarized by Susie Miles, "CBR is both a philosophy and a strategy for providing rehabilitation services in the community in a more equitable, sustainable and appropriate way than can be provided in a health or educational institution."[179] By emphasizing local resources, CBR is ostensibly both more responsive to local contexts, and more cost efficient.[180] However, as a strategy developed in the Global North, CBR exhibited ideological commitments to individual care that were often incompatible with African community priorities. Miles argues that "focusing exclusively upon the rehabilitation needs of individuals is likely to be counter-productive unless the informal support networks and the basic needs of the whole

---

175 Bezzina, "Disabled People's Organizations," 7.
176 Muyinda and Whyte, "Displacement, Mobility, and Poverty in Northern Uganda," 125–126.
177 Eide and Loeb, "Data and Statistics on Disability," 4.
178 Bezzina, "Disabled People's Organizations," 8.
179 Susie Miles, "Engaging with the Disability Rights Movement: The Experience of Community-Based Rehabilitation in Southern Africa," *Disability & Society* 11, no. 4 (1996): 502.
180 Eric van Diessen et al., "Community-Based Rehabilitation Offers Cost-Effective Epilepsy Treatment in Rural Guinea-Bissau," *Epilepsy & Behavior* 79 (2018): 23.

community are recognised and addressed."[181] Additionally, CBR programs are rarely integrated with DPO activity since "CBR workers tend to have more contact with the families of disabled people than with the disability rights movement, especially in programmes which prioritise the needs of children, and therefore do not necessarily feel that they should be accountable to DPOs."[182] Moreover, CBR funding is largely dependent on Global North donors, who typically lack the patience required to forge sustainable partnerships with DPOs.[183]

International funders and transnational organizations often remain the best-resourced approaches for addressing disability in Africa, even as they also bring their own priorities to bear upon the lives of disabled Africans. As Ingstad argues, "Universalism as advocated through the global NGO network of persons with a disability is important and necessary to raise national and global awareness, but it may work contrary to the good intentions if not complimented by the necessary understanding of—and adjustment to—the local cultural context."[184] NGOs rely on donors who are often far removed from the realities of disability in Africa and so tend to proliferate a skewed view of disabled Africans:

> The disabled African body has gained iconic weight in the global Northern imaginary through a variety of development-related media. North to South development projects, including small-scale missions and entrepreneurial ventures, increasingly draw for their legitimacy upon images of docile African bodies in need of care and rehabilitation. They distribute images not only of impaired bodies in need, but also of a crippled, ignorant Africa and its benevolent, knowledgeable Northern rescuers.[185]

NGOs tend to give assistance to DPOs rather than individuals, and DPOs largely rely on NGOs for funding, which allows NGOs to dictate how DPOs and their members ought to operate. Berghs observes how activists in Sierra Leone alter their behavior to cater to NGO expectations: "Social activism and experiences of disability were being commodified through the INGOs and media, as it became increasingly important to access 'tragic', 'victim' or

---

181 Miles, "Engaging with the Disability Rights Movement," 503.
182 Miles, "Engaging with the Disability Rights Movement," 510.
183 Miles, "Engaging with the Disability Rights Movement," 514.
184 Ingstad, "Seeing Disability and Human Rights in the Local Context," 256.
185 Nepveux and Beitiks, "Producing African Disability through Documentary Film," 237–238.

'survivor' identities to access resources and in this way people were also kept dependent."[186] When NGOs invariably cut their programs or end them entirely, DPOs who have grown dependent upon them become dispirited and often end their own operations.[187] The vast resources of international humanitarian organizations could certainly do much to transform the lives of disabled people in Africa, but more effort needs to be devoted to collaborating with DPOs and local governments to determine how best to distribute their assistance.

Chapter Descriptions

The first section of this volume, "Theorizing Disability in Africa," addresses the challenges of defining and operationalizing conceptions of disability in African contexts, as well as reconciling African approaches to disability with the field of globalized disability studies. Medical sociologist Maria Berghs argues that global public health institutions dictate pathologized practices onto Africans with disabilities. However, rather than merely accepting these impositions, disabled Africans synthesize local and global realities to create more effective approaches. Historian Fikru Negash Gebrekidan offers a historical materialist account of disability in Africa, distinguishing among the contrasting approaches taken by foragers, pastoralists, and agriculturalists across the continent. He argues that the cultural values disabled Africans contend with are primarily dependent on historically contingent socioeconomic conditions. Religious scholar Mary Nyangweso points to how disability's perceived divine connections in both indigenous and Christian religious traditions render stigmas that are particularly insidious. She suggests that universalist appeals to human rights and African communalist ethics are best suited to counter cultural misconceptions. Anthropologist Kathryn Linn Geurts considers how the multiplicity of meaning-making spaces continues to complicate and marginalize Africans with disabilities. Various sources of misfortune, as well as the challenges of seeking and managing therapy and belonging each provide complex challenges for disabled people, who meet them with creative adaptations and revisions of meaning.

---

186 Berghs, *Embodied Memory*, 195.
187 Bezzina, "Disabled People's Organizations," 8.

In the volume's second section, "Representation and Cultural Expressions," the authors utilize artistic and popularized depictions of disability to explore the ideological approaches that influence the treatment of disabled Africans. Literary scholar Ernest Cole explores how literature, cinema, and individual testimonies narrate the legacy of punitive amputations in Sierra Leone. He argues that amputation in this context operates both as a physical mark of control and as a sign of resistance. In his chapter on the plays of Wole Soyinka, performance scholar Nic Hamel argues that postcolonial Yoruba cosmologies, performance traditions, and recent histories of conflict create a complex context for portrayals of disability. He argues that approaches from traditional literary disability studies might lead to erroneously dismissive interpretations of Soyinka's depictions of disability. Kolawole Olaiya, a scholar of drama, examines how Nollywood films create and sustain stigmatized representations of mental illness. He argues that spiritualized and demeaning depictions tend to supersede any consideration of sociopolitical disability contexts. Linguist Saloua Ben Zahra offers a close reading of how J. M. Coetzee's novel *Waiting for the Barbarians* employs intersecting allegories to demonstrate disability's sociopolitical complexity. She argues that Coetzee utilizes fluid narratives of colonialism, gender, and disability to signify conceptual anxieties of identity in his characters.

The volume's third section, "Education, Community, and Caregiving," addresses practical and localized approaches to disability inclusion, empowerment, and care. Legal scholar Serges Djoyou Kamga evaluates theories of inclusive education and their potential for alleviating poverty among Africans with disabilities. He argues that inclusive education policy may be successfully implemented when framed in language of diversity and legal rights and engaged with local communities. Educational researchers Angi Stone-MacDonald and Ozden H. Pinar Irmak explore how the capability approach may be used to evaluate inclusive education initiatives in East African countries. Their case studies in Tanzania suggest that community integration is a central component for successful education of children with disabilities. Community development scholars Ntombekhaya Tshabalala, Elizabeth Ladjer Bibi Agbettor, and Theresa Lorenzo report on community-based employment programs for young blind people in Ghana and South Africa. Their case studies demonstrate program successes but also indicate that CBR priorities need to be expanded to account for more flexibility in the lives of disabled Africans. Psychologist Frances Emily Owusu-Ansah provides a firsthand account of the challenges in caring for the aging disabled in informal family caregiving environments. She argues that care for caregivers is vital, but since external support structures for this kind of care in western Africa are severely lacking, caregivers and their communities may draw on indigenous knowledge and practices.

The fourth and final section of this volume deals with "Activism and Barriers to Inclusion," where the authors illustrate practical challenges to addressing disability faced by activists and policymakers, as well as a variety of strategies taken to address them. Occupational therapist Denise Nepveux examines the experiences of four women in leadership positions with DPOs in Ghana. She finds that women face significant structural challenges but also develop their own productive engagement strategies based on humility, transparency, accountability, and engagement. Sociologist Emmanuel Sackey examines the sluggish implementation of Ghana's enacted disability policies and the fissures within disability activist groups that helped enable the government's inaction. He suggests that a lack of pragmatism by the disability movement partly led to unsuccessful policy implementations. International politics scholar Desire Chiwandire documents the status of disability inclusion in sports and recreation in South African higher education. He argues for a strong link between sports participation and community integration and finds current implementation to be significantly lacking. Kamga explores how the Convention for the Rights of People with Disabilities affected the community-based rehabilitation approach in the African legal and disability policy environments. He advocates for an inclusive form of CBR that emphasizes the importance of human rights in addition to health and welfare.

The volume concludes with a series of recommendations for future academic engagements, with Toyin Falola and Anna Lee Carothers's chapter "A Research Agenda for African Disability Studies." Also included is a follow-up to this introduction intended for scholars with little exposure to the field of traditional disability studies, entitled "Disability Studies: A Disciplinary Overview," by Carothers, Falola, and Hamel. By engaging with a wide swath of issues and scholars who encompass the breadth of practices and approaches of African disability studies, this volume argues that this is an interdisciplinary field of study worthy of consideration in its own right.

Chapter Two

Disability Studies

A Disciplinary Overview

Toyin Falola, Anna Lee Carothers, and Nic Hamel

Currently an estimated 15 percent of the global population (or one billion people) are classified as having one or more disabilities,[1] thus making those with disabilities the world's largest minority group.[2] Common characterizations of disability tend to resemble that of the US Centers for Disease Control and Prevention (CDC), which define disability as "any condition of the body or mind (impairment) that makes it more difficult for the person with the condition to do certain activities (activity limitation) and interact with the world around them (participation restrictions)."[3] Under this view, a disability may affect a person's mental health, relationships of various kinds, hearing, thinking, vision, learning, movement, remembering, or communicating.[4] Such definitions, typically referred to as pertaining to the "medical

---

1 *The World Bank*, "Disability Inclusion," *World Bank*, October 2, 2019, https://www.worldbank.org/en/topic/disability.
2 *Columbia Center for the Study of Social Difference*, "The Future of Disability Studies," *Columbia University Center for the Study of Social Difference*, n.d., https://www.socialdifference.columbia.edu/projects-/the-future-of-disability-studies.
3 *Centers for Disease Control and Prevention*, "Disability and Health Overview," *CDC*, n.d., https://www.cdc.gov/ncbddd/disabilityandhealth/disability.html.
4 *Centers for Disease Control and Prevention*, "Disability and Health Overview."

model,"[5] have been roundly denounced by scholars and activists in disability studies (sometimes referred to as "critical disability theory"),[6] for focusing too heavily on the body and mind while largely ignoring disability's various social dimensions. Alternatively, disability studies advocates for a primarily "socio-political-cultural" approach to the concept of disability.[7] This often involves distinguishing between "impairments," which are conditions that affect the body or mind, and "disabilities," which are environmental conditions that affect the well-being of people who have (or are thought to have) impairments.[8] Disability activists and scholars frequently emphasize the fluid, contingent, and temporal natures of disability, which are unavoidable for any individual, for long-term aging and exposure to basic life dangers will cause every individual to experience disability at some point.[9] Consequently, before one encounters one's disability, one is often said to be merely "temporarily able-bodied."[10]

Early scholarship on disability studies adopted the medical/social distinction developed by the 1960s and 1970s activist movements in the United Kingdom and the United States, coining what is called the "social model."[11] Essentially, the social model makes the claim that disability is a social con-

---

5   Lennard J. Davis, "Crips Strike Back: The Rise of Disability Studies," *American Literary History* 11, no. 3 (1999): 506.
6   Melinda C. Hall, "Critical Disability Theory." *Stanford Encyclopedia of Philosophy*, September 23, 2019, https://plato.stanford.edu/entries/disability-critical/.
7   Simi Linton, *Claiming Disability: Knowledge and Identity* (New York: New York University Press, 1998), 133.
8   Davis's definition of the impairment/disability distinction emphasizes the difference between biological fact and social impediment: "An impairment involves a loss or diminution of sight, hearing, mobility, mental ability, and so on. But an impairment only becomes a disability when the ambient society creates environments with barriers—affective, sensory, cognitive, or architectural," 506–507.
9   Cecilia Capuzzi Simon, "Disability Studies: A New Normal," *New York Times*, November 1, 2013, https://www.nytimes.com/2013/11/03/education/edlife/disability-studies-a-new-normal.html; and Robert McRuer, "Crip Eye for the Normative Guy: Queer Theory and the Disciplining of Disability Studies," *Modern Language Association* 120, no. 2 (2005): 586–92.
10 Simon, "Disability Studies."
11 Michael Oliver, "Social Policy and Disability: Some Theoretical Issues," *Disability, Handicap & Society* 1, no. 1 (1986): 13.

struction, and therefore when social barriers are removed and universal access is achieved, disability would cease to exist. As a rallying cry, the social model was effective for disabled people both because it identified forms of discrimination and barriers to access and "also because it provided the basis for a stronger sense of identity."[12] However, as a theoretical maxim, a strict social model approach was difficult to defend, even as it was emerging as an organizing principle of the nascent field of disability studies,[13] which was initially dominated by scholars trained in the social sciences.[14] Drawing on sociological considerations of deviance and stigma,[15] the field developed social construction critiques of rehabilitative, religious, and charitable approaches to disability. Later, humanities scholars incorporated concepts from postmodernism, psychoanalysis, and cultural studies into the field, resulting in a consensus definition of disability as something that "[confers] pain, disease, suffering, function, limitation, abnormality, dependence, social stigma, and economic disadvantage and [limits] life opportunities and quality."[16]

Scholars in disability studies consider the cultural, political, and societal spheres of disability to be important because disability, by its very nature, exists outside of the "norm" of the able-bodied or typically minded. In essence, then, disability studies examines how disability is viewed within cultures, politics, and societies. It also examines the experiences of individuals with disabilities. Perhaps most importantly, it also encourages others to question what is actually considered "normal" and whether those with disabilities should be labeled "abnormal."[17] According to prominent gender and disability scholar Rosemarie Garland-Thomson, disability studies has two aims:

---

12 Tom Shakespeare, *Disability Rights and Wrongs Revisited*, 2nd ed. (Abingdon, UK: Routledge, 2014), 20.

13 Tom Shakespeare and Nicholas Watson, "Defending the Social Model," *Disability & Society* 12, no. 2 (1997): 293.

14 Michael Oliver and Colin Barnes, *The New Politics of Disablement* (London: Palgrave Macmillan, 2012), 43.

15 See Michel Foucault, *Discipline and Punish: The Birth of the Prison* (New York: Vintage, 2012); Robert B. Edgerton, *Deviance: A Cross-Cultural Perspective* (San Francisco: Cummings, 1976); Erving Goffman, *Stigma: Notes on the Management of Spoiled Identity* (New York: Simon and Schuster, 2009).

16 Rosemarie Garland-Thomson, "The Case for Conserving Disability," *Bioethical Inquiry* 9 (2012): 340.

17 Davis, "Crips Strike Back," 504.

first, to bring interdisciplinary attention to disability and, second, to bring people with disabilities themselves into the critical conversation.[18]

Disability studies as a discipline has examined the history of the stereotyping and ridiculing of those with disability. In the United States in the 1800s, those with disabilities were deemed unable to conform to regular society. They were identified as pitiable and even monstrous, and they were often subjected to forced sterilization or confined to asylums to live out the rest of their days. Yet they were also considered morbidly fascinating entities. They were even displayed in circuses or exhibitions so that others could ogle and laugh.[19] Of course the stigma and social grievances tied to disability still exist and not just in the United States. According to Garland-Thomson, this is because of "eugenic logic," which claims that disability should be eradicated in order to make a better world.[20] This logic is ingrained in individuals of all cultures. For instance, it is common for able-bodied and neurotypical individuals to separate themselves from those with disabilities and ignore them because of their perceived differences.[21] Additionally, those with disabilities around the world are statistically more likely to receive less education and experience more poverty. Much of this is due to the barriers that those with disabilities may experience on a daily basis, such as access to health care, education, or inadequate resources for transportation.[22]

Disability categorization is nearly always bound up with some kind of stigma, even when it emphasizes elements beyond those related to a medicalized focus on bodily limitations. Paradoxically, however, discussion and identification of stigma may fall into a trap "of perpetuating the problem it investigates by focusing on individual physical signs . . . and ignoring the

---

18   Brenda Jo Brueggemann, Rosemarie Garland-Thomson, and Georgina Kleege, "What Her Body Taught (Or, Teaching About and with a Disability): A Conversation," *Feminist Studies* 31, no. 1 (2005): 27.

19   *Anti-Defamation League*, "A Brief History of the Disability Rights Movement," ADL, 2018, https://www.adl.org/education/resources/backgrounders/disability-rights-movement.

20   Garland-Thomson, "The Case for Conserving Disability," 339–340.

21   Hélène Ouellette-Kuntz et al., "Public Attitudes towards Individuals with Intellectual Disabilities as Measured by the Concept of Social Distance," *Journal of Applied Research in Intellectual Disabilities* 23, no. 2 (2010): 132–142.

22   *The World Bank*, "Disability Inclusion."

social structures that produce the perception."[23] Literature and disability scholar Tobin Siebers refers to these structural oppressions as "the ideology of ability," which he describes as "at its simplest the preference for able-bodiedness. At its most radical, it defines the baseline by which humanness is determined, setting the measure of body and mind that gives or denies human status to individual persons."[24] By contrast, disability studies promotes cultural modes of production (arts, literature, social organizations, etc.) that expose ableist discrimination and emphasize the humanity and complexity of people with disabilities.

While some activists and scholars encourage the proliferation of salient disability subcultures, others emphasize the value of disability integration into the mainstream. This can become a point of contention. For instance, the Deaf community (members of which often consider themselves to be a linguistic minority rather than people with disabilities) has opposed inclusive educational initiatives favored by many disability activists.[25] While many disabled people find value in cultural affirmations of pride, others find this tactic difficult to embrace, particularly people with painful and/or debilitating impairments, which often produce ambivalent self-perceptions.[26]

Since the last half of the twentieth century, those with disabilities and their nondisabled allies have fought for disability rights.[27] Perhaps most influential was the disability rights movement that began in the United States in the 1960s, which followed similar patterns to the women's rights and civil rights movements in that it challenged stereotypes and lobbied for change.[28] The disability rights movement truly gained momentum in the 1970s, however, when disability rights activists marched to Washington, DC, and eventually

---

23   Jan Grue, "The Social Meaning of Disability: A Reflection on Categorisation, Stigma, and Identity," *Sociology of Health & Illness* 38, no. 6 (2016): 960.
24   Tobin Siebers, *Disability Theory* (Ann Arbor: University of Michigan Press, 2008), 8.
25   Colin Barnes and Geoff Mercer, "Disability Culture: Assimilation or Inclusion?" in *Handbook of Disability Studies*, ed. Michael Bury, Katherine D. Seelman, and Gary Albrecht (Thousand Oaks, CA: SAGE, 2001), 527.
26   Barnes and Mercer, "Disability Culture," 530–531.
27   Anti-Defamation League, "A Brief History of the Disability Rights Movement."
28   Anti-Defamation League, "A Brief History of the Disability Rights Movement"; Joseph P. Shapiro, *No Pity: People with Disabilities Forging a New Civil Rights Movement* (New York: Broadway, 1994).

helped pass the Rehabilitation Act of 1973,[29] which prohibits discrimination against those with disabilities[30] and provides programs for those with disabilities through federal funding (particularly for health-care programs).[31]

Disability studies emerged from the disability rights movement and its successes in the 1970s. The concept of disability studies came into prominence after the formation of the Union of the Physically Impaired against Segregation (UPIAS) in 1972 in the United Kingdom, which spread awareness of the need for those with physical disabilities to gain equal rights around the world. Meanwhile, in the United States, those in the disability rights movement advocated for civil rights laws related to equal employment and education, as well as accessible transportation, for Americans with disabilities. In 1982 American disability activists created the Society for Disability Studies (SDS)—which was originally called the Section for the Study of Chronic Illness, Impairment, and Disability (SSCIID).

In 1990 a sociologist with disabilities named Michael Oliver published *Politics of Disablement: A Sociological Approach*, thus offering disability studies a distinctly academic platform. In this book, Oliver examined how the social issue of disability can often be mischaracterized as solely a medical issue and only relevant to disabled individuals. For Oliver, disability issues are just as important to nondisabled individuals because they participate in a society where disability exists, and they could eventually become disabled, too.[32] In 1994, the disability studies program at Syracuse University emerged as the first to critically examine disability not as a medical study but rather as a social study. The program was revolutionary also because it argued that an unforgiving, prejudiced society is what needs to be fixed—not people with disabilities.[33] Disability scholars and activists often draw comparisons among ableism, racism, sexism, and homophobia, both to help clarify forms of discrimination and to seek common cause with other civil rights

---

29 Anti-Defamation League, "A Brief History of the Disability Rights Movement."
30 Jennifer Berry and Antonis Katsiyannis, "Service Animals for Students with Disabilities Under IDEA and Section 504 of the Rehabilitation Act of 1973," *Intervention in School and Clinic* 47, no. 5 (2012): 312–315.
31 Bianca G. Chamusco, "Revitalizing the Law that 'Preceded the Movement': Associated Discrimination and the Rehabilitation Act of 1973," *University of Chicago Law Review* 84, no. 3 (2017): 1287–1288.
32 Nancy E. Rice, "Disability Studies," *Encyclopaedia Britannica*, December 5, 2018, https://www.britannica.com/topic/disability-studies.
33 Simon, "Disability Studies."

activists.[34] This rhetoric was not always responsibly employed, as illustrated when the field was embarrassed by the publication of Chris Bell's satirical essay, "Introducing White Disability Studies: A Modest Proposal."[35]

Today, disability studies continues to grow as an academic field worldwide, especially in the United States, in part because the population continues to age, and disability will become more "relevant" globally. Also, generations born after the successes of the disability rights movement are naturally more aware of the importance of inclusion and accessibility in society. Since disability studies entered the academic world, scholars have analyzed disabled individuals' narratives and voices. Specifically, among other things, those who research disability studies have written about the history of disability: how disability has been portrayed in art, literature, politics, and media; philosophies of how those with disabilities can receive more justice from society; lack of disability representation among academics; and the intersectionality of disability with race, gender, and class.[36] What follows is a brief overview of major concepts and issues in contemporary disability studies.

Access and Accessibility

Disability rights activists and disability studies scholars understand the words "access" and "accessibility" to refer not only to environmental barriers being lifted for those with disabilities but also to what extent those with disabilities are included in society at large.[37] This distinction is important because lifting barriers does not always mean that those with disabilities are truly able to engage as active participants in their community.[38] In addition, laws put in place to lift barriers may not be readily enforceable or with enough

---

34 Tom Shakespeare, "Disability: Suffering, Social Oppression, or Complex Predicament?" in *The Contingent Nature of Life: Bioethics and Limits of Human Existence*, ed. Marcus Düwell, Christoph Rehmann-Sutter, and Dietmar Mieth (New York: Springer, 2008), 240.

35 Chris Bell, "Introducing White Disability Studies: A Modest Proposal," in *The Disability Studies Reader*, ed. Lennard Davis, 2nd ed. (Abingdon, UK: Routledge, 2006), 275–282.

36 Rice, "Disability Studies."

37 Bess Williamson, "Access," in *Keywords for Disability Studies*, ed. Rachel Adams, Benjamin Reiss, and David Serlin (New York: New York University Press, 2015), 145–148.

38 Williamson, "Access," 145.

specifications.[39] This means that even if ramps for wheelchairs exist, there can still be other physical barriers that hinder the mobility of people with disabilities (for instance, when navigating sidewalks or curb cuts). Consequently, then, "access" is not a term referring to individual abilities (or lack thereof) but rather to adequate legal and social assistance. This understanding of access fits the "social model of disability." Indeed, for truly positive change to take place, lawmakers must consider how people with disabilities can fully integrate into civic life.[40]

Even though accessibility laws were originally developed in the United States, similar laws have been replicated in other regions like the United Kingdom; Australia; Ontario, Canada; and South Africa. While this is good news, there are still difficulties in some of these areas. For example, not all of these regions have an infrastructure like that of the United States (e.g., centralized transportation systems or paved sidewalks). This means that some of these other regions will have to work doubly hard to reinvent their societies as disabled-friendly places.[41] Globally as well (not just in specific regions), stigma is an important barrier to accessibility. Some claim that those with disabilities are asking for too much and are selfishly requesting infrastructural changes that only benefit them and not the whole of society.[42] These claims contribute to "rituals of shame"[43] and do not acknowledge how an infrastructural change that helps marginalized citizens will also help society at large.

Naming and Language

Few topics are as acrimonious within the disability community as those that touch on the use of proper language for describing disability. Perhaps this is because, as Irving Zola suggests, language about disability inherently

---

39   Elizabeth F. Emens, "Disabling Attitudes: US Disability Law and the ADA Amendments Act," *The Disability Studies Reader*, ed. Lennard Davis, 4th ed. (Abingdon, UK: Routledge, 2013), 42.
40   Williamson, "Access," 146–147.
41   Williamson, "Access," 147.
42   Williamson, "Access," 148.
43   Williamson, "Access," 147.

implicates identity in a way that is simultaneously personal and political.[44] Historically, most of the terms used to refer to impairments, disabilities, and the people affected by them were overwhelmingly negative. Many people have endured difficult life experiences associated with such words, and consequently the use of certain commonly used terms is discouraged in disability studies. However, the refusal to use terms that have historically been harmful may also have consequences for disability activism, with the risk of blunting claims for public consideration.[45] Consequently, some activists have sought to reclaim pejorative terms like "mad" or "crip" to resignify pride in positive minoritarian identity categories.[46]

How people refer to themselves and the way in which they would like to be referred to are perennial points of contention in disability studies. The most identifiable fault line is between advocates of "person-first" and "identity-first" language.[47] Examples of person-first language would be "a person with disabilities," "a person with a mobility impairment," or "a person with intellectual disabilities." Whereas identity-first language would include labels such as "a disabled person," "a blind person," or "an autistic person." Advocates of person-first language include the American Psychological Association, many disability care practitioners, and people who interact regularly with the disabled. This group argues that by emphasizing the person rather than the disability, such language affirms the humanity of the individual who is often dehumanized for their disability status.[48] Advocates of identity-first language include the National Federation of the Blind, members of the autistic community, and advocacy-inclined activists. They argue that privileging the disability-related word implies that disabilities and impairments should not be stigmatized and affirms people as autonomous subjects who cannot be separated from particular attributes.[49] Use of both approaches may be found

---

44   Irving Zola, "Self, Identity, and the Naming Question: Reflections on the Language of Disability," *Social Science & Medicine* 36, no. 2 (1993): 167.
45   Zola, "Self, Identity, and the Naming Question," 170.
46   Carrie Sandahl, "Queering the Crip or Cripping the Queer? Intersections of Queer and Crip Identities in Solo Autobiographical Performance," *GLQ: A Journal of Lesbian and Gay Studies* 9, no. 1–2 (2003): 27.
47   Dana S. Dunn and Erin E. Andrews, "Person-First *and* Identity-First Language: Developing Psychologists' Cultural Competence Using Disability Language," *American Psychologist* 70, no. 3 (2015): 256.
48   Dunn and Andrews, "Person-First *and* Identity-First Language," 258.
49   Jim Sinclair, "Why I Dislike 'Person First' Language," *Autonomy, the Critical Journal of Interdisciplinary Autism Studies* 1, no. 2 (2013): 255–264.

throughout this volume (and indeed within this chapter), in deference to context and the particular preferences of individual authors.[50]

Independent Living and Institutionalization

Much of the emphasis of disability activism in the 1960s had to do with advocating for environments where disabled people could live, work, and go to school on their own terms. British poet and activist Simon Brisendon articulates how normalizing ideologies push disabled people into "a conditioned uselessness" where they are simultaneously reliant upon and demeaned by external forms of care: "It teaches us to be passive, to live up to the image of ourselves as objects of charity that we should be grateful to receive, and to ignore the possibility that we may be active people who have something to contribute to society."[51] In the face of such dehumanization, Brisendon advocates "independence" for disabled people, though he is keen to emphasize that the term means "someone who has taken control of their life and is choosing how that life is led."[52] He contrasts this with people living in institutions, where most life decisions are made by medical professionals rather than disabled people themselves.

Much has been accomplished toward the goal of independent living, particularly after the 1990 passage of the ADA in the United States and the 1995 Disability Discrimination Act in the United Kingdom. However, even as the basic principles of independent living were embedded in these and other legislation, implementation has often been far from comprehensive.[53] This is especially true for people with intellectual disabilities, whose access needs are often considered by organizations to be too "high level" to cost-effectively

---

50 Our own practice is to employ identity-first language in circumstances that imply a political situation, and to use person-first language when referring to individuals outside of an explicitly political context.

51 Simon Brisendon, "Independent Living and the Medical Model of Disability," *Disability, Handicap, & Society* 1, no. 2 (1986): 175.

52 Brisendon, "Independent Living and the Medical Model of Disability," 178.

53 Andrew Power, "Understanding the Complex Negotiations in Fulfilling the Right to Independent Living for Disabled People," *Disability & Society* 28, no. 2 (2013): 215.

implement.[54] Prevailing care practices for people with intellectual disabilities tend not to emphasize employment, independence, or mainstreaming;[55] however, there are indications that contemporary care workers do prioritize choice individual decision making.[56]

Institutions have a long and sordid relationship with disability. As criminologist Liat Ben-Moshe suggests, "Institutional life, whether in a prison, hospital, mental institution, nursing home, group home, or segregated 'school,' has been the reality, not the exception, for disabled people throughout North American history (and globally)."[57] Indeed carceral practices across all of these institutions have often been strikingly similar, despite their wide-ranging goals. Deinstitutionalization movements began for people with mental illnesses in the 1950s, while the process started benefiting people with developmental disabilities in the 1970s.[58] While disability activists have largely approved of these measures and promoted "abolition" of institution-style care, they were often not paired with sufficient community-based supports. Consequently, "Closure of large institutions has not led to freedom for disabled people, nor has it resulted in the radical acceptance of the fact of difference amongst us."[59]

Invisible Disabilities and the "Healthy Disabled"

Many of the most prominent activists in the disability movement were and are physically disabled. The International Symbol of Access, used "to represent purposely facilitated access, has become ubiquitous throughout the

---

54 Jenny Morris, "Independent Living and Community Care: A Disempowering Framework," *Disability & Society* 19, no. 5 (2004): 430.
55 Edward Hall, "Spaces of Social Inclusion and Belonging for People with Intellectual Disabilities," *Journal of Intellectual Disability Research* 54, no. 1 (2010): 52.
56 Roy McConkie and Suzanne Collins, "The Role of Support Staff in Promoting the Social Inclusion of Persons with an Intellectual Disability," *Journal of Intellectual Disability Research* 54, no. 8 (2010): 694.
57 Liat Ben-Moshe, "'The Institution Yet to Come'": Analyzing Incarceration Through a Disability Lens," *The Disability Studies Reader*, ed. Lennard Davis, 4th ed. (Abingdon, UK: Routledge, 2013), 132.
58 Ben-Moshe, "'The Institution Yet to Come,'" 135.
59 Ben-Moshe, "'The Institution Yet to Come,'" 140.

world,"⁶⁰ features the image of a person in a wheelchair. This has led to a common misconception that all people with disabilities are visibly identifiable as such, which excludes some people whose impairments might include fatigue, pain, or whose disabilities are psychological, intellectual, or intermittent. These conditions are sometimes referred to as "invisible disabilities" because they are usually not identifiable without a disclosure. It is important to emphasize that there is not a clear line between what disabilities qualify as visible or invisible, and indeed these categories can be fluid depending on the situation.⁶¹ This may give rise to practices that require individuals to repeatedly (and sometimes embarrassingly) prove their disabilities when receiving public accommodations, as in the example of aggressive policing of disability-reserved parking spots.⁶²

A related issue has to do with what feminist disability scholar Susan Wendell refers to as the "unhealthy disabled," which refers to a person with a debilitating or aggravated impairment due to illness.⁶³ This may prevent them from regularly or reliably participating in activities such as traditional work schedules, meetings, correspondence, or political demonstrations.⁶⁴ With an activist disability movement traditionally dominated by the "healthy disabled," impairments due to illness may ironically create barriers to participation in a movement for increased social inclusion. Both invisible and unhealthy disabilities problematize disability studies' typical notions of individualized impairment, as well as the idea of a "typical" disabled person being healthy and rational.⁶⁵ Each category also pushes conceptual boundaries of who qualifies as a person with disabilities and who does not.

---

60   Liat Ben-Moshe and Justin J. W. Powell, "Sign of Our Times? Revis(it)ing the International Symbol of Access," *Disability & Society* 22, no. 5 (2007): 489.
61   Margaret Price, "Defining Mental Disability," *The Disability Studies Reader*, ed. Lennard Davis, 4th ed. (Abingdon, UK: Routledge, 2013), 304.
62   Ellen Samuels, *Fantasies of Identification: Disability, Gender, Race* (New York: New York University Press, 2014), 132.
63   Susan Wendell, "Unhealthy Disabled: Treating Chronic Illnesses as Disabilities," *The Disability Studies Reader* ed. Lennard Davis, 4th ed. (Abingdon, UK: Routledge, 2013), 163.
64   Wendell, "Unhealthy Disabled," 167.
65   Price, "Defining Mental Disability," 301.

Bioethics and Euthanasia

In the essay "Recognizing Death while Affirming Life: Can End of Life Reform Uphold a Disabled Person's Interest in Continued Life?," Adrienne Asch considers the saying that it is "better to be dead than to be disabled," as well as the bioethical conflicts surrounding end-of-life societal attitudes and medicinal practice.[66] Asch notes that when a recently disabled patient (or their family) must choose between assisted suicide or medical assistance, using parlance like "quality of life" versus "sanctity of life" often does not get to the heart of end-of-life issues. Ultimately, this shortsighted distinction fails to recognize the very real problematic factors that may influence a patient's life or death.[67]

For instance, it is essential to discuss how society generally fears and thus stereotypes those with disabilities. People may assume that when one receives some measure of permanent medical assistance that this is a condemnation to a life devoid of any meaning or autonomy. However, this view inherently acknowledges only what disabled individuals have lost and fails to acknowledge what they have retained.[68] Asch explains this as follows:[69]

> Using the services and skills of a personal assistant who helps them get into and out of bed, eat their meals, or travel to their next appointment is no more shameful or embarrassing than it is for a nondisabled person to work closely with an administrative assistant or to value the expertise of a mechanic, plumber, or the magician who restores data after a computer crash.

Additionally, Asch argues that society feels inherently uncomfortable with disability because images of disability are uncomfortable reminders of our own frailties.[70] It is this very perception that concerns Asch the most.[71] Data have consistently shown that recently disabled individuals seek assisted suicide not because they fear loss of autonomy or the prospect

---

66 Adrienne Asch, "Recognizing Death While Affirming Life: Can End of Life Reform Uphold a Disabled Person's Interest in Continued Life?" *Hastings Center Report* 35, no. 6 (2005): S31–S36.
67 Asch, "Recognizing Death While Affirming Life," S31.
68 Asch, "Recognizing Death While Affirming Life," S32.
69 Asch, "Recognizing Death While Affirming Life," S33.
70 Robert Burt, *Taking Care of Strangers* (New York: Free Press, 1979), quoted in Asch, "Recognizing Death While Affirming Life," S33.
71 Asch, "Recognizing Death While Affirming Life," S33–S34.

of constant pain but because they fear being a burden on others.[72] Given this data, it is important for clinicians and the public at large to ask themselves whether the worst part about a person's disability is actually the disability itself or the emotional isolation from loved ones who may treat them with pity or disgust.[73] In Asch's words: "To anyone with the capacity to perceive the difference between warmth, toleration, and coldness in how he or she is treated by others, the thought of days, months, or years of life subject to resentful, duty-filled physical ministrations may be a fate worse than death."[74]

Ultimately, Asch argues that as long as a human being has cognitive ability and can still potentially benefit from meaningful relationships with others, a life of dignity for them means having the chance to maintain closeness with important people. Moreover, medical professionals must recognize this truth and no longer enforce isolation for disabled individuals. They must instead offer the sort of medical and emotional support for the patient and their loved ones that will enable them to maintain and strengthen their preexisting bond.[75] In Asch's view, the issue of disabled individuals who no longer have the cognitive ability and potential to benefit from meaningful relationships with others is more complicated, but to neglect those with intact cognitive abilities would mean an even harsher form of neglect for those without intact cognitive abilities. This is incredibly dangerous and inhumane.[76]

Lastly, Asch recommends that advanced directive forms be more specific. They should "describe the various medical scenarios that might occur in certain situations and encourage people to consider what they would or would not want done in each instance."[77] For example, they could ask the patient to reflect more on the essential things that are most meaningful for them (cognitive capacities, activities, etc.). In this way, the patient will be able to think more clearly about their desires rather than just assume that any disability should lead to assisted suicide.[78]

---

72   Asch, "Recognizing Death While Affirming Life," S34.
73   Asch, "Recognizing Death While Affirming Life," S34.
74   Asch, "Recognizing Death While Affirming Life," S34.
75   Asch, "Recognizing Death While Affirming Life," S34.
76   Asch, "Recognizing Death While Affirming Life," S34.
77   Asch, "Recognizing Death While Affirming Life," S36.
78   Asch, "Recognizing Death While Affirming Life," S36.

Eugenics and Abortion

Today, throughout much of Europe (including the United Kingdom), more than 90 percent of fetuses that test positive for Down syndrome are aborted. Furthermore, between the years 1995 and 2011 in the United States, about 75 percent of women whose fetus tested for Down syndrome chose to abort.[79] According to Marsha Saxton, a lecturer at the University of California at Berkeley and the director of research and training at the World Institute on Disability (WID)[80]: "Fetuses that are wanted are called 'babies.' Prenatal screening results can turn a 'wanted baby' into an 'unwanted fetus.'"[81] Arizona State philosopher and professor Bertha Alvarez Manninen draws similar conclusions. The issue of aborting a fetus predicted to have a disability (specifically Down syndrome) became deeply personal for Manninen when one of her friends (pseudonym Jackie) discovered her unborn child would have Down syndrome. According to Jackie, almost all of her friends and family told her that she should abort "it." This quick conclusion and use of the word "it" disturbed Manninen because, while she is pro-choice, she could not help but notice how the default response in society is to assume that abortion is the appropriate response to discovering that a fetus has a disability like Down syndrome.[82] For Manninen, this scenario presented extreme cognitive dissonance because prior to the diagnosis, family and friends had lavished attention on Jackie and the hypothetical person her fetus would become, "But now, at the *mere prospect* of being diagnosed with Down syndrome, [the person] was stripped of her ascriptive personhood and had become an abort-able, easily replaceable, fetus."[83]

Undoubtedly, argued Manninen, stripping a fetus of its personhood (or at least potential personhood) just because it might be disabled comes with

---

79 Jaime L. Natoli et al., "Prenatal Diagnosis of Down Syndrome: A Systematic Review of Termination Rates (1995–2011)," *Prenatal Diagnosis* 32, no. 2 (2012): 142–153.

80 *Othering & Belonging Institute*, "Marsha Saxton: Lecturer in Disability Studies," *Othering & Belonging Institute*, https://belonging.berkeley.edu/marsha-saxton.

81 Marsha Saxton, "Disability Rights and Selective Abortion," in *The Disability Studies Reader*, ed. Lennard Davis (Abingdon, UK: Routledge, 2010), 126.

82 Bertha Alvarez Manninen, "The Replaceable Fetus: A Reflection on Abortion and Disability," *Disability Studies Quarterly* 35, no. 1 (2015), https://dsqsds.org/article/view/3239/3831#endnote01.

83 Manninen, "Replaceable Fetus."

moral complications. While society can debate whether the growing tissue in a uterus is in fact a person, it is difficult to deny that this tissue is part of the human race. In Manninen's view, while a woman (or person with a uterus) is never obligated to participate in such an intimate act of carrying a life form (even for the sake of life itself), this does not mean that all abortions are morally equal—some motivations are sounder than others. All abortions should be carefully thought through, but there should be no moral exception for a fetus with a disability. After all, argues Manninen, a disability does not dictate what life will be like for a fetus once it is born. Not all disabilities are equal, and to automatically abort a fetus just because it has a disability is not a reflection of thoughtfulness but rather of prejudice toward those with disabilities.[84]

As disability studies scholars and disability advocates constantly show, an impairment does not lead to suffering in all cases. The CDC has consistently claimed and demonstrated that having a disability does not mean one is unhealthy. For both able-bodied and disabled people, being healthy is defined as "getting and staying well so [they] can lead full, active lives. . . . That means having the tools and information to make healthy choices and knowing how to prevent illness."[85] For people with disabilities, making healthy choices and preventing illness means having the knowledge that side effects of disabilities (like pain or depression) can be treated. But, just as with able-bodied individuals, disabled individuals should be treated for their whole selves and not just for their disabilities. While it may sometimes be more difficult for disabled individuals to stay healthy, people with disabilities should do what any person without disabilities should do: be physically active, eat healthily (and in healthy portions), drink in moderation, regularly attend health check-ups, and maintain contact with family and friends.[86] The CDC seems to suggest, therefore, that it is important to realize that quality of life for those with disabilities can be maintained and that the able-bodied and disabled have more similarities than differences.

Disability studies scholars like Garland-Thomson also argue that countereugenic logic should be valued over eugenic logic so that disability can be conserved rather than eradicated. According to the countereugenic

---

84 Manninen, "Replaceable Fetus."
85 *Centers for Disease Control and Prevention*, "Disability and Healthy Living," *CDC*, September 4, 2019, https://www.cdc.gov/ncbddd/disabilityandhealth/healthyliving.html.
86 *Centers for Disease Control and Prevention*, "Disability and Healthy Living."

logic, disability is "generative" rather than an "unequivocally restricting liability."[87] Disability is generative in that it demonstrates how the body can interact with and respond to the environment over time. Since most people will develop some form of disability over time, disability is inherently part of human evolution. This means that disability is part of humanity's very essence and should not be destroyed, lest humanity as we know it is also destroyed.[88]

Feminist Disability Studies

According to Garland-Thomson in her essay "Feminist Disability Studies," feminist disability studies asks society to reimagine what disability means and consider how disabled individuals, along with women and people of color, have been relegated to a subordinate class. Nirmala Erevelles and Alison Kafer aptly summarize this concept: "The ideology of disability has been used to justify the racial and gendered division of labor based on heteronormative notions of the family and, in doing so, organizes class relations in a capitalist society."[89] Feminist disability scholars contend that disability in societal terms is not so much a medical phenomenon as a sociological phenomenon, whereby a culture interprets a disabled person as a fearful, pitiable "other" outside of a classified norm. In other words, disability is not an innately inferior trait, but heteronormativity makes it so.[90]

Feminist disability scholars study how disability is not merely an attribute that individuals have. It is a classification (a system) that was constructed to condemn attributes that are aberrations of a physical and cognitive norm (based upon the majority).[91] While feminist disability scholars recognize a whole range of disabilities, society labels people with any disability as simply "disabled." The word "disability," then, becomes a collective term and a social

---

[87] Garland-Thomson, "Case for Conserving Disability," 341.
[88] Garland-Thomson, "Case for Conserving Disability," 342.
[89] Nirmala Erevelles and Alison Kafer, "Committed Critique: An Interview with Nirmala Erevelles," in *Deaf and Disability Studies*, ed. Susan Burch and Alison Kafer (Washington, DC: Gallaudet University Press, 2010), 206.
[90] Rosemarie Garland-Thomson, "Feminist Disability Studies," *Signs* 30, no. 2 (2005): 1557.
[91] Garland-Thomson, "Feminist Disability Studies."

identifier—like race, gender, class, or sexuality.[92] Moreover, to label someone as "disabled" is to inflict a power system upon them and make them societally "othered"—much like what can happen to people in marginalized groups such as women, persons of color, working-class individuals, or those who identify as LGBTQ+. [93]

Feminist disability scholars also challenge society to reconsider the language surrounding those with disabilities. For instance, rather than saying "disability," we could instead say "the traits we think of as a disability." Or rather than referring to a body as disabled, we could instead refer to a body as one that violates "the normative standards and expectations of bodily form and function." These changes more accurately reflect the "phenomenon of disability" as a cultural, arbitrary designation that is stigmatized and feared. Accordingly, some feminist disability scholars even advocate for person-first language in order to demonstrate how disability or lack thereof does not ever fully encompass anyone's entire identity.[94]

Intersectionality

Related to feminist disability research is how disability intersects with other social categories like race, gender, class, and sexuality. Disability studies scholars want to emphasize how disability is an essential part of intersectionality because those with disabilities have rich cultures and lives—in part because of their societally prescribed "otherness"—that deserve acknowledgment. Moreover, understanding how disability relates to intersectionality allows for disability to be seen more as a political and social phenomenon rather than a purely medical phenomenon: this way, one is less inclined to say that disability is an inherent wrong that needs to be righted. One is also better able to see how the social category of "disabled" privileges the able-bodied and persecutes the disabled with regard to civic life, the law, and medical assistance.[95] Indeed, this very act of oppression based on disability intersects with oppression based on race. Margaret Sanger, in her influential

---

92 Garland-Thomson, "Feminist Disability Studies," 1557–1558.
93 Garland-Thomson, "Feminist Disability Studies."
94 Garland-Thomson, "Feminist Disability Studies," 1558.
95 Jennifer C. James and Cynthia Wu, "Editors' Introduction: Race, Ethnicity, Disability, and Literature: Intersections and Interventions." *MELIUS* 31, no. 3 (2006): 3.

and now infamous 1922 book *The Pivot of Civilization*, said that those with disabilities were "biological and racial mistakes."[96] According to disability studies historian Douglas Baynton:

> While [d]isability has functioned historically to justify inequality for disabled people themselves, the concept of disability has been used to justify discrimination against other groups by attributing disability to them . . . [N]on-white races were routinely connected to people with disabilities, both of whom were depicted as evolutionary laggards or throwbacks.[97]

In the early twentieth century, Sanger misled American black women to accept abortions or sterilizations as part of the Negro Project. This initiative was undoubtedly meant to depopulate the black race and whatever "defects" were thought to have come with it.[98] Happily, however, those with disabilities have recognized how their positionality intersects with other categories, including race, and have consequently formed powerful, positive alliances. This means, then, that intersectionality can exist in empowering as well as stigmatizing terms.[99]

Intersectionality of race and disability does not imply that being disabled is "just as bad" as being a person of color[100]— saying this creates a hierarchy of oppression, which is difficult (if not impossible) to assess. However, intersectionality of race and disability does mean that being disabled can result in a sort of oppression, just as being a person of color can result in a sort of oppression. In addition, being a person of color and a person with disabilities can create a doubling of oppressions. Finally, the intersectionality of color and ability also makes a distinction between people who are white and able-bodied, white and disabled, of color and able-bodied, and of color and disabled. Making these distinctions is important because they challenge

---

96 Margaret Sanger, *The Pivot of Civilization* (1922; repr. Amherst: Humanity, 2003), 6, as quoted in James and Wu, "Editors' Introduction," 5.
97 Douglas Baynton, "Disability and the Justification of Inequality in American History," *The New Disability History: American Perspectives*, ed. Paul K. Longmore and Lauri Umansky (New York: New York University Press, 2001), 36, as quoted in James and Wu, "Editors' Introduction," 4.
98 James and Wu, "Editors' Introduction," 5.
99 Rosemarie Garland-Thomson, *Extraordinary Bodies: Figuring Physical Disability in American Culture and Literature* (New York: Columbia University Press, 1997), as cited in James and Wu, "Editors' Introduction," 5.
100 James and Wu, "Editors' Introduction," 6.

the notion that all experiences of disability are the same. These important distinctions culminate into a politics of representation.[101]

It is also particularly useful to highlight here the intersectionality of femaleness and disability. Aristotle himself said that women were incomplete and "deformed" versions of men—and consequently were "inferior [beings]."[102] Aristotle also said that monstrosity, by definition, was "a graduated scale of imperfection falling away from . . . the intended perfect form: that of man."[103] As a result, particularly in Western cultures, male bodies have been considered "the norm," and female bodies have been seen as monstrous and therefore disabled or deformed by default.[104] With this logic, it can be stated that if an "able-bodied" female is already inherently disabled by virtue of her female parts, a female with other features considered to be further deviations from maleness or able-bodied femaleness is even more stigmatized and criticized. In other words, a female who has more "deformities" other than her femaleness is, in a sense, doubly disabled.

Queer and Crip Critiques

While not exclusively referring to sexuality, disability studies has employed a variety of methods and critiques from queer theory, particularly the conceptual fluidity of normalcy and deviance. Disability scholars who engage with queer theory often describe their approach as "crip," a reclaimed form of the pejorative term "cripple." Robert McRuer offers a sexual identity analogy to explain how the "crip" relates to the "normal":

> Able-bodied identity and heterosexual identity are linked in their mutual impossibility and in their mutual incomprehensibility—they are incomprehensible in

---

101 James and Wu, "Editors' Introduction," 5.
102 Cynthia Freeland, "Nourishing Speculation: A Feminist Reading of Aristotelian Science," in Engendering Origins: Critical Feminist Readings in Plato and Aristotle, ed. Bat-Ami Bar On (Albany: State University of New York Press, 1994), 145–146.
103 Zakiya Hanafi, *The Monster in the Machine: Magic, Medicine and the Marvellous in the Time of the Scientific Revolution* (Durham, NC: Duke University Press, 2000), 8.
104 Julie Joy Clarke, "Doubly Monstrous? Female and Disabled," *Essays in Philosophy: A Biannual Journal* 9, no. 1 (2008): 1; Rosemarie Garland-Thomson, "Integrating Disability, Transforming Feminist Theory," *NWSA Journal* 14, no. 3 (2002): 6.

that each is an identity that is simultaneously the ground on which all identities supposedly rest and an impressive achievement that is always deferred and thus never really guaranteed.[105]

For McRuer, disability, like queerness, is an outsider concept that fundamentally rests on insiders' (able-bodied people) anxiety about maintaining people's own power. Further, a crip reaction to ableism may employ traditionally queer strategies, as identified by performance theorist Carrie Sandahl: "Both queering and cripping expose the arbitrary delineation between normal and defective and the negative social ramifications of attempts to homogenize humanity, and both disarm what is painful with a wicked humor, including camp."[106] The process of cripping, for Sandahl, resembles the performatively satirical playfulness also expressed in queer communities, "to challenge oppressive norms, build community, and maintain the practitioners' self-worth."[107]

Alison Kafer expands the scope of crip theory to encompass a variety of future-oriented concerns, by which she seeks to critique "everything from reproductive practices to environmental philosophy, from bathroom activism to cyberculture."[108] Like McRuer, Kafer suggests that the concept of disability is based on fear and anxiety, but she emphasizes the temporal element to make the point that "a future with disability is a future no one wants."[109] Calling into question the status of the disabled body as temporally static, Kafer advocates a political stance that seeks to imagine and implement alternative futures. Sami Schalk expands the concept of crip even further, suggesting that it may serve as a symbol of solidarity among oppressed identity categories.[110] Through "claiming crip," Schalk suggests that people who are oppressed because of their nonnormative bodies can claim a kinship with one another across traditional identity categories of race, gender, sexuality, and disability.

---

105 Robert McRuer, *Crip Theory: Cultural Signs of Queerness and Disability*, 9.
106 Carrie Sandahl, "Queering the Crip or Cripping the Queer?," 37.
107 Sandahl, "Queering the Crip, or Cripping the Queer?," 38.
108 Alison Kafer, *Feminist, Queer, Crip* (Bloomington: Indiana University Press, 9).
109 Kafer, *Feminist, Queer, Crip*, 2.
110 Sami Schalk, "Coming to Claim Crip: Disidentification with/in Disability Studies," *Disability Studies Quarterly* 33, no. 2 (2013).

Disabilities in Academia

While many academic institutions in the United States have not reported how much of their faculty is considered disabled, there is evidence that very few academics are disabled.[111] For instance, at the University of California at Berkeley in 2017, it was reported that only about 1.5 percent of the full-time faculty members were disabled.[112] This is especially concerning for academics who are both women and disabled since women in general make up only 38 percent of tenured faculty positions in academia overall across the United States.[113] Thus, academics who are both women and disabled are doubly underrepresented in academia. Indeed, the default academic is white, male, and able-bodied.[114]

For this reason, "What Her Body Taught (Or, Teaching about and with a Disability): A Conversation"[115] by Brenda Jo Brueggemann, Rosemarie Garland-Thomson, and Georgina Kleege is significant in the disability studies literature. All three women are academics with physical disabilities who are professors at major US universities and who have extensive publications in disability studies as well as other fields. In their article, these three academics record their insightful discussion on their experiences as female scholars with disabilities, as well as their opinions on how disability should be recognized in academia and society at large.

One topic of great significance covered by these academics is how they want students to see them as professors and as individuals with disabilities in the classroom. This question ultimately amounts to how much disability should be acknowledged in general (or how much disability should be

---

111 Aleksaundra (Sasha) Konic et al., "Researchers with Disabilities in the Academic System," *American Association of Geographers*, September 1, 2018, http://news.aag.org/2018/09/researchers-with-disabilities-in-the-academic-system/.

112 Joseph Grigely, "The Neglected Demographic: Faculty Members with Disabilities," *Chronicle of Higher Education*, June 27, 2017, https://www.chronicle.com/article/The-Neglected-Demographic-/240439.

113 Colleen Flaherty, "More Faculty Diversity, Not on Tenure Track," *Inside Higher Ed*, August 22, 2016, https://www.insidehighered.com/news/2016/08/22/study-finds-gains-faculty-diversity-not-tenure-track.

114 Simi Linton, "Reassigning Meaning," in *Claiming Disability*, ed. Simi Linton (New York: New York University Press, 1998), 14–15.

115 Brueggemann, Garland-Thomson, and Kleege, "What Her Body Taught," 13–33.

invisible in general).[116] In Garland-Thomson's view, "forgetting" about a disability has positive and negative repercussions. On the one hand, it means that those with disabilities are considered neutral. On the other hand, this is to ignore very real complications that can limit disabled people's full integration into society. According to Garland-Thomson: "We don't want [students] to forget [that we have disabilities], but what we do want, I think, is for them to realize that our impairments no longer have the determining force of a master status. We want to redefine, to reimagine, disability—not make it go away."[117]

However, this question of disability recognition in the classroom also relates to disabled people's personal feelings about disclosing information about their disabilities. How open should they be, and how much pressure is too much? On the one hand, for Brueggemann, discussing disability too openly can feel "too personal in a classroom space." On the other hand, perhaps this is what classroom space is for: to wonder about things and to be authentic with one another.[118] Ultimately, to Garland-Thomson, even though disabled professors' discussion of their disabilities "breaks a dam," this allows for disability to no longer "have this status as a thing that you don't talk about and the thing that you can't look at and the thing that's so tragic . . . foreign . . . and so horrific," according to Kleege.[119] This means that while disabled professors should take care to preserve the privilege of a private life, they should also keep in mind that discussing their disability (or disabilities) to a reasonable extent can destigmatize disability in society. Admittedly, however, this comes with an unavoidable necessity to purposefully structure the conversation; otherwise, true student epiphany can become mere pity from students. Indeed, the point of discussing disability is not to make students (or any individual) feel sorry for those with disabilities. The point, rather, is to reveal the valuable experiences of those with disabilities.[120]

Furthermore, in many cases discussing disability is necessary for professors due to the nature of how their disability (or disabilities) will affect students'

---

116 Brueggemann, Garland-Thomson, and Kleege, "What Her Body Taught," 13–15.
117 Brueggemann, Garland-Thomson, and Kleege, "What Her Body Taught," 15.
118 Brueggemann, Garland-Thomson, and Kleege, "What Her Body Taught," 15.
119 Brueggemann, Garland-Thomson, and Kleege, "What Her Body Taught," 16.
120 Brueggemann, Garland-Thomson, and Kleege, "What Her Body Taught," 17–18.

interactions with them. For these three academics, it is useful and almost essential to disclose their disabilities to their students on the first day of class since they will already have been discussing the syllabus and their expectations for the course. For instance, Kleege must tell her students that she cannot see them when they raise their hand, and Garland-Thomson must ask her students not to send long emails. This information is essential to disclose because it will help students know how to best communicate with their professor.[121] On the first day of class, Brueggemann also must reveal she is deaf, but she chooses to turn this revelation into a joke: "But hey, *don't* call me! I don't even have a cell phone—so there!"[122] For Brueggemann, keeping a sense of lightness in the conversation allows her to feel less afraid, and it helps her cope with the unfortunate possibility that there could always be a student who drops the class because they or their parents do not want a deaf professor.[123]

In a similar vein, these three academics use various forms of technology and alternative teaching methods to help them and their students navigate the classroom. For Brueggemann, visual aids help her ascertain her students' knowledge and assess their work. PowerPoint is one such aid, and she has found that it helps students better engage with the course material as well. Web-based discussions are also helpful for Brueggemann and other students to process one another's thoughts.[124] Kleege requests that her students tape record their work, and she, like Brueggemann, has found that this sort of classroom accommodation not only helps her but also her students because it offers another style of learning.[125] According to Kleege: "There is something about the experience of just reading the text out loud, having had that language in your mouth that in many cases opens them up in a way that doesn't always happen when they write a paper."[126] Consequently, it is quite serendipitous that accommodating disabilities also opens up students to new

---

121 Brueggemann, Garland-Thomson, and Kleege, "What Her Body Taught," 17–18.
122 Brueggemann, Garland-Thomson, and Kleege, "What Her Body Taught," 18.
123 Brueggemann, Garland-Thomson, and Kleege, "What Her Body Taught," 18.
124 Brueggemann, Garland-Thomson, and Kleege, "What Her Body Taught," 24–25.
125 Brueggemann, Garland-Thomson, and Kleege, "What Her Body Taught," 25.
126 Brueggemann, Garland-Thomson, and Kleege, "What Her Body Taught," 25.

forms of learning and expression. The classroom, therefore, becomes more inclusive and engaging.[127]

Globalization and Debility

As should be evident by this point, most traditional and contemporary disability studies are performed by and about people living in the comparatively wealthy and privileged countries of the minority world. The field has recently started to recognize this limitation, and a variety of prominent disability scholars advocate for approaches that engage more directly with disability and disabled subjects in the Global South. Helen Meekosha highlights the importance of "social suffering" to disabled subjects in the majority world, which she contends "does not equate with the concept of personal tragedy as critiqued by disability scholars."[128] Further, the causes of disabled people's social suffering are often the result of globally oppressive behaviors and systems:

> The idea of racial and gender supremacy of the Northern Hemisphere is very much tied to the production of disability in the global South and racialized evolutionary hierarchies constructed the colonized as backward, infantile, and animal-like. We cannot meaningfully separate the racialised subaltern from the disabled subaltern in the process of colonisation.[129]

Attention to the global dimensions of disability requires a more complex approach than disability studies has traditionally been able to provide. Nirmala Erevelles utilizes a historical materialist approach to argue that the forces of transnational capitalism have resulted in a situation where "it becomes almost impossible to claim the sovereign subject, now mutually constituted via race, disability, and gender as a dehumanized commodity."[130] The concerns of an autonomous individual with disabilities whose civil rights were advocated in terms of independent living or accessibility make little difference when confronted with these multiple valences of oppression.

---

127 Brueggemann, Garland-Thomson, and Kleege, "What Her Body Taught," 26.
128 Helen Meekosha, "Decolonising Disability: Thinking and Acting Globally," *Disability & Society* 26, no. 6 (2011): 671.
129 Meekosha, "Decolonising Disability," 673.
130 Nirmala Erevelles, *Disability and Difference in Global Contexts: Enabling a Transformative Body Public* (London: Palgrave Macmillan, 2011), 42.

Jasbir Puar draws attention to the importance of considering the causes of disability and thus distinguishes the importance of debilitation, or the process by which people may become impaired. She claims that contemporary ableist processes are oppressive because they force bodies into a position where they are no longer recognizably human: "The distinctions of normative and nonnormative, disabled and nondisabled do not hold up as easily. Instead, there are variegated aggregates of capacity and debility."[131] In the global context, debility is produced in complexly material ways that often intersect with disability but not exclusively. Puar claims that unequal distributions of capacity and debility partly function to "control societies," whose purpose is to regulate all lives, and so "all bodies are being evaluated in relation to their success or failure in terms of health, wealth, progressive productivity, upward mobility, enhanced capacity. And there is no such thing as an 'adequately abled' body anymore."[132]

While this chapter by no means represents an exhaustive exploration of the concepts and controversies explored by traditional disability studies, we hope that it may provide a basic orientation to readers unfamiliar with the field.

---

131 Jasbir Puar, "The Cost of Getting Better: Ability and Debility," in *The Disability Studies Reader*, ed. Lennard Davis, 4th ed. (Abingdon, UK: Routledge, 2013), 181.

132 Puar, "Cost of Getting Better," 182.

Part Two

Theorizing Disability in Africa

Chapter Three

An African Ethics of Social Well-Being

Understanding Disability and Public Health

Maria Berghs

Introduction

The *World Report on Disability*[1] states that around 15 percent of the world's population have a disability, and between 2 and 4 percent have "significant difficulties in functioning." Increasingly, evidence indicates that most of these people are located in middle- and low-income countries in the Global South and that disability is associated with multidimensional poverty, lower educational attainment, lower employment rates, and higher medical costs.[2] A long-standing obstacle to understanding disability has been the lack of robust statistical data, especially for countries in large continents like

---

1   World Health Organization, *World Report on Disability* (Geneva: World Health Organization, 2011).
2   Sophie Mitra, Aleksandra Posarac, and Brandon Vick. "Disability and Poverty in Developing Countries: A Multidimensional Study," *World Development* 41 (2013): 1–18.

Africa.[3] In Africa, Groce[4] relates that in different domains such as health, education, employment, and social protection a disability gap in terms of development now also exists, and this must be tackled by both disability-specific and inclusive policies. Generally, in development discourses disability correlates with what will exacerbate risks in terms of social determinants of health, with inequalities significantly linked to not only individual determinants but also sociopolitical and environmental factors.[5] The seventeen UN Sustainable Development Goals (SDGs) outline this more explicitly, noting links between equity and increasing environmental sustainability.[6] Disability is also correlated more strongly to well-being and mental health, but the focus is on "prevention" and "eradication" of morbidity overall.[7] Significant challenges for many countries are linked to the heterogeneity of development issues as well as greater prosperity, such as multidimensional poverty in the lowest income countries;[8] the short- and long-term disabilities linked to conflict, wars, famine, migration, and infectious diseases;[9] and middle-income countries dealing with rises in communicable and noncommunicable diseases, challenges of rapid urbanization, substance abuse issues; as well as further complexities of both rising youth and aging populations.[10] Additionally, there is the shameful legacy of colonialism and racism in many countries, like South Africa, which continues to have an impact in terms of

---

3   Nora Groce et al., "Disability and Poverty: The Need for a More Nuanced Understanding of Implications for Development Policy and Practice," *Third World Quarterly* 32, no. 8 (2011): 1493–1513.

4   Nora Groce, "Bridging the Gap: Examining Disability and Development in Four African Countries," *Impact*, no. 4 (2018): 73–75.

5   Michael Marmot et al., "Closing the Gap in a Generation: Health Equity Through Action on the Social Determinants of Health," *Lancet* 372, no. 9650 (2008): 1661–1669.

6   United Nations, *Transforming Our World: The 2030 Agenda for Sustainable Development* (New York: United Nations, n.d.), https://sustainabledevelopment.un.org/content/documents/21252030%20Agenda%20for%20Sustainable%20Development%20web.pdf.

7   United Nations, *Transforming Our World*.

8   Groce, "Disability and Poverty," 1493.

9   Maria Berghs and Nawaf Kabbara, "Disabled People in Conflicts and Wars," in *Disability in the Global South*, ed. Shaun Grech and Karen Soldatic (New York: Springer, 2016), 269–283.

10 Shaun Grech and Karen Soldatic, *Disability in the Global South* (New York: Springer, 2016).

health inequalities, and how they are lived as intersectionality to ethnicity, gender, age, and socioeconomic status.[11]

Globalization and the economic policies of the World Bank (WB) and International Monetary Fund (IMF) have also had contested influences on public health systems in many countries in Africa and how they were funded. Countries in economic crisis seeking loans have to go to the WB and IMF, and loans often have structural conditions attached to them. The structural adjustment program from the 1980s had an adverse effect, and the newer structural adjustment programs typically have neoliberal economic characteristics, such as limiting the role of the state and increasing commercialization of health and social care services.[12] While newer programs emphasize the mainstreaming of disability organizations and stakeholders, in terms of Poverty Reduction Strategy Papers (PRSPs), it is unclear how inclusion and mainstreaming in policy papers trickles down to actual practices and real social change. The fact that persons with disabilities (PWDs) are being included and mainstreamed in policy development practices is a sign of disability activism's success and rights enshrined in the UN Convention on the Rights for Persons with Disabilities (CRPD).[13] However, Swartz[14] argues that while much agenda-setting work has been done on a global policy level, this has not trickled down to actual local practices to ensure the full privileges of citizenship.

---

11 Hoosen Coovadia et al., "The Health and Health System of South Africa: Historical Roots of Current Public Health Challenges," *Lancet* 374, no. 9692 (2009): 817–834; Brian Watermeyer, Judith McKenzie, and Leslie Swartz, *The Palgrave Handbook of Disability and Citizenship in the Global South* (New York: Springer, 2018).

12 Alexander E. Kentikelenis, "Structural Adjustment and Health: A Conceptual Framework and Evidence on Pathways," *Social Science & Medicine* 187 (2017): 296–305; Maria Berghs, "The Global Economy of Care," in *Disabling Barriers-Enabling Environments*, ed. John Swain et al. (London: SAGE, 2013), 270–276; Kentikelenis, "Structural Adjustment and Health"; and Bergs, "The Global Economy of Care."

13 Assembly, UN General, "Convention on the Rights of Persons with Disabilities," *Ga Res* 61 (2006): 106.

14 Leslie Swartz, "Disability and Citizenship in the Global South in a Post-Truth Era," in *The Palgrave Handbook of Disability and Citizenship in the Global South*, ed. Brian Watermeyer, Judith McKenzie, and Leslie Swartz (London: Palgrave Macmillan, 2019), 57–65.

Furthermore, despite inclusion of local and global stakeholders in poverty reduction processes and global health initiatives, most agendas and health frameworks affecting disability are set by institutions and funding priorities in the Global North.[15] This gives a skewed vision of what disability is, associated only with poverty and abuse in the African context.[16] The dominant health frameworks for understanding various forms of mental, physical, and sensory states of being are typically termed versions of "disability"—a global English-language medical signifier that becomes institutionalized and localized.[17] In global medical frameworks, these states of being are predicated in terms of something other than the able-bodied norm that can be quantified in measurements of prevalence or using metrics, such as the World Health Organization's (WHO) Disability Adjusted Life Year (DALY) or Years Living with Disability (YLD).[18] Certainly understanding the prevalence, incidence, and progression of disease as well as the effects of injury, chronic pain, and other sensory and mental health conditions is important in terms of health and social care services planning.[19] But it is unclear why this has to be in terms of "burden" or risk, or indeed, if services for disability are then implemented accordingly in anticipation of disability.[20] In most African cultures, a plurality of medical systems and resources exist. The quality of medical care

---

15 Helen Meekosha, "Decolonising Disability: Thinking and Acting Globally," *Disability & Society* 26, no. 6 (2011): 667–682.

16 Leslie Swartz, "Representing Disability and Development in the Global South," *Medical Humanities* 44, no. 4 (2018): 281–284.

17 Maria Berghs, *War and Embodied Memory: Becoming Disabled in Sierra Leone* (London: Routledge, 2016); Maria Berghs, "Ethical (Dis)enchantment, Afflictive Kinship and Ebola Exceptionalism," in *Disability, Normalcy and the Everyday*, ed. Gareth Thomas and Dikaios Sakellariou (London: Routledge, 2018), 160–182.

18 Maria Berghs et al., "Implications for Public Health Research of Models and Theories of Disability: A Scoping Study and Evidence Synthesis," *Public Health Research* 4, no. 8 (2016).

19 Theo Vos et al., "Global, Regional, and National Incidence, Prevalence, and Years Lived with Disability for 301 Acute and Chronic Diseases and Injuries in 188 Countries, 1990–2013: A Systematic Analysis for the Global Burden of Disease Study 2013," *Lancet* 386, no. 9995 (2015): 743–800.

20 Rayna Rapp and Faye Ginsburg, "Making Disability Count: Demography, Futurity, and the Making of Disability Publics," *Somatosphere.net*, May 11, 2015, http://somatosphere.net/2015/making-disability-count-demography-futurity-and-the-making-of-disability-publics.html/.

systems varies widely, depending on what medicines people can access and what formal and informal caring systems can be relied on and are available.

Another issue that will impact how disability is understood and treated in the future is the immense power and control that large multinational companies, pharmaceutical companies, and philanthropic organizations based in the Global North are accumulating in terms of research, capacity, and control over public health agendas. While arguments have often been made in terms of rethinking the responsiveness requirement for international research—and how "morally reprehensible" it is that 90 percent of research funding is directed at 10 percent of the population[21]—such moral arguments were ignored until the West African Ebola epidemic was linked to global biosecurity. While funding collaborations and research platforms have changed, research trends and priorities are still set by the Global North.[22]

Similarly, despite calls for decolonization linked to "disability" in Africa, these have not affected global institutions or their definitions of disability. I take a different trajectory and begin with an understanding of disability in moral terms and investigate if that understanding can be translated in terms of public health ethics, practices, and policy. This chapter will illustrate how disability becomes linked to morality and how we need to reconceptualize our ethical basis and understanding of public health. To effectively address disability in Africa, we need to reconceptualize how we think of ethics in public health. I begin by investigating what an African morality and ethics would look like, why it is linked to conceptions of personhood and kinship, and how that figures into multiple local and global understandings of disability. Secondly, I note how African ontologies and epistemologies have been linked to "cultural" or "traditional" understandings of disability and frame those arguments in terms of understanding "the good" or social well-being. Thirdly, I argue that neither ethics nor disability have been integrated into public health approaches in many African contexts. Lastly, I note some of the future challenges that the continent will face and why reconceptualizing ethics, disability, and public health should be a priority.

---

21 Rebecca Wolitz, Ezekiel Emanuel, and Seema Shah. "Rethinking the Responsiveness Requirement for International Research," *Lancet* 374, no. 9692 (2009): 847–49; and Kathryn M. Chu et al., "Building Research Capacity in Africa: Equity and Global Health Collaborations," *PLoS Medicine* 11, no. 3 (2014): e1001612.

22 Maria Berghs, "Neoliberal Policy, Chronic Corruption and Disablement: Biosecurity, Biosocial Risks and the Creation of 'Ebola Survivors?,'" *Disability & Society* 31, no. 2 (2016): 275–79.

African Moralities and Understanding Disability

African conceptions of morality are usually given primacy of place in African ethics and philosophical thinking, but they have not influenced other fields, especially the field of disability studies, where the academy tends to be influenced by researchers from the Global North either infantilizing, overcomplicating, or ignoring ideas of postmodern creolization, plurality, and hybridity.[23] Similarly, it is the southern African philosophical ideas of *ubuntu* that dominate African disability studies despite the fact that many other African traditions come into play, as well as influences such as globalization and the major world and indigenous religions. I argue that in order to understand disability we need to understand what morality means: this becomes important in understanding African ontologies and epistemologies for the public good and social well-being. This entails processes of decolonization and moving away from understanding disability in negative metrics as risk or burden while still being inclusive of an anticipatory disability (bio)politics[24] of diversity.

African conceptions of disability are all too often included in terms of culture or traditional beliefs that are outdated or something that service providers need to "work with" to provide rehabilitative or other services.[25] This has also been conceptualized as a cultural model of disability, in the sense that it is culture that will unlock cross-cultural understandings of "disability," but such models often foreground anthropological knowledge or positioning as the go-between for indigenous understandings.[26] Another conception of "culture" has been to equate it with the reasons for hatred, abuse, abandonment,

---

23   Swartz, "Representing Disability and Development in the Global South," 281–84; and Leslie Swartz, "Five Challenges for Disability-Related Research in Sub-Saharan Africa," *African Journal of Disability* 3, no. 2 (2014).

24   Gina Jae, "The Anticipatory Politics of Improving Childhood Survival for Sickle Cell Disease," *Science, Technology, & Human Values* 43, no. 6 (2018): 1122–1141.

25   Patrick Devlieger, "Disability and Community Action in a Zimbabwean Community: Priorities Based on a Biocultural Approach," *Journal of the Steward Anthropological Society* 22 (1994): 41–57.

26   Benedicte Ingstad and Susan Reynolds Whyte, eds., *Disability and Culture* (Berkeley: University of California Press, 1995); Benedicte Ingstad and Susan Reynolds Whyte, eds., *Disability in Local and Global Worlds* (Berkeley: University of California Press, 2007); and Patrick Devlieger, "The 'Why' of Disability: From an Existential to a Transmodern Perspective," in *Rethinking*

violence, and deaths of people with various forms of impairment without investigating the underlying structural and social inequalities that lie at the origins of those processes. Swartz and Marchetti-Mercer[27] rightly bring up violence against disabled people as an issue that must be addressed but note that such discussions are rarely nuanced and all too often reflect dominant racist stereotypes about Africa and Africans. Almost twenty years ago, Ingstad[28] called such stereotypes from the Global North, such as the belief that disabled people in Africa are hidden away from public view, "myths" linked to disability. For example, Ingstad takes issue with the stereotype that disabled people are hidden and neglected, noting how: (1) impairment does not define a person's worth; (2) the origins of impairment are attributed to witchcraft and cures are sought for community imbalances; and (3) when families or communities cannot cope with caring for a disabled child or aging relative it is due to poverty, lack of education, and lack of institutional and other support.[29] The same myths become operationalized in terms of understanding how disease, impairment, and disability are defined and become linked to "cultural" or traditional explanations.

In order to understand how an impairment becomes categorized, discursively formed, and ascribed a positive or negative value, this is linked to understandings of local and global morality.[30] We can take as an example the West African country of Sierra Leone where among various different ethnic groups impairments are given physical, sensory, cognitive, or even spiritual descriptions. Yet impairment is interpreted in many different ways and is also linked to the local and global. How people's impairments are interpreted is constructed based on social as well as spiritual criteria using amalgams of the colonial past and neoliberal present. Examples are accusations that someone comes from the "kingdom of witches of vast riches," which they fly to in an

---

Disability: World Perspectives in Culture and Society, ed. Patrick Devlieger et al. (Antwerp: Grant, 2016), 389–397.

27 Leslie Swartz and Maria Marchetti-Mercer, "Disabling Africa: The Power of Depiction and the Benefits of Discomfort," *Disability & Society* 33, no. 3 (2018): 482–86.

28 Benedicte Ingstad, "The Myth of Disability in Developing Nations," *Lancet* 354, no. 9180 (1999): 757–758.

29 Ingstad, "Myth of Disability in Developing Nations," 757–758.

30 Berghs, "Ethical (Dis)enchantment," 160–82.

airplane at night, or that they use a "witchgun."[31] People can be viewed as having an impairment arising from spiritual conditions instead of physical, mental, or cognitive causes. It is entrenched community beliefs that the past or present ascription of misfortune, bad luck, and/or moral defect that has physical or spiritual ramifications and needs remedying.

As Ingstad[32] argues, if a person becomes ill or a child is born with an impairment, it is the illness or impairment itself that needs to be treated via formal and informal medical and/or social remedies. Illness, disease, and impairment are signifiers and located within local and global moral economies where action is required. For example, "disability" is constructed as a global institutional signifier linked to impairment that demands medical and rehabilitative action and becomes linked to medical categories and bureaucratic social identities. By contrast, an impairment or illness in Sierra Leone also falls within moral categories indicating that a moral fault has occurred and needs repair.[33] Actions thus become associated with a particular kinship group or misappropriation of land, resources, or animal totem connected to the ancestors that necessitates embodied actions of social and thus spiritual repair. This posits an understanding of what constitutes a disability that transcends Western understanding, because concepts of goodness and the collective are both material and immaterial.

The witchcraft accusation functions as a means of pinpointing where the moral fault or tension lies in terms of moral ambivalence that is felt locally and globally. It often focuses on bodily sacrifices given or taken by illicit means for good fortune, political power, or resources. This mimics the neoliberal present and past colonial histories of Sierra Leone in terms of exploitation and use of the body.[34] Accusations of witchcraft tend to focus on outsiders to a community, people with unexplained riches, young children one cannot care for or who may die, or wives outside the patrilineage who move to their husband's house. In terms of why kinship or familial relationships are in disorder, Van de Grijspaarde et al.[35] found that distribution of witchcraft accusations was also connected to the rise of neoliberalism

---

31   Rosalind Shaw, *Memories of the Slave Trade: Ritual and the Historical Imagination in Sierra Leone* (Chicago: University of Chicago Press, 2002).
32   Ingstad, "Myth of Disability in Developing Nations," 757–758.
33   Berghs, "Ethical (Dis)enchantment," 160–182.
34   Rosalind Shaw, "The Production of Witchcraft/Witchcraft as Production: Memory, Modernity, and the Slave Trade in Sierra Leone," *American Ethnologist* 24, no. 4 (1997): 856–876.
35   Huib van de Grijspaarde et al., "Who Believes in Witches? Institutional Flux in Sierra Leone," *African Affairs* 112, no. 446 (2013): 22–47.

and affected communities where male patriarchal power was under threat. Similarly, very ill children whose lives are threatened are called *obanje* (a Nigerian term for those who come and go) spirits. Schneider found this term applied to a young man, but that element of uncertainty in his life was explained as punishment of the misdeeds of female members of the kinship group.[36] Thornhill[37] found a similar dynamic in Liberia, where child rape was linked to witchcraft's: 1) accumulative power, 2) criticism of neoliberal power, and 3) a metaphysical theft of female power. Lastly, what Thornhill does not mention is that rape is also a source of spiritual pollution and prompts a change in one's moral luck in terms of altering the well-being and future riches of the person affected; it is an action that needs a moral opposite and reversing action.[38] In this way, witchcraft is physically, socially, and spiritually disabling, but the links between witchcraft, morality, and disability are often misunderstood.

In many rural areas in Sierra Leone, when people do not understand the medical cause of visibly disabling conditions such as poliomyelitis (polio) or sickle cell, they link the cause of the condition to witchcraft through an object such as snake or witch gun. This allows the family to engage in actions directed at the object of the witchcraft or parts of the body affected by witchcraft (not the condition or person) to ensure better relationships and healing of the person through native medicine or indigenous healers. Yet witchcraft also functions as a means by which people can justify the abandonment of children or people they cannot care for because of poverty of lack of resources, which is often the case with children with disabilities. Research has indicated that reasons for lack of social inclusion of children with disabilities often correlate with limitations of social belonging exacerbated by poverty.[39] This is differential ethics.

If the witchcraft accusation is a sign that there has been a moral breakdown or fissure, moral deflection and moral actions become important to resolve that tension from the relationship. It is important that a carer, family,

---

36 Luisa T. Schneider, "The Ogbanje Who Wanted to Stay: The Occult, Belonging, Family and Therapy in Sierra Leone," *Ethnography* 18, no. 2 (2017): 133–152.
37 Kerrie Thornhill, "Power, Predation, and Postwar State Formation: The Public Discourse of Ritual Child Rape in Liberia," *Third World Thematics: A TWQ Journal* 2, no. 2–3 (2017): 229–247.
38 Berghs, "Ethical (Dis)enchantment," 160–182.
39 Femke Bannink, Richard Idro, and Geert Van Hove, "'I Like to Play with My Friends': Children with Spina Bifida and Belonging in Uganda," *Social Inclusion* 4, no. 1 (2016): 127–141.

or community is viewed as behaving morally in terms of addressing the social causes of moral breakdown of which illness, disease, and disabilities are signs. If those actions do not resolve the cause of impairment, a moral ambivalence in terms of identity can be created. This is the case for people with polio, who because of their condition's visibility and what it implies morally in terms of kinship relationships, are often abandoned. Szanto[40] found that this moral ambivalence is linked to why they are still often involved in activities like blacksmithing or in begging. Historically, in West Africa, blacksmithing signifies a liminal identity in that blacksmiths are intermediaries to the material and immaterial worlds through their craftsmanship.[41] This is why many people with polio prefer globalized medical identities, as people with "polio" or newer social identities predicated on rights as citizenship, such as persons with disabilities. They draw on a plurality of moral identities and worlds in which their identities are understood.

I hope that the above elucidates how important morality is to understanding local and global conceptions of disability and how morality lies at the heart of why impairment becomes discursively defined as negative or positive. Morality also explains why what is disabling may be broadly understood in terms of environmental and spiritual consequences of moral luck, and thus African ontologies and epistemologies need more reflection.

African Ontologies and Epistemologies for the Good and Social Well-Being

To understand how ethics and disability become interlinked, I argue that African societies have to develop ethics as a mission statement of their own public health approaches. Taking African ontologies and epistemologies seriously means that we understand how African sociality and human values are broader than concepts from the Global North. As I have discussed elsewhere, "when you ask people in Sierra Leone who have an impairment what that means for them, they will typically not use the term 'disability' or 'disabled' but say something linked to explaining feelings of moral abjection (akin to

---

40 Szántó Diána, "Where Parallel Worlds Meet: Civil Society and Civic Agency" (PhD diss., University of Pecs, 2015).

41 Patrick R. McNaughton, *The Mande Blacksmiths: Knowledge, Power, and Art in West Africa* (Bloomington: Indiana University Press, 1993).

Fatmata) or abandonment, like stating, 'I am useless.'"[42] Despite the long tradition of African philosophy and how it has been translated cross-culturally and in relation to Western and Arabic philosophical systems,[43] it has not been taken seriously in the realm of public health.

African ontologies and epistemologies have tended to be linked to "cultural" or "traditional" understandings of disability, which are usually negatively framed, but as we have seen, they are linked to understanding the good and are signifiers of why social well-being does not function in terms of kinship. Most African ontologies and epistemologies are framed with the intention of acting for the common good or in terms of virtues of character expressing good that will lead to such behavior. Yet witchcraft also elucidates areas in which the collective has moral issues and how local and global resources are used to resolve those ambiguities, such as the changing status of people in society, impact of inequalities, or the growing power of women. Witchcraft acts as historical memory and a present moral barometer to give expression to the destructive forces that people live with but cannot control.[44]

There are a multitude of ontological and epistemological positions in a vast continent like Africa, but what is important is the shift to taking such positions epistemologically seriously in order to develop the ethical grounding for health-care practice and policy.[45] For example, Nicolson[46] argues for a global African ethics in terms of *ubuntu* for the well-being of the group but does not question in whose interest that well-being is framed, how it becomes linked to certain institutions, or why it has to be South African. Yet in Metz's[47] overview of sub-Saharan African ethical positions he considers that much of African ethics has a normative focus in explaining how we should act. Furthermore, such an ethics posits that this action should

---

42 Berghs, "Ethical (Dis)enchantment," 164.
43 Dismas A. Masolo, *African Philosophy in Search of Identity* (Bloomington: Indiana University Press, 1994).
44 Shaw, "Production of Witchcraft," 856–876.
45 Boaventura de Sousa Santos, *Epistemologies of the South: Justice against Epistemicide* (London: Routledge, 2015).
46 Ronald Nicolson, *Persons in Community: African Ethics in a Global Culture* (Scottsville: University of KwaZulu-Natal Press, 2008).
47 Thaddeus Metz, "An Overview of African Ethics," in *Themes, Issues and Problems in African Philosophy*, ed. Isaac E. Okpokolo (Cham, Switzerland: Palgrave Macmillan, 2017), 61–75.

be for the common good in terms of communitarian or vitalist approaches. Communitarian approaches link to understandings of the importance of kinship, caring, and virtues of character that are linked to social well-being. Vitalist approaches consider the different ontological and epistemological understandings that ground how different ethnic groups understand the origins and foundations of their world: this can be inclusive of animals, ancestral lands, and the spiritual realm.

Communitarian and vitalist approaches could easily accommodate a number of African ontological and epistemological positions such as *ubuntu* among others. These can be translated into institutional priorities, for example, in terms of sustainability and the UN SDGs and how those would fit within communitarian or vitalist philosophies or ethical approaches. As I have argued, *ubuntu* politically links disability, human rights, and ecology, none of which have received enough attention in the African context.[48] Ethical communitarian and/or vitalist approaches also have implications in terms of how those theories could be translated realistically into developing public health services, practice, and policy. A communitarian approach could also be applied in terms of the CRPD and how assurances of individual rights are illustrated of the greater public good.

Developing public health framework based on communitarian or vitalist ethical approaches founded in the ontological and epistemological positions of the ethnicities that live in African countries would be a first step in decolonizing and also prioritizing African philosophies. The above also illustrates how much southern theory and culture has to teach us in terms of disability[49] and how they may act to reframe public health theories and institutional concepts that guide our conceptions of health and well-being. This entails a move toward southern theory[50] and what that can teach us about personhood, humanity, and by extension how we should live: this would mean addressing some of the ethical misgivings about research and inequalities in how public health agendas are currently being set. If we are going to act ethically in terms of the group or ecosystem, what would this

---

48 Berghs, "Practices and Discourses of Ubuntu," 6.
49 R. Connell, *Southern Theory: Social Science and the Global Dynamics of Knowledge* (Cambridge: Polity, 2007).
50 Jean Comaroff and John L. Comaroff, "Theory from the South: Or, How Euro-America Is Evolving toward Africa," *Anthropological Forum* 22, no. 2 (New York and London: Routledge, 2012), 113–131.

correctly imply in terms of public health ethics? Would this necessitate the development of new ethical approaches to inform public health?

Ethics and Disability: New Public Health Approaches

In order to formulate new public health approaches, models of disability can be informative, such as providing indications of where future challenges will be. They can also give answers to how to respond to those challenges in terms of informing new public health approaches. I argue that African societies have to develop African-based ethics mission statements for their own public health understandings. This should not just be a "hermeneutical exercise"[51] but encompass a disability biopolitics for diversity. Taking African ontologies and epistemologies seriously means understanding how African sociality and human values are broader than concepts from the Global North and encourage development of communal ethics, ethics of sociality or vitalist ethics accordingly.[52] This in turn means that we do not view disability as individual but as discursive social creation and imbedded in social responsibilities toward disabling conditions and practices. While creation of an African ethics of social well-being has not been adequately funded in terms of development practices or in terms of African (bio)ethical approaches,[53] I give some concrete examples of how such approaches could fit into development of public health.

An ethics of social well-being would easily fit into existing public health theories but also determine how social well-being could also encompass ideas about well-being in the wider ecosystem. This requires that the definition of the social determinants of health of "the conditions in which people are born, grow, live, work and age" and "the fundamental drivers of these conditions" is also viewed in terms of structural inequalities that affect this wider

---

51   Albert Mark E. Coleman, "What Is 'African Bioethics' as Used by Sub-Saharan African Authors: An Argumentative Literature Review of Articles on African Bioethics," *Open Journal of Philosophy* 7, no. 1 (2017): 31.

52   Subrata Chattopadhyay et al., "A Question of Social Justice: How Policies of Profit Negate Engagement of Developing World Bioethicists and Undermine Global Bioethics," *American Journal of Bioethics* 17, no. 10 (2017): 3–14.

53   Chattopadhyay et al., "A Question of Social Justice."

ecosystem.[54] Arguments have already been made to examine the underlying causes of the social determinants of health of, for example, epigenetic risks that begin within the structural and social inequalities that some communities live with[55] or syndemics.[56] Similarly, those risks can also be understood in terms of expressing inequalities as genetic, physical, and other forms of disablement and understanding the fundamental drivers of those conditions. In order to address the social determinants of health for an ethics of social well-being, concrete structural investments would have to be made not only in accessibility and affordability of health and social care but also in terms of ensuring the health of the local and global environment and social care for the community. This would have far-reaching consequences in thinking about lack of infrastructure such as electricity and roads, social investments such as education, and ensuring, for example, training of nurses in terms of African ethics of care, which might be more communitarian in nature.[57] This would be broader than a right to health: it would extend the concept of rights to the right to live well in an African ecosystem or a communal and/or vitalist right to health. So, while a common response to disability and poverty is implementation of welfare programs—or, for instance, disability grants in South Africa—[58] this does not improve overall communal living conditions; it simply addresses poverty of resources at an individual level.

If we take as a concrete example the concept of equity and how that links to the financing and development of universal public health-care coverage in African countries, such a concept would have to be predicated on ethics of social well-being and tie into the UN SDGs as well. In terms of ethics of social well-being, defining equity in communitarian terms would mean

---

54 Michale G. Marmot and Ruth Bell, "Action on Health Disparities in the United States: Commission on Social Determinants of Health," *Jama* 301, no. 11 (2009): 1661.

55 Paula Braveman and Laura Gottlieb, "The Social Determinants of Health: It's Time to Consider the Causes of the Causes," *Public Health Reports* 129, no. 1 (2014): 19–31.

56 A. C. Tsai et al., "Co-Occurring Epidemics, Syndemics, and Population Health," *Lancet* 389 (2017): 978–982.

57 Mitchell Loeb et al., "Poverty and Disability in Eastern and Western Cape Provinces, South Africa," *Disability & Society* 23, no. 4 (2008): 311–321.

58 Thaddeus Metz, "The Western Ethic of Care or an Afro-Communitarian Ethic? Specifying the Right Relational Morality," *Journal of Global Ethics* 9, no. 1 (2013): 77–92.

ensuring that everyone had a right to health as well as ensuring that communities had access to health care. This would likely have wider implications of assurances of, for example, that there are adequate health-care resources for everyone. In terms of disability and thinking about how disablement is socially constructed and how to address assurances of equity, one would have to think about disability as communal creation of its prevention: this would also mean global corporate responsibilities and local institutional responsibilities toward those with impairments.

This could also be restorative in nature in that people with impairments will begin advocating for a transformational disability politics in claims against multinationals, institutions, or African states that do not ensure well-being and social justice. That would also encompass ecosystem loss of environment and disablement linked to loss of ancestral lands or totemic animals: this could also include genomic or epigenetic detriment linked to dangerous working or living conditions. I want to illustrate some of the practical consequences of how social justice claims could become linked to ethics and reappropriation of concepts such as "rights" so they reflect African public health priorities. I argue that an African ethics would mean a public health perspective that is more diverse and more respectful of communal health and well-being.

The development of African ethics is thus crucial to future advancement of African public health approaches. And African understandings of the "good" and its links to well-being should inform health and social care. I have tried to illustrate how understanding morality and its links to disability means that disability is not understood through the individual but discursively of social ethics and well-being of the group.

African Challenges: African Ethics for African Futures

In the previous section, I have illustrated some of the challenges that the continent will face correlated to public health and disability. I have also illustrated through the use of theory, how many of these future challenges are linked to historical and present inequalities and in turn lead to future forms of disabilities that are broader in public health scope than those related to chronic ill health, mental health, infectious diseases, and aging. While many of the answers for addressing ill health, disease, and other impairments have been found in the social organising, biosociality, and kinship found in identity politics,[59] I have shown why an approach focusing on political organization or ascription of "disability" as identity is actually illustrative of local and global morality. Hence, in order to properly address disability and public health, it is imperative to develop an African ethics for social well-being. Most public health discourses are medicalized and focus on prevention or promotion of health—but typically in terms of health risks on an individual level. The individual is the focus in health, healing, and caring; thus, an African ethics of social well-being could create some balance of locating an individual not just within the community but across wider ecosystems. This would move the focus from individuals with ill health, biosociality, or disability to be viewed as part of the kind of diversity that we should advocate for environments of well-being. The responsibility for the well-being and diversity of the individual is a collective one.

---

59   Susan Reynolds Whyte, "Health Identities and Subjectivities," *Medical Anthropology Quarterly* 23, no. 1 (2009): 6–15.

Chapter Four

Rethinking African Disability Studies

From the Cultural-Deficit Model to a Socioeconomic Perspective

Fikru Negash Gebrekidan

Introduction

The CRPD has been met with mixed reactions. While the framing of disability rights through human rights discourse has been universally applauded, questions have been raised about its enforceability in middle- to low-income countries.[1] Equally uncertain has been the role of the social model of disability, which was the philosophical underpinning of the 2006 convention. Despite the social model's emancipatory ethos, its foundational premise for disability studies worldwide remains compromised by its preoccupation with postindustrial social priorities.[2] Nowhere is this more evident than in

---

1   Raymond Lang, "United Nations Convention on the Rights and Dignities for Persons with Disabilities: A Panacea for Ending Disability Discrimination?" *Alter: European Journal of Disability Research* 3 (2009): 266–285.

2   For a critique of the social model from multiple global perspectives see Shaun Grech, "Decolonizing Eurocentric Disability Studies: Why Colonialism Matters in the Disability and Global South Debate," *Social Identities* 21, no. 1

the budding field of African disability studies, where the social model continues to cohabit with the local equivalent of the dated medical paradigm: the cultural-deficit perspective. In 2016, for example, the United Nations Department for Economic and Social Affairs (UNDESA) prepared a training manual entitled *Toolkit on Disability for Africa*. One of its modules, headed "Culture, Beliefs and Disability," incorporated some discussion of the social model theory. Yet like the proverbial old wine in a new bottle, its explanation of stigma and ostracism rested primarily on cultural attitudes, saying nothing of the role of socioeconomic structure through which such collective beliefs were produced and perpetuated.[3] The cultural-pathology approach is built on two assumptions. First, disability is a by-product of backward beliefs and harmful traditional practices. Second, such disabling environments can be reversed through modernization, secularism, and disability-awareness education.[4] The flaws in this prognosis, in some ways reminiscent of the nineteenth-century civilizing mission, are too many to enumerate. African belief systems, unlike the major world religions, are infinite and unscripted. For every cherrypicked anecdote of a greater humanistic insight, one can cite a counterexample of overwrought ableism and outright rejection. On this ground alone, the cultural paradigm lacks universal articulation, privileging local distinctiveness over broader patterns or trends. Likewise, preoccupation

---

(2015): 6–21; and Helen Meekosha and Karen Soldatic, "Human Rights and the Global South: The Case of Disability," *Third World Quarterly* 32, no. 8 (2011): 1383–1398.

3   United Nations, "Culture, Beliefs, and Disability," *United Nations*, November 18, 2016, www.un.org/esa/socdev/documents/disability/Toolkit/Cultures-Beliefs-Disability.pdf.

4   For sample essays on the role of culture in African disability worldviews see Benedicte Ingstad and Susan Reynolds Whyte, eds., *Disability and Culture* (Berkeley: University of California Press, 1995); Chomba Wa Munyi, "Past and Present Perceptions towards Disability: A Historical Perspective," *Disability Studies Quarterly* 32, no. 2 (2012), http://dsq-sds.org/article/view/3197/3068; Angi Stone-MacDonald and Gretchen Buttera, "Cultural Beliefs and Attitudes About Disability in East Africa," *Review of Disability Studies* 8, no. 1 (2014), www.rdsjournal.org/index.php/journal/article/view/110; Hebron L. Ndlovu, "African Beliefs Concerning People with Disabilities: Implications for Theological Education," *Journal of Disability & Religion* 20: no. 1–2 (2016): 29–39; and Edwin Etieyibo and Odirin Omiegbe, "Religion, Culture, and Discrimination against Persons with Disabilities in Nigeria," *African Journal of Disability* 5, no. 1 (2016): a192.

with the role of the supernatural or the maleficent, a theme so pervasive in African disability literature, reinforces the primordial view of society as simple, static, and without agency. Even when a positive practice like *ubuntu* is identified and hailed as a role model, without sociohistorical context its virtues become so essentialized that critics are tempted to raise the red flag of cultural racism.[5]

This chapter proposes a socioeconomic matrix, or mode of production, as a more appropriate analytical tool in African disability studies. Besides revealing the intimate connection between means of livelihood and the attendant disability worldview, socioeconomic analysis facilitates the type of Pan-African perspective that the cultural approach has been lacking. Finally, in light of the global trends of urbanization, population explosion, and fast-changing technology, a socioeconomic orientation would help not only in addressing contemporary realities but also in anticipating new scenarios and possibilities.[6]

At the global level, attention to socioeconomic structure places African disability studies on a par with disability studies elsewhere. For over three decades now, North American and European disability theorists have gravitated toward a consensus. From welfare to immigration to eugenic laws, they agree on the economic rationale of capitalism as having shaped a modern disability worldview.[7] Victor Finkelstein was the first to trace the evolution

---

[5] See Alana Lentin, "Replacing Race: Historicizing Culture in Multiculturalism," *Patterns of Prejudice* 39, no. 4 (2005): 379–96.

[6] African societies are a poor example for a disability worldview shaped by a major world religion, although exemptions might be made in the case of Islamic West Africa and Christian Ethiopia. One has to turn to their European and Asian counterparts to better appreciate the connection between transnational disability worldviews and world religions. For example, see Henri-Jacques Stiker, *A History of Disability* (Ann Arbor: University of Michigan Press, 1999); Sara Scalenghe, *Disability in the Ottoman Arab World: 1500–1800* (New York: Cambridge University Press, 2014); and M. Miles, "Disability in an Eastern Religious Context," *Journal of Religion, Disability & Health* 6, no. 2–3 (2002): 53–76.

[7] See Douglas C. Baynton, "'These Pushful Days': Time and Disability in the Age of Eugenics," *Health and History* 13, no. 2 (2011): 43–64; Bill Hughes, "Bauman's Strangers: Impairment and the Invalidation of Disability in Modern and Postmodern Cultures," *Disability and Society* 17, no. 5 (2010): 571–584; and Hugh Gregory Gallagher, "Holocaust: The Genocide of Disabled Peoples," in *Century of Genocide: Critical Essays and Eyewitness*

of Western construction of disability in terms of historical materialism.[8] Finkelstein's conceptualization of three phases, each corresponding with a distinct era in European economic history, was later refined by Michael Oliver in accordance with the more conventional Marxist developmental stages.[9] In the feudal past, where labor was not regimented and mechanical skills were the exception, the disabled were integrated into the workforce directly or indirectly. Alienation from production began with the advent of industrialization, during which efficiency and speed became the new economic sine qua non. The nineteenth century represented the peak of that trend, not just economically but also socially. Away from family and invisible to the outside world, an ever-growing number of persons with disabilities languished sequestered in "workhouses, asylums, colonies and special schools."[10]

In precolonial Africa, at least three distinct modes of production resonate with Finkelstein's and Oliver's paradigm of economic functionalism. They consist of foragers, nomadic pastoralists or herders, and agriculturalists. Despite their egalitarian values, foragers developed few coping mechanisms against infirmity, and incapacitation was often tantamount to a premature death. Mortality because of injuries and insufficient care might have declined among pastoralists, but transhumant movements and the harsh environment still resulted in one of the poorest accommodations of disability. In contrast to pastoralism or foraging was the advantage offered by farming, whose surplus harvest ensured a more stable food supply. Transition to agriculture did not represent a leap forward in every respect, but it did allow the relative integration of the disabled into socioeconomic life. Thus, this chapter is organized in three sections, each focusing on a particular economic way of life and its concomitant disability worldview. The final section concludes on mendicancy as a form of agency, again relying on the socioeconomic model to explain the presence of a conspicuous class of disabled beggars in Christian Ethiopia and Islamic West Africa.

 Accounts, ed. Samuel Totten and William S. Parsons (New York: Routledge, 2009).

8 Victor Finkelstein, *Attitudes and Disabled People: Issues for Discussion* (New York: World Rehabilitation Fund, 1980), 6–9.

9 Michael Oliver, *The Politics of Disablement: A Sociological Approach* (New York: St. Martin's Press, 1990), 26–28.

10 Oliver, *Politics of Disablement*, 28.

Foragers

In its refined stage, the Paleolithic mode of production combined hunting, gathering, and fishing, herein collectively referred to as foraging. It took tens of thousands of years for the practice to spread from Africa and to other parts of the globe through migration. Homo sapiens, the force behind these innovations, evolved into "behaviorally modern human beings" during the late stone age of fifty to forty thousand years ago. While still in Africa they developed the use of spoken language, began the ritual of burying their dead, and tended to their infirm and aging populations. A bigger brain size and the opposable digits were responsible not only for the making of refined hunting tools and ornaments but also for the production of abstract cultural expressions such as cave paintings. When viewed through the grand evolutionary scheme, Africa was thus where Homo sapiens first recognized the utilitarian value of the human body as a means of production. The significance of this claim to disability studies cannot be overstated. Among other things, it demonstrates why the temporal depth of disability studies should extend to Paleolithic Africa, where the pecking order of primates based on male muscle power and female fertility was to mutate into a quintessentially modern human behavior.[11]

There is an even more immediate reason why the intermarriage between disability studies and African studies matters. In the same way that postcolonial thought has revealed the false universalism of Eurocentric knowledge,[12] a nexus between disability studies and African studies is well situated to disrupt the hegemonic privilege of ableist epistemology.[13] A case in point is the academic invention of the myth of a primitive golden age. Human beings have been hunter-gatherers for 99 percent of their evolutionary history, most

---

11 Eric Gilbert and Jonathan Reynolds, *Africa in World History: From Prehistory to the Present*, 3rd ed. (Upper Saddle River, NJ: Pearson Education, 2012), chapters 2–3. Also see Richard G. Kleine, "Anatomy, Behavior, and Modern Human Origins," *Journal of World Prehistory* 9, no. 2 (1995): 167–198.

12 See Dipesh Jakrabarty's *Provincializing Europe: Postcolonial Thought and Historical Difference* (Princeton, NJ: Princeton University Press, 2000); and Richard Delgado and Jean Stefancic, *Critical Race Theory: An Introduction*, 3rd ed. (New York: New York University Press, 2017).

13 See Douglas C. Baynton, "Disability in History," *Disability Studies Quarterly* 28, no. 3 (2008): 1–4; and Catherine Kudlick, "Disability History: Why We Need Another 'Other,'" *American Historical Review* 108, no. 3 (2003): 763–793.

of that lived in Africa. In the aftermath of the unprecedented scale of human carnage of World War II grew a soul-searching preoccupation with the meaning of modernity among social scientists. Paleolithic societies, untainted by the original sin of greed and ego, provided the answer. Allegedly idyllic, stress free, and with plenty of leisure time, Stone Age people came to epitomize a tranquil lifestyle that their twentieth-century descendants could only dream of. A bountiful environment, limited wants, and aversion to hoarding ensured their contentment with few material possessions. This was what came together in a paper presented at a symposium in 1966, during which anthropologist Marshall Sahlins introduced the phrase "original affluent society."[14]

To its merit, the "original affluent society" thesis drew attention to the self-serving hubris of modernism, or what Sahlins called "bourgeois ethnocentrism."[15] Since the eighteenth century, scientists had believed that early human beings had lived in a Hobbesian state of wanton desperation survived into modern times by the quintessential African hunter-gatherer, which often went by the pejorative name of "Bushman."[16] The functionalist explanation that Sahlins popularized helped correct that stereotype, showing that foraging was a lifestyle of preference and not of deprivation. The theory succeeded, perhaps even far beyond what Sahlins had initially envisaged. For several decades, hunter-gatherers would play the role of humanity's Horatio Alger, a pervasive if naïve myth, and their untainted holism a source of fascination to many a social scientist.[17]

It was not until disease, disability, and premature deaths factored into the equation that the romantic appeal of primitivism began to fade. One such study that took a revisionist look at Stone Age cornucopia was Steven Pinker's

---

14 Richard B. Lee and Irven DeVore, *Man the Hunter* (Chicago: Aldine, 1968), 3 and 85; Marshall Sahlins, *Culture in Practice: Selected Essays* (New York: Zone, 2000), 95–135.
15 Sahlins, *Culture in Practice*, 98.
16 See Andrew Bank, "Evolution and Racial Theory: The Hidden Side of Wilhelm Bleek," *South African Historical Journal* 43, no. 1 (2000): 163–178; Clifton C. Crais and Pamela Scully, *Sara Baartman and the Hottentot Venus: A Ghost Story and a Biography* (Princeton, NJ: Princeton University Press, 2009); and Robert Gordon, "The Rise of Bushman Genitalia, Germans, and Genocide," *African Studies* 57, no. 1 (1998): 27–54.
17 See John M. Gowdy, ed., *Limited Wants, Unlimited Means: A Reader on Hunter-Gatherer Economics and the Environment* (Washington, DC: Island, 1998).

Better Angels of Our Nature. In his 2011 bestseller, the Harvard scholar presented the first comprehensive study of the long history of violence, demonstrating a steady downward trajectory through the ages. The two world wars, for which the twentieth century became infamous, destroyed about 3 percent of the earth's population. In routine intergroup warfare of the pre–Neolithic Age, by contrast, death per a hundred ran in the double digits, a ratio even more sanguine and difficult to fathom. Compared to modern times, in other words, ancient societies lived in a constant cycle of retributive bloodletting such that war, instead of peaceful coexistence, was the accepted norm.[18]

Because subsistence living demanded that hunter-gatherers constantly shed excess populations, ancient societies were also accustomed to a variant of intragroup homicide in the form of sanctioned killing. Although primary victims comprised those unable to fend for themselves because of infirmity or old age, in certain circumstances even healthy infants could not be spared. Since a woman could not shift camp as easily with more than one child in tow, and since she could not supplement breastfeeding with cow milk or gruel, she applied natural contraceptives to intersperse her pregnancies. In the case of unwanted conception, infanticide served as a standard recourse, its legitimacy resting on the fact that initiation rites to personhood were not held until several years after birth, normally until the child was old enough to have been weaned. With this delayed endowment of membership status early humans stripped infanticide of its social taboo, a practice to which the rejection of twins in some parts of the modern world could still be traced.[19]

This is not to say that pre-Neolithic ancestors left no positive imprints on the evolution of disability worldview. Foraging societies that transitioned to sedentary life could tap into their egalitarian ethos to build a culture of caregiving that was relatively more sustainable and all embracing. For the chronically homebound, newly acquired longevity could even enrich their social capital and agency. The Baka of southeastern Cameroon, pejoratively known as "pygmies" because of their diminutive stature, have been drawn to the semisedentary life of agricultural work since the 1950s. If the dry

---

18   Steven Pinker, *The Better Angels of Our Nature: Why Violence Has Declined* (New York: Viking, 2011), 48–50.
19   Jared Diamond, *The World Until Yesterday: What Can We Learn from Traditional Societies?* (London and New York: Viking, 2012), 214–217, 177–279.

unemployment season forced the Baka back into the rainforest for months of hunting and gathering, individuals with disabilities and their families would stay in the permanent settlement raising small gardens and doing remunerative chores for the more prosperous Bantu neighbors. Thus, those deemed too frail to migrate were not only presented with a choice, but their continuous presence in the village also helped nurture a harmonious relationship between the foraging Baka and the agriculturalist Bantu.[20]

Likewise, among the Ju/'hoansi of the Kalahari, Harriet Rosenberg discovered exclusive aging privileges. Since society was structured across a horizontal axis, Ju/'hoansi seniors experienced less social anxiety and personal insecurity. They spoke their minds freely without the fear of reprisal; and communal ceremonies were not complete without their special participation and blessing.[21] In one waterhole community, Rosenberg counted four visually impaired elders who served as spirit mediums officiating a healing ritual. In another, she observed a half-conscious patient receive round-the-clock care by members of his extended family. His relatives did this not because of the dying man's social status or as a final goodwill gesture, but because of the belief that every member of the community mattered.[22]

Still, long-term care remained a relatively recent development in the Kalahari, which Rosenberg hastened to attribute to the rise of permanent or semipermanent settlements.[23] For contrast, one only needed to look back a couple of generations to the time when hunting and gathering was the sole source of livelihood in the arid region. Death-hastening measures were frequently applied then, even in instances when demise was not imminent. After all, to a group on the go, sometimes no more than a few dozen strong including women and children, the logistics for transporting and caring for the chronically bedridden simply did not exist. One of Rosenberg's elderly informants thus remembered the practice of abandoning such victims in the bush, or what the Ju/'hoansi themselves called *n/a a tsi*:

---

20 Mikako Toda, "Disability and Charity Among Hunter-Gatherers and Farmers in Cameroon," *How Do Biomedicines Shape People's Lives, Socialities, and Landscapes?*, ed. Akinori Hamada and Mikako Toda, Senri Ethnological Reports, no. 143 (December 2017), https://pdfs.semanticscholar.org/1754/a7ee79c90c97380e4c20da93411eeaae8a4c.pdf.

21 Harriet Rosenberg, "Complaint Discourse, Aging and Caregiving Among the Ju/'hoansi," in *The Dobe Ju/'hoansi*, ed. Richard B. Lee, 4th ed. (Belmont, CA: Wadsworth, 2012), 104–105.

22 Rosenberg, "Complaint Discourse," 115–118.

23 Rosenberg, "Complaint Discourse," 103.

They'd leave him/her and go off, because they didn't know what to do with him/her. . . . Sometimes they'd try to carry the person where they were going. Someone else would carry the person's things, if there were many people. But if the people were few, or if there was only one man, they didn't know what to do with the old person. They would admit defeat, leave him/her, and go.[24]

This causal relationship between way of life and caregiving (or the lack thereof) was corroborated by a study of foragers from another part of Africa. The Mbuti of the Ituri Forest of northeastern Congo replicated the lifestyle of the West African Baka, living in small bands and moving routinely in search of game and edible plants. Colin Turnbull, a pioneering ethnographer, has recorded Mbuti folklores in which themes of abandonment featured centrally. Turnbull wrote that the Mbuti took good care of the senescent. However, he admitted "to having seen no complete cripples, and to having heard disquieting stories about cripples that just happened to disappear, or who suddenly just 'died completely.'"[25]

Turnbull was later to encounter an Mbuti girl who could not move on her own because of a paralytic leg. This was ten-year-old Lizabeti, whose story the British anthropologist told in the final chapter of his widely read classic *The Forest People*. Turnbull and his assistant built Lizabeti a makeshift crutch from a tree branch: it was the first crutch the community had ever seen. The girl mastered the technique and began to walk unassisted, and her potential as a would-be mother and a productive member of the band was restored. The story had a more-than-happy ending. Hobbling on a crutch gained social acceptance when both children and adults alike adopted it as a popular pastime. What began as an adaptive device (and a crude one at that) became a symbol of communal bonding, quite unlike the stigmatic or othering effects of modern prosthetics.[26]

Two points can be extrapolated from the scenarios above. First, far from being idyllic, the life of foraging was quite Darwinian, at least from a disability studies point of view. Incapacitation either led to an untimely death because of insufficient care, or it resulted in an induced death under deliberate neglect or exposure. Senilicide, infanticide, and invalidicide were

---

24　Rosenberg, "Complaint Discourse," 113.
25　Colin M. Turnbull, "Legends of the BaMbuti," *Journal of the Royal Anthropological Institute of Great Britain and Ireland* 89, no. 1 (1959): 52, 55–56.
26　Colin M. Turnbull, *The Forest People* (New York: Simon and Schuster, 1961), chap. 15.

thus as typical among the dwellers of the Kalahari and the Congo Forest, as they were among the hunter-gatherers of the Arctic Inuit, the Australian Aborigines, or the South American Yanomamo.[27]

The second point builds on the first. Foragers had sporadic brushes with severe infirmities since few could last long in such conditions. Because of that, foragers did not develop a complex disability worldview, whether in material culture or in social stigmatization. In fact, that Lizabeti's improvised crutch was soon duplicated by others for purposes of sport could be read as evidence that the Mbuti lacked an entrenched prejudice. That such less stratified societies harbored few stigmas toward the disabled, in contrast to their purgative practices, is reinforced by what anthropologist Clifford Geertz observed among the Pokot of Kenya. Geertz wrote that those with birth defects were customarily disposed of by the Pokot, while some were allowed to survive as a matter of pure chance. "The lives they live are miserable enough, but they are not pariahs—merely neglected, treated with indifference as though they were mere objects, and ill-made ones at that."[28]

Pastoralists

Pastoralists often engaged in mixed modes of production: sometimes looking more like farmers than foragers and sometimes having more in common with foragers than farmers. Some left lasting imprints on world history as long-distance traders and empire builders. Others never outgrew their "cattle complex," which was what drove their cyclical seasonal movements. Transhumant pastoralists, as the latter came to be differentiated from the nomadic type, dominated the traditional economies of eastern and southern Africa after farming. Compared to foragers, pastoralists possessed a superior material culture in the form of livestock and pack animals. Such advantages did not necessarily translate into a more conducive disability worldview, their migratory lifestyle being a major deterrent factor.[29]

---

27 See Diamond, *World Until Yesterday*, 177–179, 214–217, 286–292; and Rolf L. Wirsing, "The Health of Traditional Societies and the Effects of Acculturation," *Current Anthropology* 26, no. 3 (1985): 305.

28 Quoted in Robert Garland, *Eye of the Beholder: Deformity and Disability in the Graeco-Roman World* (Ithaca, NY: Cornell University Press, 1995), 16.

29 For a general discussion on pastoralism see Alan H. Jacobs, "African Pastoralists: Some General Remarks," *Anthropological Quarterly* 38, no. 3 (1965): 144–154; Monique Borgerhoff Mulder et al., "Pastoralism and

In 1856 Sir Richard Burton became the first European to reach the eastern highlands of Ethiopia from the Somali coast. The journey from the Red Sea port of Zeila to the walled city of Harar took the Victorian explorer across a territory traversed by the cattle-herding Issa. Much of it covered a ragged and sparsely populated semidesert landscape, including a haunting site where "the sick and decrepit were barbarously left behind, for lions and hyenas to devour."[30] Suffice it to say that travel anecdotes of this nature have to be approached with caution because of their inherent Eurocentric bias. However, worth noting is also that variations of Burton's claim would persist into the twentieth century and beyond. Writing in a medical journal in 1955, for example, Leon Brotmacher attributed to the Oromo pastoralists of eastern Ethiopia the custom of letting their chronically sick die in the wild.[31] In 2004, likewise, Aneesa Kassam and Ali Balla Bashuna documented the presence of "token infanticide" among the Waata of northern Kenya, also an Oromo-speaking nomadic subgroup.[32]

While the pioneering generation of African social historians focused on challenging colonially constructed myths, the effort to unravel the deeper significance of such aberrant phenomena fell on cultural anthropologists. Yet owing to the blurred boundaries between cultural relativism and cultural romanticism, anthropologists, too, presented controversial interpretations. In East Africa, few societies have had their disability worldviews dissected in the manner that the pastoralist Maasai did, a Nilotic-speaking population that sprawled across southern Kenya and northern Tanzania. It all began with the dissertation fieldwork by Aud Talle: "The 'disabled person', with whom we are so familiar in a Western context, is a phenomenon not encountered among the Maasai," argued the Norwegian social anthropologist.[33]

Wealth Inequality: Revisiting an Old Question," *Current Anthropology* 51, no. 1 (2010): 35–50; and Melville J. Herskovits, "The Cattle Complex in East Africa," *American Anthropologist New Series* 28, no. 1 (1926): 230–272.

30 Richard Francis Burton, *First Footsteps in East Africa* (London: Routledge, 1966), 116.

31 Leon Brotmacher, "Medical Practice Among the Somalis," *Bulletin of the History of Medicine* 29, no. 3 (1955): 202.

32 Aneesa Kassam and Ali Balla Bashuna, "Marginalisation of the Waata Oromo Hunter-Gatherers of Kenya: Insider and Outsider Perspectives," *Journal of the International African Institute* 74, no. 2 (2004): 200.

33 Aud Talle, "A Child Is a Child: Disability and Equality Among the Kenya Maasai," in Ingstad and Whyte, *Disability and Culture* (Berkeley: University of California Press, 1995), 56.

Egalitarian ethos dictated that the Maasai treat their disabled children with respect and equality: "That is to say, they are neither mistreated nor neglected nor particularly favored. They are given the same diet as other children and are subjected to the same prescribed ritual blessings and ceremonial procedures while growing up."[34]

Talle's conclusion was taken at face value for a couple of decades, affirming her trailblazing stature in East African disability studies. The high rate of infant mortality among pastoralists, which a German officer in colonial Tanganyika had attributed to the widespread practice of infanticide, was now explained in terms of a fatalistic mindset conditioned by a harsh environment. Among the Maasai, in fact, the special value they attached to fertility encouraged the raising of large families regardless of physical status. Moreover, their disabled men and women were expected to marry as well as to play active social roles, including serving as the leader of one's age group (*olaiguenani*).[35]

As it turned out, not all the fieldwork data supported Talle's revisionist premise. A case in point was the story of Parmeleu, the troubled Maasai youth whose multiple disabilities were documented. Parmeleu was born as a result of his mother's extramarital affairs with a man younger than her husband's age group, which was a violation of sexual taboo in Maasai culture. Because of his cognitive disability, the boy grew up being treated like a "fool," which he rebelled against by resorting to acts of petty theft. In his teen years, Parmeleu's degenerating sight rendered him practically blind, which the community believed was a sign of the power of his father's curse. Parmeleu periodically ran away from home and came back. Then he was seen no more, although five years later his parents remained unmoved by news of their son being spotted in a town outside Maasailand.[36] Given Parmeleu's visual and mental disabilities, his desertion was more likely to have been orchestrated with the complicity of his family. Yet since acknowledging that fact would have weakened Talle's egalitarian thesis, she chose to explain the misfortune in terms of social stigma. "Through his bad eyesight, Parmeleu is definitely physically impaired," she insisted, "but his true disability within the Maasai society derives from his unfortunate fate of being the product of a sinful relation that has marginalized him as a person."[37]

---

34   Talle, "A Child Is a Child," 67.
35   Talle, "A Child Is a Child," 67–69.
36   Talle, "A Child Is a Child," 65–66.
37   Talle, "A Child Is a Child," 66.

A monograph on disability edited by Sheryl Feinstein and Nicole D'Errico in 2010 presented stories of disabled Tanzanian women in their own words, allowing a nuanced appreciation of their life journeys as wives, divorcees, employees, spinsters, as well as outright victims.[38] That Talle's pioneering work did not appear even in a footnote was indicative of how much the ethnographic pendulum had moved away from cultural relativism. Feinstein recalled seeing two children at a local rehabilitation center who had the fortune of being rescued alive after they were abandoned. She further mentioned that most of her sixty-eight Maasai informants, while denouncing the willful killing of the disabled as sinful, agreed that death from neglect, denial of food, and abandonment was acceptable. "We hide them in the house and leave them when we migrate" was how one of them put it. Tellingly, the words "hide" and "kill" are used interchangeably in the local vernacular, according to Feinstein.[39]

Feinstein's findings would resonate with grassroots perspectives that have since sounded the death knell on pastoral romanticism. In the Maasailand of Tanzania, wrote Kaganzi Rutachwamagyo, disabled girls and boys continue to be killed by their parents "with the excuse that such children cannot endure long treks in search of pastures especially in the dry season."[40] If the congenital disability is detected earlier, added disability rights activist Alex Munyere, the child would have an even shorter lifespan. The unwanted life was often brought to a premature end in one of three ways: leaving the infant at the gate of the compound through which the cattle were to enter, exposing it to the elements, and denying it breast milk.[41] A Maasai born with albinism, Munyere himself was spared of that fate only by luck. As a survivor, his life experience would lead him to study social work at university, after which he held various positions in the disability rights movement, including chairperson of the Albinism Society of Kenya.[42]

---

38 Sheryl Feinstein and Nicole C. D'Errico, *Tanzanian Women in Their Own Words: Stories of Disability and Illness* (Lanham, MD: Lexington, 2010).

39 Sheryl Feinstein, "A Research Study on Individuals with Disabilities in the Maasai Tribe of Tanzania," *Review of Disability Studies* 5, no. 4 (2009): 3–10.

40 Kaganzi Rutachwamagyo, "A Profile of Tanzanians with Disabilities," in *Disability, Society, and Theology: Voices from Africa*, ed. Samuel Kabue and Ester Mombo (Limuru: Zapf Chancery, 2011), 365.

41 Alex Munyere, "Living with a Disability That Others Do Not Understand," *British Journal of Special Education* 31, no. 1 (2004): 31–32.

42 Information given by Alex Munyere during a taped interview with author, June 9, 2011.

Finally, lest this section appears unduly critical of pastoralists and foragers, some global perspective is in order. The discarding of the most vulnerable members of society was a widespread phenomenon. Ancient Greeks and Romans practiced it, with the Spartans leading the way with the least tolerance for disabled infants. So entrenched is the legend of Oedipus in modern folklore that it has captured the attention of a revisionist classicist. According to Martha Rose, the decision to abandon Oedipus in the bush was not related to his deformity but rather with the circumvention of a patricidal prophecy,[43] which is to say that the myth of infanticide is a backward projection of present-day ableist death wish.[44]

However one may question the frequency of the practice of infanticide in the ancient Mediterranean world, one thing is clear: since Rome and Greece were agricultural societies capable of supporting some surplus population, removal of the disabled had little to do with the logistics of survival. Their exterminatory preoccupation was, instead, an early form of eugenics, driven by the desire to breed a superior military race in the case of the Spartans. What happened among foragers and pastoralists, by contrast, was dictated by socioeconomic exigencies. Even then, the African practice of neglect and abandonment was relatively the most passive, primitive societies' version of euthanasia. A comparative study with some of the hunter-gatherers in Australia and the Americas would reveal much more aggressive measures of doing away with the disabled, such as throwing them off a cliff, stabbing them, strangling them, and even burying them alive.[45]

Agriculturalists

Barring unexpected environmental calamities, the Neolithic revolution ensured a steady source of food security, at least until the next round of harvest. There was also the longue durée effect. Over time, food production catalyzed massive social transformation, whose cumulative advantages mutated into "farmer power," in the words of Jared Diamond.[46]

---

43   Martha L. Rose, *The Staff of Oedipus: Transforming Disability in Ancient Greece* (Ann Arbor: University of Michigan Press, 2003), 29.
44   Rose, *Staff of Oedipus*, 49.
45   Diamond, *World Until Yesterday*, 214–217.
46   Jared Diamond, *Guns, Germs, and Steel: The Fates of Human Societies* (New York and London: Norton, 1997), 85–92.

Agriculturalists saw frequent births not as an incumbrance but as an incubator of more fieldhands, the first line of defense against destitution for aging parents. Just as consequential was the impact on disability. Sedentary settlement, division of labor, and improved material culture made it possible for dependents to be offered more sustainable care, even to be integrated into socioeconomic life. Much of that unfolded in a rather roundabout way. Dense settlements and poor hygiene exposed Neolithic societies to periodic outbreaks of contagion. Since this multiplied the possibility of contracting temporary or lifelong debility, communities grew accustomed to the quotidian presence of infirmity in their midst. Customary law in the form of taboo and social shame ensued, protecting the vulnerable against excessive forms of abuse and negligence. Likewise, there evolved imaginative means of accommodation, such as the attribution of metaphysical powers to survivors of certain types of affliction.[47]

In the African context, such an embrace of human interdependence has been attributed to the communal ethos of *ubuntu*, or to its many variants in the Bantu languages. The 1993 South African constitution made explicit references to *ubuntu*, relating it to the country's homegrown quest for restorative justice and collective peace.[48] *Ubuntu* has since gained a place in African disability studies, suggesting a symbiosis between the well-being of the individual and the integrity of the social whole: "a person is a person through other persons."[49]

Shortly after World War II, the British government dispatched a team of experts to Africa to study how blinded ex-servicemen in the colonies could be best rehabilitated. It turned out that many of the societies visited already had an inbuilt social safety net. The group recommended that the rehabilitation work proceed or be tailored in line with this rich tradition of *ubuntu*. "Where the system of family and group responsibility remains intact, as in most parts of Colonial Africa," its report noted, "the blind are ensured of

---

47 Diamond, *Guns, Germs, and Steel*, 89–90.
48 Camilla Hansen, "Ability in Disability Enacted in the National Parliament of South Africa," *Scandinavian Journal of Disability Research* 17, no. 3 (2013): 261.
49 Maria Berghs, "Practices and Discourses of Ubuntu: Implications for an African Model of Disability?" *African Journal of Disability* 6, no. 1 (2017): 1–8; Moeketsi Letseka, "In Defence of Ubuntu," *Studies in Philosophy and Education* 31, no. 1 (2011): 47–60; Gubela Mji et al., "An African Way of Networking Around Disability," *Disability and Society* 26, no. 3 (2011): 365–368.

food, shelter, clothing and a position in society which is not disadvantageous by native standards."[50] Cultural superstitions and "pampering" did force individuals into a vegetative lifestyle, the group recognized, adding that some were still able to rise above that fate with their own ingenuity: "The wonder is, not that most blind Africans are helpless and inert, but that a few, despite every discouragement, live actively."[51]

This was not without global parallels. If there was any era in European history during which corporeal boundaries fluctuated the most, it was in the Middle Ages.[52] The deaf, who faced exclusion in family gatherings and similar social settings, could assimilate with little trouble into the toiling lot of the peasantry. The blind and the crippled, who counted on family to have their plots cultivated and harvested, could specialize in indoor crafts such as rope making, basket weaving, and pottery. Many altogether required no special accommodation and lived ordinary lives; for agricultural routines, unlike the regimented industrial workforce, could be modified and managed according to one's pace.[53]

In this regard, *ubuntu* stood out not because it was uniquely African, but because it represented holistic social relations of a preindustrial era. Still, accustomed to the individualistic worldview of the time, nineteenth-century European travelers found it remarkable that African rulers reached out to their needy subjects. Among the Swazi of southern Africa, for example, it was up to the chief to look after the less fortunate, hence the saying "the goods of the king are the goods of the nation."[54] In the south-central African kingdoms of Kuba, Bulozi, and Bemba, rulers maintained special granaries for the public good. Particularly notorious for his largesse was Msiri, master of a vast empire in southeastern Congo in the second half of the nineteenth century, whom David Livingstone saw offer food and shelter to the needy, including lepers and the elderly.[55]

---

50   Douglas F. Heath, *Blindness in British African and Middle East Territories* (London: Colonial Office, 1948), 24.
51   Heath, *Blindness*, 23.
52   Finkelstein, *Attitudes and Disabled People*, 6–8; Oliver, *Politics of Disablement*, 26–28.
53   Oliver, *Politics of Disablement*, 27.
54   John Iliffe, *The African Poor: A History* (Cambridge: Cambridge University Press, 1987), 71.
55   Iliffe, *African Poor*, 50–59.

But kinship cooperation was not without a flaw. An obvious setback was that it could fall apart in times of resource scarcity. This was demonstrated in Colin Turnbull's ethnographic work on the Ik of northeastern Uganda, a society that had recently converted from hunting and gathering to subsistence farming before falling on hard times.[56]

Unlike his experience with the well-endowed Mbuti of the Ituri forest, Turnbull's stay with the Ik in 1966 coincided with the outbreak of a severe famine. Foreign food aid arrived not only too late, but it was never sufficient enough to stop routine fights over food. In his 1972 *Mountain People*, Turnbull drew a nihilistic picture of a society whose entire social fabric had collapsed: the strong preying on the weak, stealing or snatching their food rations, even taking a sadistic pleasure in their suffering.[57] A controversial bestseller, the book was met by mixed and emotionally charged reactions. Anthropologist Fredrik Barth found it so denigrating of a culture he raised the possibility of a libel suit, while the Ugandan government went as far as declaring Turnbull persona non grata. Environmentalists, on the other hand, saw in the Ik tragedy a Malthusian prophecy coming to pass, and British stage director Peter Brook even converted *Mountain People* into a highly sensational live performance.[58]

Another scenario for the decline of *ubuntu* was the rise of competitive societies, namely societies with a greater exposure to market economy. Since Africa was a continent of chronic underpopulation in relation to its vast landmass, labor was in constant shortage. Market-driven cultivators overcame this challenge by actively mobilizing extra fieldhands, even by acquiring slaves. A bigger workforce cleared and planted more virgin land, ensuring

---

56 Colin M. Turnbull, *The Mountain People* (New York: Simon and Schuster, 1972).

57 A certain Lo'ono, an old woman who had been thrown out by her son, embodied the type of victim that could be found scattered across the pages of *Mountain People* showing the extreme depravity to which the community had sunk. "She too had been abandoned, and had tried to make her way down the mountainside," Turnbull wrote in one of his most graphic depictions. "But she was totally blind and had tripped and rolled to the bottom of the *oror a pirre'i*, and there she lay on her back, her legs and arms thrashing feebly, while a little crowd standing on the edge above looked down at her and laughed at the spectacle." See Turnbull, *Mountain People*, 226.

58 See Peter J. Wilson et al., "More Thoughts on the Ik and Anthropology," *Current Anthropology* 16, no. 3 (1975): 343–358; and John Knight, "The Mountain People as Tribal Mirror," *Anthropology Today* 10, no. 6 (1994): 1–3.

a richer yield of surplus. This so-called primitive accumulation of capital in turn guaranteed better provision for dependents including the sick, the aging, pregnant and nursing women, as well as for oneself in case of incapacitation. Benefits came with social cost. The predatorial labor system created an unequal society, between the free and the unfree, while those unfit for agricultural work were declared pariahs and physically segregated. Thus began the collective identification of the latter with perennial poverty, ostracism, and social pollution, which were phenomena little known among foragers and pastoralists.[59]

Such were the conditions under which some societies gravitated toward the charity model of disability. Under this coping mechanism, accommodation became a haphazard solitary affair, a stark departure from when it was a kinship mandate. Nor was access to food and shelter a birthright, but something that had to be negotiated consistently and adeptly. And if disability once belonged within the family homestead, it now jockeyed for attention in public spaces such as the marketplace and the village square. In other words, disability took on the form of a personal tragedy as opposed to being a collectively shared life course, and the reaction to it moved away from the *ubuntu* model of empathy to individualized expressions of sympathy.

Belonging to this category were fledgling urban centers such as the Yoruba towns of Abeokuta and Ibadan, whose relatively dense populations and flourishing commerce could support a large dependent underclass even by nineteenth-century standards. Along with war refugees and economic immigrants from the countryside, the towns attracted a wide variety of stragglers, among them widows, orphans, lepers, the blind, the deaf, and the chronically sick and aging.[60] Yet, the West African towns were all but a recent sideshow in the history of African beggary. For a longer and deeper history of public largesse one would have to turn north to the Sahel belt. Extending from the West African savannah to the Ethiopian plateau, the drought-prone ecozone stood out for its early embrace of the monotheistic faiths of Islam and Christianity. Here, random acts of charity enjoined by religious duty coalesced into a de facto welfare institution, in some instances giving rise to distinct social classes akin to caste or guild of beggars.[61]

According to historian John Iliffe, in the Hausa town of Kano, a center of Islamic learning and an inland trade entrepôt, thrived Africa's most

---

59 See Iliffe, *African Poor*, 4–6.
60 Iliffe, *African Poor*, 82–85.
61 Iliffe, *African Poor*, chapters 1–2.

conspicuous and enterprising underclass.⁶² Religious beggars of Kano, *Mai-bara*, congregated in walled neighborhoods, where each group was organized into a guild governed by an appointed chief or *Sarki*. Caste association instilled a sense of community and self-worth among the deserving poor, and among the deaf it even led to the birth of the Hausa sign language: *Maganar Hannu*.⁶³

The guild of the blind, which had about thirteen hundred members by late nineteenth-century estimates,⁶⁴ was recognizable enough so as to have had a special mention in the Kano Chronicle. As the chronicler noted, under the reign of Yaji (1349–1385), the unbelievers among the Hausa, both men and women, were struck blind for their defilement of a mosque. "Yaji turned the chief of the pagans out of his office and said to him, 'Be thou Sarki among the blind,'" and thus emerged Kano's historic blind community in a separate part of town and with its own leader.⁶⁵ What began as an allegory on the spiritual state of *Jahiliyyah* (or nonbelievers) would take on the more literal appellation of an intergenerational curse. In 1953, for example, Kano's guild of blind beggars attracted the attention of some British visitors. When the guests asked if they could take pictures of the chief, the chief's interpreter is said to have responded: "The King will allow you to take his photograph so long as you don't use it to restore his sight. Allah has made him blind; it is not for men to interfere."⁶⁶

Indeed, disability agency in the form of religious mendicancy pervades the historical literature of monotheistic Africa. One could even argue that it provides a rare transnational theme that cuts across the Islamic and Christian divide. In the monastery of Aba Gerimma in northern Ethiopia, famed for its miracle workings, Father Francisco Alvarez reported of the congregation of "more than three thousand cripples, blind men and lepers."⁶⁷ In 1841,

---

62   Iliffe, *African Poor*, 32–33.
63   Constanze Schmaling, *Maganar Hannu, Language of the Hands: A Descriptive Analysis of Hausa Sign Language* (Hamburg: Signum Verlag, 2000); and Ruth Zilla Morgan, *Sign Language Studies* 2, no. 3 (2002): 335–341.
64   Iliffe, *African Poor*, 31.
65   H. R. Palmer, trans., "The Kano Chronicle," *Journal of the Anthropological Institute of Great Britain and Ireland* 38 (1908): 71.
66   John Wilson, "Blindness in Colonial Africa," *African Affairs* 52, no. 207 (1953): 141.
67   Francisco Alvarez, *Narrative of the Portuguese Embassy to Abyssinia during the Years 1520-1527*, trans. Lord Stanley of Alderly (New York: Burt Franklin, 1970), 89.

three centuries after the Portuguese priest penned the above observation, the situation was not much different. English traveler Cornwallis Harris described a throng of Ethiopian alms-seekers near the king's compound in Ankober, Shewa, and among which included "the palsied, the leprous, the scrofulous. . . . the old, the halt, the deaf, the noseless, and the dumb, the living dead in every shape and form."[68]

Harris could have included the most conspicuous caste of Ethiopian alms seekers, the *Hamina*, whose claim of disability through a leper ancestor could best be described as fictive. Faces veiled for anonymity, Hamina beggars walked from door to door in the predawn hours, singing haunting songs that lamented the vanity of the flesh in rhyming couplets. Patrons gave so as to be spared the mendicants' allegedly potent curse and much less out of compassion.[69]

According to Mesele Terecha Kebede, Hamina were perhaps remnants of an extinct pre-Christian community in the Shewan highlands, who when dispossessed of land by the expanding Christian state in the thirteenth and fourteenth centuries resorted to a nomadic life of beggary. Folklore traditions sanctioned their pariah status by painting them with a hereditary curse of leprosy, thanks to an ancestor who touched and defiled the holiest church relic: the Ark of the Covenant.[70] Without alternative forms of livelihood because of a high rate of unemployment and rural overpopulation, many Hamina still maintain the itinerant lifestyle bequeathed by their fictive disability. When interviewed by a recent researcher about the role of beggary as a cleanser, Hamina informants responded affirmatively: "If we do not move from place to place and from door to door singing our songs; if we don't suffer under the chilly/frosty nights and under attacking and barking dogs, we will definitely be struck by leprosy."[71]

Mutually recognizable disability worldviews across Sahel Africa rested on two grounds. First, agricultural harvests were susceptible to recurrent

---

68 William Cornwallis Harris, *Highlands of Ethiopia*, vol. 2 (London: Longman, 1844), 244.

69 Mesele Terecha Kebede, "Society Unhealed: Leprosy and Identity in Twentieth-Century Ethiopia" (PhD diss., University of Oslo, 2017), 105–128. Also see Mesele Terecha Kebede, "Origin and Transformation of the Hamina Song-Mendicant Tradition," *African Studies Monograph* 41 (2010): 63–79.

70 Kebede, "Origin and Transformation," 73.

71 Timkehet Teffera, "Mendicancy and Oral Poetry in Ethiopia: The Case of the Hamina," https://zemaafrica.files.wordpress.com/2013/01/mendicancy-and-oral-poetry-in-ethiopia-the-case-of-the-hamina-5.pdf.

droughts, facilitating a culture of vagrancy among those who could no longer subsist on farming. Second was the unique role of geography through which beggary was exposed to global influences. Because the Sahel was where black Africa overlapped with the southern fringes of the Mediterranean world and the Middle East, it was not long before certain social and cultural adaptations accompanied its embrace of the monotheistic faiths, among them religious mendicancy. Likewise emerged integrated centers of religious learning, Koranic as well as monastic, whose emphasis on oral literacy allowed those with vision impairment to excel equally. In theory, therefore, disability agency in Sahel Africa covered a much broader spectrum, from the lowly village pauper to the learned court cleric—and to the life of the wandering leper.

Finally, mention must be made of two literary icons whose examples once again attest to the malleability of African disability agency. First is the warrior king Sundiata, who according to oral tradition grew up as a severely "crippled child." In embellished recitals of his laurels by storytellers, or griots, were some insights into how physical variations were understood. "People had seen one-eyed kings, one-armed kings, and lame kings, but a stiff-legged king had never been heard tell of," according to one oral tradition.[72] Regardless of whether such extraordinary individuals actually reigned, the passage underscores a popular point in critical disability studies. Medieval West African imagination, like that of the rest of the medieval world, entertained wide-ranging corporeal possibilities. In the ambiguous representations of Sundiata both as disabled and warrior, disability scholar Lennard Davis would argue, was one more proof that preindustrial societies did not lump humankind into statistical binaries of normal versus abnormal, or standard versus deviant.[73]

The other icon is Scriptural. He is black Africa's first convert to Christianity, whom the Acts of the Apostles perfunctorily identify by his reproductive disability: the Ethiopian Eunuch. Owing to the Eunuch's sacral role in the spread of apostolic evangelism, the Ethiopian church took a relaxed view of Leviticus and its strict physical requirements for the priesthood. As a result, Ethiopian Orthodoxy showed little opposition to the ordination of persons with visible physical impairments, some of whom rose above the rank

---

72 D. T. Niane, *Sundiata: An Epic of Old Mali*, trans. G. D. Pickett (London: Longman, 1965), 18.

73 Lennard J. Davis, "Disability, Normality, and Power," in *Disability Studies Reader*, ed. Lennard J. Davis (New York: Routledge, 2013), chap. 1.

of ordinary clergy. Jeronimo Lobo, a seventeenth-century Jesuit visitor to Ethiopia, remembered breaking bread with a blind monk who was "a man of learning . . . fairly conversant and knowledgeable in the Scriptures, with which knowledge he caused himself to be respected."[74] Lobo might as well have been talking of the eighteenth-century Mamher Esdros who, although blind from childhood, also lived an iconic monastic life. Unsettled questions of Christology, or debate over the nature of Christ, led Esdros to study and analyze hundreds of manuscripts scattered in various monasteries, prompting a contemporary to describe his works of synthesis as the "meeting point of all traditions."[75]

Coincidentally, the integration of the disabled into the Ethiopian clergy resonated with a special tradition of the Islamic world, where the blind were considered ideal candidates for the role of muezzin. From the height of a minaret top only a blind crier could not pry into the private lives of the neighborhood below. In men with sensory restrictions was thus found the ideal qualification for an office,[76] hence why a disability historian on the Ottoman Arab world was to describe blindness as the "noblest impairment."[77]

Muslim Africans also honored the tradition. Gaspard Mollien, an early nineteenth-century traveler in the West African hinterlands, commented that a blind muezzin was the norm in the "Fouta country," adding that "everyone was eager to fill the calabash of the muezzin with millet or flour."[78] Among the remarkable individuals that caught Mollien's attention in the course of his sojourn was a certain Abdoulai. Mollien first took notice of Abdoulai at a literary gathering as he was leading a group of Marabouts, or holy men, through some intricate religious texts. "One of these Marabouts was

---

74   Donald Lockhart, trans., *The Itinerario of Jeronimo Lobo* (London: Hakluyt Society, 1984), 221.

75   Ronald Cowley Watford, "Mamher Esdros and His Interpretations," in *Proceedings of the 6th International Ethiopian Studies Conference, Tel-Aviv, 14–17 April 1980*, (Boston: A. A. Balkema: 1986), 41–42.

76   Mohammed Ghaly, *Islam and Disability: Perspectives in Theology and Jurisprudence* (New York: Routledge, 2010), 107–108.

77   Scalenghe, *Disability in the Ottoman World*, 52–58.

78   Gaspard Mollien, *Travels in the Interior of Africa, to the Sources of the Senegal and Gambia*, trans. E. Bowdich (London: Henry Colburn, 1820), 103.

reading aloud; some young men attentively followed him in their books; and Abdoulai, who was blind, explained the difficult passages," Mollien wrote.[79]

Conclusion

The prominent role of blind clerics in the Ethiopian Orthodox church or of the blind muezzins in Islamic West Africa is, indeed, an ideal place to look for African disability agency. However, such historical investigations should delve beyond the search for ableist role models. As much if not more attention should be given to those whose life is part of the daily toil and drudgery. Beggars have much to offer in this. Mendicancy used to be a full-time vocation, and for this reason alone it debunks the entire myth of the disabled as passive dependents. Across many farming societies the communal spirit of *ubuntu* provided the basis of a social safety net. In the West African savannah and the Ethiopian highlands, however, living off public charity meant shuffling between market towns, royal courts, and pilgrimage sites. Viewed from this angle, agency of the deserving poor would become all the more compelling, as life with impairment depended on negotiated environments and the constant juggling of survival techniques.

At a deeper level, beggary provides some insight into the connection between the mode of production and coping mechanisms of disability. That beggars always appeared in large-scale societies was by no means accidental. These were societies whose complex economy supported a perennial underclass and whose large populations made it possible for individuals to live anonymously without a sense of family shame or fear of reprisal. Segregated quarters and guilds initially may have been about protecting the able-bodied from social pollution. Yet they had the unintended result of promoting a sense of community among renegades, a coping mechanism that the tightly knit village life did not allow.

Among pastoralists and foragers there were no beggars and only rarely were persons with disabilities noticed by outside observers. Cultural anthropologist Marshall Sahlins had even coined the phrase "original affluent society" to describe what he believed was the most idyllic lifestyle in the prehistoric past. From a disability studies point of view, such a golden age never existed. Foragers, even more so than pastoralists, possessed few of the material and social conditions on which a dependent population could be supported. And

---

79 Mollien, *Travels*, 251.

with a negligible population of such persons, these societies never shared the agriculturalists' complex worldview of disability, including biases and coping strategies.

It is true that agricultural societies, especially large-scale ones, lacked the tightly knit social fabric of pastoralists or foragers. However, in their division of labor were opportunities that enabled many of the disabled to engage in specialized crafts. The chief blacksmith in the court of Sundiata's father, we are told, was an old blind man, Nounfairi, who foretold the coming of Mali's warrior king.[80] Then again, opportunities did not come without a cost. Nonagricultural occupations were relegated to low-caste status, and the social stigma associated with them forced many to join the anonymous life of the urban underclass. In fact, if there has been a continuum in African disability history through the precolonial, colonial, and postcolonial times, it is this quest for a more accommodating mode of existence. Behind the present-day influx from rural areas into urban centers, where the disabled continue to eke out a living as hawkers, laborers, and beggars, is a long history of struggle for personal autonomy, access to opportunities, social acceptance, and better means of livelihood.

Finally, what such everyday struggles say to the cultural premise of disability studies should be clear. In and of themselves, cultural values and practices are responses to socioeconomic imperatives. In the postindustrial Global North, the social model of disability has become prevalent because of the legal and technological benefits generated by surplus wealth and its concomitant middle-class values. Likewise, disability realities in the Global South are shaped by either preindustrial or semi-industrial modes of production. Thus, as the medical model has fallen out of vogue in Western disability studies, so should the cultural-deficit rationale in African disability studies give way to a new paradigm focusing on socioeconomic contingencies. At the macro level, therefore, critical African disability discourse should frame itself around the overarching themes of economy, politics, technology, and environment, as well as their intertwined impact on policymaking, social relations, human rights, and activism.

---

80   Niane, *Sundiata*, 6.

Chapter Five

Disability in Africa

A Cultural/Religious Perspective

Mary Nyangweso

Introduction

Disability is part of the human condition, and most human beings are likely to experience disablement at some point in their lives. Those with disabilities represent a significant proportion of the world's population. According to *the World Report on Disability*, more than a billion people worldwide experience some form of disability.[1] This is about 15 percent of the world's population. About 80 percent of them live in developing countries, while 20 percent of those reside in the poorest of these countries. According to WHO, about 40 percent of Africa's population live with disabilities: that is, more than half a billion people. Of these, about 15 percent are school-age children.[2] The central questions explored in this study are (1) Why is disability considered a problem in many societies in Africa? (2) What is the origin or justification of perceptions and behavior toward people with disabilities? (3) What are the moral implications of attitudes and behavior toward those with disabilities?

---

1   World Health Organization, *World Report on Disability* (Geneva: World Health Organization, 2011), https://www.who.int/publications/i/item/world-report-on-disability.
2   SIDA, "Disability Rights in Sub-Saharan Africa," *SIDA*, January 2015, www.sida.se.

It is argued that perceptions about disability are complex, influenced as they are by sociocultural and biomedical factors.

On November 20, 1975, around 10 a.m., Idi Amin, then dictator and president of Uganda, drove into Kampala's main car park. He was accompanied by some of his ministers and bodyguards. He got out of his car and found a group of men playing *ajua*, a locally popular game. Amin asked to join the game, and one of the players gave up his position for the president. It was soon apparent that Amin was good at *ajua*. He was cheered by the crowd as he beat one man after another. As the word got around that the president was playing *ajua*, the crowd grew. In the middle of these scenes of jubilation, there came a crippled man by the name of Wandera Maksini. Wandera, who was quite popular in Kampala, pushed his way through the crowd with his crutches and collapsed in front of Amin. He glared at Amin and started insulting him. He called the president names and told him that he should not have banished Asians from Uganda because the "common man" was now suffering. "We don't have commodities in the shops, yet you call yourself president, son of a bitch! Kill me if you want—" Wandera dared the president.

One of Amin's bodyguards raised his pistol to strike Wandera, who then cried out, "I hear you are a murderer and that you shoot people with guns. Shoot me now!" Amin quietly got to his feet and left the crowd with his ministers and bodyguards. Three days later, Wandera was seen being hauled into a military vehicle. The same day, it was announced on Radio Uganda that anybody with disabilities who needed help should report to the nearest police station. The government announced that it would offer free accommodation and free food to people with disabilities in Jinja, a city envisioned to be the next capital city of Uganda. The following morning, thousands of people with disabilities turned up at Kampala police stations. They were loaded onto military trucks and driven to Jinja, where on arrival they were all unloaded into the Nile River. All people with disabilities on the trucks fell into the crocodile-infested river and drowned. Those who clung to the trucks were shot down until they fell into the river.[3]

While Amin's actions seem extreme, abnormal, or radical, they are not necessarily unique. They reflect common attitudes and behavior displayed toward people with disabilities in Africa and indeed the world over. A few examples suffice to illustrate this. On Friday, December 12, 2014, Cyriaque

---

3 *Drum Magazine*, "Shocking: How Amin Got Rid of All the Disabled People," *Drum Magazine*, February 17, 2017.

Minani, a twenty-seven-year-old man with albinism was ritually murdered in the province of Makamba in the town of Kayogoro. In March of 2015, 220 "witchdoctors" and traditional healers were arrested in Tanzania in a crackdown on the murder of an albino. The latest victim included a one-year-old albino boy killed in northwestern Tanzania.[4] This murder was attributed to the beliefs surrounding albinism, who most myths associate with ghosts, magical beings or curses, while others describe them as "deified" "gods." In 2011, four people were remanded for killing Ifeoma Agela Igwe for ritual purposes in a southern Nigeria court in Nigeria. Ifeoma, a hunchback woman, was kidnapped, beheaded, butchered, and then her hunchback was removed. In her community, it is believed that the hunch contains a magical substance resembling mercury that can make people rich.

In Zimbabwe, Masimba Kuchera, who was born blind, recounts the challenges he faced due to his disability. He explains how many in his situation do not realize their dreams or even go to school. "They are very few government schools for children with disabilities," he said. He went on to explain that most children with disabilities do not go to school because the government does not invest in this area and that people with disabilities face various challenges such as accessing public amenities, education, and information. "Access to public transport buildings and public gathering is very difficult," says Kuchera. He explains how in the streets of Harare, hundreds of people with disabilities beg for alms. Most are dressed in dirty clothes and in makeshift wheelchairs or are on crutches, with some dragging themselves on their hands and knees. Lucky ones are cared for in special homes like the *Jairos jiri* center.[5] Cases of disability-related violence abound in Africa.

These narratives not only illustrate that disability is a disadvantage but also exemplify perceptions and behavior toward people with disabilities in Africa. Perceptions about disability are not only varied in cultures around the world, but there are also various rationales and beliefs used to justify such behavior. It is common in some communities to perceive people with disabilities as

---

4   "Tanzania's Alibo Community: 'Killed Like Animals,'" *BBC News*, December 9, 2014, https://www.bbc.com/news/world-africa-30394260#:~:text=%22We're%20being%20killed%20being%20killed%20like,in%20the%20last%203%20years&text=People%20with%20albinism%20face%20prejudice,tiny%20community%20of%20about%2030%2C000.

5   Kwenda, Stanley, "Africa's Disabled Will Not Be Forgotten," *Africa Renewal*, April 2010, https://www.un.org/africarenewal/magazine/april-2010/africa%E2%80%99s-disabled-will-not-be-forgotten.

hopeless and helpless, while other communities have treated them as extraordinary human beings who deserve respect and even adoration.[6] Africa, as a vast continent with varied cultural and religious values, both local and foreign, offers a variety of perceptions of disability. Some perceptions lead to inexplicable contradictions. While some communities believe that disabilities are caused by witchcraft, *juju*, sex-linked factors, God, gods, ancestors, or some supernatural force, others consider people with disabilities to be special and even sacred.[7] The central question is whether the negative treatment of people with disabilities is a way of avoiding the influence of evil in society. This chapter presents an exploration of perceptions, attitudes, and behavior toward people with disabilities while highlighting cultural and religious explanations of this behavior. Drawing examples from Africa, perceptions, attitudes, and behavior toward disabled people are interrogated within their sociocultural context. Explored as well are moral questions regarding basic human rights of those with disabilities and how the African ethic that is embedded in the *ubuntu* and modern values of human rights can inform perceptions, attitudes, and behavior toward disabled people through empowerment. It should be noted here that examples discussed in this chapter, while they may allude to commonalities with regard to perceptions of people with disability across Africa, do not reflect the perceptions of all communities on the continent.

In Nigeria, for instance, negative perceptions of children with disabilities are rooted in varying beliefs. Disabilities can be viewed as caused by a curse from God for perceived gross disobedience to God's commandments); ancestral violations of social norms (e.g., stealing); offenses against the gods of the land (e.g., fighting); breaking of laws and family sins such as stealing and lying about it; misfortunes as in the case of incest; witches and wizards; adultery; are a warning from the gods of the land due to supposed pollution of water and the environment; including arguing and fighting with the elders; criminal misdeeds in a previous life; illegal or unapproved marriage by the societal elders; and possession by evil spirits, among others.[8]

---

6   D. Desta, *Needs and Provisions in the Area of Special Education: The Case of Ethiopia* (Uganda: 2nd South-North Workshop, 1995).
7   C. O. Abosi and E. D. Ozoji, *Educating the Blind: A Descriptive Approach* (Ibadan: Spectrum, 1985).
8   S. Marten, "Prejudice or Ambivalence? Attitudes towards Persons with Disabilities," *Disability and Society* 5, no. 3 (1990): 227–241; M. Eskay, "Disability Within the African Culture," *U.S-China Education Review* B4

In Ghana, among the Ashanti, children with physical deviations were rejected. For instance, an infant born with six fingers would be murdered at birth.[9] Children with severe special needs were sometimes described as being "animal-like" and would often be abandoned by the riverbanks or near the sea so they could return to what was believed to be "their own kind." People with disabilities were precluded from becoming chiefs, and a chief who acquired a debilitating illness such as epilepsy would be destooled.[10] In some communities in Kenya and Zimbabwe, a child with a disability was believed to symbolize a "curse" that had befallen her family. Such a child was considered a "shame." [11]

Although there are common negative perceptions, attitudes, and behavior toward people with disabilities, there are positive views as well. Some communities perceive and treat people with disabilities as special beings. Among the Igbo of Nigeria, for instance, people with disabilities were cared for in some cases and rejected in others. The Ga from Accra, Ghana, treated feeble-minded individuals with awe. They believed that those with disabilities were a reincarnation of a deity. They were always treated with great kindness, gentleness, and patience.[12] Among the Chagga of East Africa, the physically handicapped were perceived as pacifiers of the evil spirits. For this reason, care was taken not to harm them. Among the Benin of West Africa, children born with disabilities were revered because of the belief that they were protected by supernatural forces. As such, they were accepted in the community because they were believed to bring good luck.[13]

Among the Yoruba of Nigeria, one myth presents an elaborate description of the origin of the disability. According to this myth, Obatala, one of the Orisha deities, is believed to be the patron of people with disabilities. The mythology describes how the supreme god, Olodumare, the creator of

---

(2012): 473–484; and P. O. Nwogu, *The Provision of the National Policy on Special Education in Nigeria* (Ibadan: Foundation, 1988).

9   R. S. Rattray, *Ashanti Proverbs* (London: Clarendon, 1952).

10 Rattray, *Ashanti Proverbs*; Peter Sarpong, *Ghana in Retrospect: Some Respects of Ghanaian Culture* (Accra: Ghana Publishing, 1974).

11 Bjorn Franzen, "Attitudes towards People with Disabilities in Kenya and Zimbabwe" (master's thesis, School for International Training, 1990), 21–26.

12 Margaret Joyce Field, *Religion and Medicine of the Ga People* (1937; repr. London: Oxford University, 1961), 183.

13 B. A. Wright, *Physical Disability: A Psychological Approach* (New York: Harper and Bon, 1960).

the universe, sent his sons Obatala and Oduduwa down to earth to assist with the creation of humans. Obatala was asked to complete the creation of humans by molding them out of clay. He was to form their bodies and give them heads, after which he would give them to Olorun (the other name of the creator god) so he would blow the breath of life into them. Obatala did as he was told, and for this reason he is regarded as the lord of human heads. Obatala, however, loved to drink palm wine, and so while forming the bodies he would take short breaks and refresh himself with this beverage. As time passed, he became intoxicated and fell into a stupor. Because of his drunken state, he would sometimes give people impairments and deformities. According to this myth, he created albinos, cripples, and blind people when he was drunk. Repentant, he forsook alcohol and became the patron of those born with disabilities. In memory of Obatala's drunkenness, worshippers are forbidden to drink palm wine, and afflicted people are considered to be sacred and special to the god. These individuals are often given positions of importance in Obatala's shrines. It is for this reason that people born with congenital defects are called *eni-orisa*, literally meaning "people of the god Obatala." While this myth is a good explanation of the origin of disabilities, the deeper meaning of the story alludes to the reality of imperfection in this world and how imperfections are sometimes expressed via physical disabilities. The moral teaching in the narrative is about the acceptance of imperfections—since God is on the side of all even those perceived to be imperfect.[14]

The experience of people with disabilities is dire not just because they are stigmatized, but because their suffering is rooted and sometimes justified by culture and religion. For instance, to be an albino in an African country like Tanzania is to live with the fear of being attacked and killed for body parts. Josephat Torner has lived with this fear his entire life. He is lucky to have evaded numerous attempts on his life because of his white skin. He explains how people would encourage his parents to poison him for fear that his albino condition is a curse. "The society does not see you as a human being," he explains.[15] Sabina Namigambo, also an albino, escaped attack after screaming and alerting her neighbors, actions which forced her attacker

---

14 Miguel A. De La Tourre, *Santarea: The Beliefs and Rituals of a Growing Religion in America* (Grand Rapids, MI: Eedermans , 2004).

15 Dann Gilgoff, "As Tanzania's Albino Killings Continue, Unanswered Questions Raise," *National Geographic*, October 10, 2013, https://www.nationalgeographic.com/news/2013/10/131011-albino-killings-witch-doctors-tanzania-superstition/.

to back off. She had gone to the lake to fish, only to be assaulted. "After jumping out of the window, they still came after me, and I was screaming for help," she explains.[16] Josephat and Sabina exemplify the plight of albinos in African communities. In several parts of Africa, albinos face discrimination and abuse because of the condition of their skin. For instance, on March 18, 2015, a ten-year-old girl by the name of Sena Mireille Tonoukouin escaped possible abduction in the town of Simwe Hounto, Benin. On August 14, 2014, a twelve-year-old boy with albinism was killed in Gaoua, Burkina Faso. His body was found with his head and genitals removed. The albinism advocacy organization, Under the Same Sun, has documented reports of 440 such incidences in twenty-five African countries since 2008.[17] According to available statistics, as many as one in five hundred people in sub-Saharan Africa and one in twenty thousand people in Europe and North America have albinism.

Albinism is a worldwide hereditary genetic condition involving the lack of melanin pigment in the hair, skin, and eyes, which causes vulnerability to sun exposure. This condition can easily lead to cancer and severe visual impairment. The term "albino" has a derogatory connotation because this condition has led to discrimination, violence, and even the murder of those with this condition. According to the 2006 BBC *Public Health Report*,[18] people with albinism face prejudice and death threats every day. From 2000 to 2013, the United Nations Human Rights Office received over two hundred reports of the murder and dismembering of people with albinism for ritual purposes in fifteen African countries. Some of these countries have been listed as being involved in crossborder trade of people with albinism and their body parts.

The albino condition is also explained in African beliefs. It is a common belief that albinos are cursed ghosts whose body parts can ward off bad luck and bring wealth and success. As Josephat explains, "Some believe that the witchcraft ritual is more powerful if the victim screams during the

---

16 "Tanzania's Alibo Community," *BBC News*.
17 Under the Same Sun, "Reported Attacks of Persons with Albinism—Most Recent Attacks Included," *underthesamesun.com*, December 17, 2020, https://www.underthesamesun.com/sites/default/files/Attacks%20of%20PWA%20-%20extended%20version.pdf.
18 Esther S. Hong and Hajo Zeeb, "Albinism in Africa as a Public Health Issue," *BMC Public Health* 6, no. 212 (2006), https://bmcpublichealth.biomedcentral.com/articles/10.1186/1471-2458-6-212.

amputation."[19] It is for this reason, body parts are often amputated from live victims, especially children. There is the belief that men who have contracted HIV/AIDS can be healed from this condition if they slept with albino girls. This erroneous belief has led to the abduction and rape of albino girls. Beliefs such as these are said to be strong around the lake zone, a populous area in Tanzania's northwest. Such beliefs make albinos vulnerable and susceptible to violence.

Another common disability worth highlighting is angular kyphosis: a condition of curvature of the upper spine. This condition, often caused by degenerative diseases such as arthritis or developmental problems, is perceived in some African communities to be the result of a curse or the work of spiritual forces.[20] In the state of Osun Nigeria, a twenty-two-year-old female named Taibat Oseni was killed for having angular kyphosis. According to Osun State Police Command, Oseni was kidnapped from her home and then taken to an abandoned building owned by a senator who was later implicated in her death. It is argued that she was murdered here, and her protrusion was removed and taken for some kind of medicinal purposes.[21] In Benin City, Edo State of Nigeria, a famous herbalist male with angular kyphosis was murdered.[22] In the same city, a man with albinism was beheaded while working on the farm.[23] Like the albinos, people with angular kyphosis have lived with discrimination and violence, and some have been trafficked or murdered.

Disability: A Matter of Perspectives

WHO defines disability as an impairment or abnormality of a psychological, physiological, or anatomical structure or function.[24] It is any restriction or lack of ability to perform an activity in the manner or within the range

---

19 Gilgoff, "Albino Killings."
20 O. Omiegbo, "Superstitious Beliefs Associated with the Handicapped in Africa," in *African Traditional Religion: A Book of Selected Readings*, ed. A. O. Orubu (Benin: Institute of Education, 2001), 26–28.
21 Gabriel Dike, "Murder of a Hunchback: Senatoe Ogunwale Moved to Abuja," *Sun News*, October 11, 2009; and Y. Kolawale, "Senator Quizzed Over Alleged Murder," *Thisday*, October 7, 2009.
22 Omiegbo, "Superstitious Beliefs."
23 Edwin Etieyibo, "Religion, Culture, and Discrimination against Persons with Disability in Nigeria," *African Journal of Disability* (2016): 2223–9170.
24 World Health Organization, *World Report on Disability*, 213.

considered normal for a human being. According to the ADA, disability is a physical or mental impairment that substantially limits one or more life activities. The emphasis here is on the disadvantage and the inability to fulfill a role that is considered normal.[25] One is disabled if he/she has a physical or mental impairment that substantially limits them from engaging in major life activities, has a record of such an impairment, or is regarded as having such an impairment.[26] The fluid nature of what it means to be disabled is reiterated in the *World Report on Disability*, which describes disability as negative aspects of interactions between the individual and higher context (environment and personal factors) and limitations and restrictions in participating in society.[27] Simply put, perspectives tend to inform notions of disability. That is why those who may be perceived as disabled may or may not consider themselves as disabled.

According to Kasnitz and Shuttleworth, disability exists when people experience discrimination based on perceived functional limitations. In other words, impairment occurs when physiological or behavioral statuses or processes are socially categorized as problems, illnesses, conditions, disorders, syndromes, medically diagnosed as such.[28] Susman defines disability as the loss or abnormality of a psychological, physiological, or anatomical structure or function.[29] To Ginsburg and Rapp, disability is a relational category that is shaped by social conditions.[30] These works reveal the complexity that surrounds what is considered disability. Misperceptions that disability is only about long-term visible conditions associated with people in wheelchairs and blind and deaf people overlook invisible impairments and disabilities that are more common than is often acknowledged. In a study conducted by the Australian National Health Survey, 40 percent of people with a severe or profound disability rated their health as good, very good, or excellent.[31]

---

25   World Health Organization, *World Report on Disability*, 213.
26   US Department of Labor Employment Standards Administration Office of Federal Contract Compliance Programs, www.dol.gov/esa/regs/statutes/ofccp/ada.
27   World Health Organization, *World Report*; M. Leonardi et al., "The Definition of Disability: What Is in a Name?" *Lancet* 368 (2006): 1219–1221.
28   Shuttleworth and Kasnitz, "Stigma," 2.
29   J. Susman, "Disability, Stigma and Deviance," *Social Science and Medicine*, 36, no. 1 (1994): 15–22.
30   Faye Ginsburg and Rayna Rapp, "Disability Worlds," *Annual Review of Anthropology* 42 (2013): 53–68.
31   National Health Survey, 2001–2008.

To fully comprehend disability, one needs to consider the various perception models, namely the medical, the social, and the biopsychosocial models, as these offer significant insights into this discourse of disability. According to the medical model, disability is a physical or mental impairment of the individual. This model, which is informed by the biomedical model used in modern health care, links disability diagnosis to an individual's physical body. According to this model, health constitutes the freedom from disease, pain, or defect. Ultimately, a healthy human condition is designated as normal. The medical model, therefore, emphasizes a therapeutic theme that views disability as a disease or illness, a view that is often adopted unreflectively by health-care professionals, bioethicists, and philosophers. As an approach, it emphasizes the biological determinants of disability, while ignoring the environment that defines people with disabilities. It presupposes that disability reduces one's quality of life.[32] Implied in this model is a mandate to "cure" people with disability, a perspective that overlooks the broad definition of disability.[33]

The social model, on the other hand, considers disability as a relation between the individual and the social environment. It holds that the inclusion and exclusion of people with certain physical and mental characteristics from major domains of social life are determined by social norms. In other words, disability is perceived as a social construction that is determined by social standards for normative bodies, behavior, and role fulfillment.[34] The recognition of disability, as a consequence of negative interactions between a person with impairment and his or her social environment, implies that this condition transcends the appearance of the body. This is because disability is about socially constructed difference. Consequently, as Senghas and Monaghan explain, disabled individuals are often marked as different

---

32   Ellen Annandale, *The Sociology of Health and Medicine: A Critical Introduction* (Cambridge: Polity, 1998).

33   J. Scheer and N. Groce, "Impairment as a Human Constant: Cross-Cultural and Historical Perspectives on Variation," *Journal of Social Issues* 44, no. 1 (1988): 22–37; and Shuttleworth and Kashnitz, "Stigma."

34   J. Armstrong and F. Maureen, "Culture and Disability Studies: An Anthropological Perspective," *Rehabilitation Education* 10, no. 4 (1996): 247–304; B. Holzer, A. Vreede, and G. Weight, *Disability in Different Cultures: Reflections on Local Concepts* (Bonn: Bielefeld, 1999); B. Ingstad and S. R. Whyte, *Disability and Culture* (Berkeley: University of California Press, 1995); and Susman, "Disability," 15.

or treated "problematically" in their societies.[35] By focusing on the social causes of disability, the model interrogates ways that society imposes limitations on people with disabilities, thus making the problem a societal issue. In other words, disability as a creation of the social and material conditions that impede the full participation of those with disabilities adds to a significant view of this condition.[36] While acknowledging the significance of the medical and social models in understanding disability, both models on their own fail to account for how intersectional and relational the issue of disability is. People with disabilities can experience problems arising from their health as well as their social conditions. Scholars who take this view have advocated a third approach: the bio-psycho-social model. This model acts as a compromise between the medical and the social model.[37] Calls for a balanced approach are based on the claim that purely medical or social approaches fail to capture the interaction between health and social factors that inform disability.

A bio-psycho-social model is more adequate because it offers a broader and more integrated approach to human behavior. Central to the model is the argument that "there may be important issues beyond purely biological factors,[38]. By recognizing disability as a social construct of intricate variables and interaction of biological, psychological, and social factors is to recognize its complexity; specifically, the intersectionality that informs disability is recognized as argued by Santrock.[39] As a model, the bio-psycho-social model emerges out of the call for a new medical model as articulated by psychiatrist George L. Engel[40], who argued that psychological factors can cause a biological effect. Engel argues that experts and practitioners who seek to be both effective communicators and ethical practitioners of medicine should embrace this model, which extends health care beyond the patient to include

---

35 R. J. Senghas and L. Monaghan, "Signs of their Times: Deaf Communities and the Culture of Language," *Annual Review of Anthropology* 21 (2002): 69.

36 H. Cervinkova, "Disability and the Other in Cultural Anthropology," *Human Mosaic* 30, nos. 1–2 (1996): 56–63; and Tom Shakespeare, "The Social Model of Disability," in *The Disability Studies Reader*, ed. Lennard J. Davis (New York, Routledge, 1998).

37 World Health, *World Report*, 4–5.

38 Imtiaz Ahmed Dogor, "Biopsychosocial Model," *A.P.M.C* 1 (2007).

39 J. W. Santrock, *A Topical Approach to Human Life-Span Development*, 10th ed. (St. Louis: McGraw-Hill, 2020).

40 George L. Engel, "The Need for a New Medical Model: A Challenge for Biomedicine," *Science* 196 (1977): 129–136.

family and the community. When utilizing the bio-psycho-social model, the emphasis is often placed on the prevention of illness/condition and the promotion of health as in the treatment of disease/condition. Despite criticism from psychiatrists like Hamid Tavakoli[41] and sociologists like David Pilgrim,[42] the successful recognition of the intersection of the scientific and ethical virtues help promote the full comprehension of disability as a health and a social reality.

Intersectionality, a term coined by Kimberlé Crenshaw, recognizes how complex reality is and how this complexity informs social conditions and social behavior.[43] It acknowledges that people's lives are defined by multiple layered identities that derive from social relations, histories, cultures, and other operations of structures of power. As a tool of analysis, intersectionality helps to understand and respond to the ways in which social issues intersect with other identities and recognizes them as unique experiences of oppression and privilege. For this reason, disability is not viewed as an independent variable but as a condition that is constructed within social norms. In revealing multiple identities and in exposing the different types of discrimination and disadvantages that occur because of the combination of identities, intersectionality helps to address the way social structural norms such as racism, patriarchy, classism, and other social systems of discrimination interconnect to create social inequalities that construct attitudes and behavior toward those who are different—such as those with disabilities. Alison Kafer argues that while intersectionality highlights how terms such as "defective," "deviant," and "sick" are constructed and used to justify discrimination against people whose bodies, minds, desires, and practices differ from the norm, it is also a paradigm through which moral values such as human rights and *ubuntu* are interpreted, as these intersect locally and

---

41 Hamid R. Tavakoli, "A Closer Evaluation of Current Methods in Psychiatric Assessments: A Challenge for the Biopsychosocial Model," *Psychiatry, (Edgmont)* 6, no. 2 (2009): 25–30.

42 David Pilgrim, "The Biopsychosocial Model in Anglo-American Psychiatry, Past, Present, and Future," *Journal of Mental Health* 11 (2001): 585–594.

43 K. W. Crenshaw, "Mapping the Margins: Intersectionality, Identity Politics, and Violence against Women of Color," in *Critical Race Theory: The Key Writings that Formed the Movement*, ed. K. W. Crenshaw et al. (New York: New Press, 1995), 357–383.

globally.[44] It is a methodology for the development and promotion of more affirming values as human rights.

Social theorists who acknowledge disability as a social construct affirm the subtle cultural standards of normality and how these define attitudes and behavior toward those who have disabilities.[45] They acknowledge that disability is created by social and historical realities such as diseases and physical injuries resulting from events such as wars and are thus significant in the interrogation of disability. They also acknowledge that cultures sometimes attach meanings to various disabilities or illnesses, and those with disabilities are excluded from meaningful activities. In some cases, cultural and religious norms are used to stereotype and stigmatize people with disabilities. Society may exclude people with impairments due to discrimination that categorizes the disabled body as different. The exclusion and segregation, which is often deliberate, is shaped by the environment and organized as social activity that precludes or restricts the participation of people seen or labeled as having a disability. The cultural attitude that physical or mental differences deviate from "normal" marginalizes people with disabilities and feeds in the fear, ignorance, and pathos surrounding disabled bodies.

The justification of these attitudes by religious values is more problematic because they evoke the power of the divine, a sacred power that is not to be rationalized or questioned. Sociologists such as Peter Berger have argued that religion has played a significant role in legitimizing social norms. In producing reality through the influence and control of the socialization process, it becomes the basis of social control.[46] According to Nancy Eisland,[47] theological themes tend to legitimize disability when they conflate this condition with punishment for wrongdoing or when they justify it as virtuous suffering. When disability is identified with suffering that must be endured to "purify" the righteous, such justifications encourage passive acceptance of disability as a condition willed by God. For instance, scriptural views of

---

44   Alison Kafer, *Feminist Queer, Crip* (Bloomington: Indiana University Press, 2013), 17.
45   Susan Wendell, *The Rejected Body: Feminist Philosophical Reflections on Disability* (New York: Routledge, 1996), 37–56; and Michael Oliver and Collins Barnes, *The New Politics of Disablement*, 2nd ed. (London: Palgrave Macmillan, 2012).
46   Peter Berger, *The Sacred Canopy* (New York: Anchor, 1969), 91.
47   Nancy Eisland, *The Disabled God: Toward a Liberatory Theology of Disability* (Abingdon, UK: Abingdon, 1994).

disability are displayed in the Bible where common diseases such as leprosy, blindness, deafness, and paralysis are explained away as a curse or forms of punishment from God for disobedience and transgressions of sin. These explanations tend to subvert justice by encouraging a continuation of treatment of people with disabilities as "other" instead of empowering them for full social economic and political participation. Eisland calls this a "disabling theology."[48] Disabling theology cites biblical verses to justify disability as a curse and a consequence of disbelief and ignorance. Leviticus 26: 14–16 reads "I will bring upon you sudden terror, wasting disease and fever that will destroy your sight and drain away from your life." A similar scriptural text that describes disability as punishment is that of Judges 14:2, which describes how Samson was struck blind because of his disobedience to God. This view of blindness as disability is further described in Proverbs 30:17, which warns that the disrespect of parents will lead to the plucking out of one's eyes by birds of prey. Paralysis is described as a punishment of God. In 1 King 13:4, the sudden paralysis of King Jeroboam is described as punishment for disobeying God. Theology such as this is not unique to the Bible. As demonstrated in narratives above, indigenous African theologies also justify attitudes and behavior toward people with disabilities through beliefs. These beliefs find reinforcement in Jewish, Christian, and Islamic values that sanction negative attitudes and behavior toward people with disability, thus reinforcing perceptions of these people as "other."

Attention must be paid, therefore, to the societal perceptions, attitudes, and behavior that determine the extent to which the personal, social, educational, and psychological needs of persons with disabilities are treated. As Hobbs[49] observes, the message a child with a disability receives about himself or herself determine their feelings of who they are and how to behave and what they are capable of. Ultimately, rejection produces inferiority, self-consciousness, and fear.[50] Because of these perceptions, attitudes, and negative behavior, people with disabilities find themselves with limited opportunities

---

48   Eisland, *The Disabled God*, 73–74.
49   M. C. Hobbs, *The Future of Children Categories and Their Consequences* (San Francisco: Jossey-Bass, 1973).
50   R. G. Baker, "Social Sciences Resource Council," in *Adjustment to Physical Handicap and Illness: A Survey of the Social Psychology of Physique and Disability*, ed. B. A. Wrights, L. Meyerson, and M. R. Gonick (New York: Social Science Research Council, 1953); G. A. Roener, "Significance of Public Attitudes in the Rehabilitation of the Disabled," *Rehabilitation Literature* 22 (1961): 66–72; and Wright, *Physical Disability*.

because they are socially rejected and discriminated against. Community attitudes affect not only self-perception, the opportunity to associate with others, and the extent of one's mobility but also lead to diminished employment opportunities. Parsons calls this process the internalization of role expectancy.[51] The assumption that disability is a personal or family problem rather than a matter of social responsibility absolves society from the moral responsibility to treat disabled people as fully human.

The Human Rights Question

The suffering of people with disabilities is reported in many societies. Throughout antiquity, people with disabilities are routinely harassed verbally, physically, and sexually and subjected to oppressive behavior that causes horror, fear, anxiety, and distrust. Also disabled people arouse pity in others that can seem overprotective and patronizing at the same time.[52] Often, the disabled suffer violence and sexual abuse in private and public institutions, in their own homes, and sometimes at the hands of family members, friends, and caretakers. Statistics indicate that the risk of physical assault, robbery, and rape is four times higher among people with disabilities compared to that of nondisabled individuals. Discrimination and violence associated with disability include (1) trafficking and murdering people with mental illness, oculocutaneous albinism, and angular kyphosis; rape of women with mental illness, and children with disabilities unethically employed for alms begging.

Gender-based violence is exacerbated among individuals with disabilities. Women with disabilities face even more difficulties in private and in public, as they not only experience gender inequality but are also at a greater risk of gender-based violence such as sexual abuse, neglect, maltreatment, and exploitation. The Center for Women's Policy Studies indicates that disabled women are raped and abused at a rate twice that of nondisabled women.[53] In addition to suffering, these individuals face a range of barriers to exercising their fundamental rights. Many people with disabilities are prevented

---

51   Talcot Parsons, *The Social System* (New York: Free Press, 1951).
52   L. Barton, "The Struggle for Citizenship: The Case of Disabled People," *Disability, Handicap and Society* 8, no. 3 (1993): 235–248.
53   M. Inglesias, *Violence and Women with Disability* (Vedras: AIDES, 1998); and The Roeher Institute, *Violence against Women with Disabilities* (Ottawa: Ottawa Public Health Agency, 2004).

from accessing basic liberties such as marriage, education, health care, voting, rehabilitation, employment, and legal representation. The *WHO World Report on Disability* reports lower employment rates of persons with disabilities relative to those without disabilities across eighteen countries, which include African countries. In South Africa, for instance, employment of people with disabilities is only 12.4 percent compared to 41.1 percent for the overall South African population.[54] In this section, ethical values influencing attitudes and behavior toward people with disabilities are examined insofar as they inform the human rights of these people.

The suffering of people with disabilities raises moral questions about social inequalities and injustices that are prevalent in African communities. The subjection of any individual to violence, abuse, involuntary sterilization, or unlawful confinement and to prejudice and disrespect—as in denying them access to health care, employment, and political participation or rendering them incompetent because of their disability—is a violation of their basic human rights. To deny any social group their autonomy just because they are different is considered a gross violation of human rights principles. Human rights principles were instituted in the 1940s to protect human beings from inhumane atrocities that violated their human dignity. The international commitment to protect human rights was instituted early in 1948 when the United Nations Commission on Human Rights adopted a draft declaration that, in turn, was adopted by the General Assembly that year as the Universal Declaration of Human Rights.[55]

According to the Universal Declaration of Human Rights, human rights are based on the "recognition of the inherent dignity and of the equal and inalienable rights of all members of the human family" as the "foundation of freedom, justice, and peace in the world."[56] Article 5 of the Universal Declaration of Human Rights cautions against the subjection of anyone "to torture, or to cruel, inhuman or degrading treatment or punishment." The United Nations Declaration of the Rights of Children, adopted in

---

54 Statistics South Africa, *Prevalence of Disability in South Africa Census* (Pretoria: Statistics South Africa, 2011); and Lieketseng Ned and Theresa Lorenzo, "Enhancing the Public Sector's Capacity for Inclusive Economic Participation of Disabled Youth in Rural Communities," *African Journal of Disability* 5, no. 1 (2016).

55 Henry J. Steiner and Philip Alston, *International Human Rights in Context: Law, Politics, Morals* (Oxford: Clarendon, 1996), 119–120.

56 Steiner and Alston, *International*, 1156.

1959, stipulates that each child should be given the opportunity "to develop physically, mentally, morally, spiritually, and socially in a healthy and moral manner and in conditions of freedom and dignity" and that he/she should be "protected against 'all forms of neglect, cruelty, and exploitation.'" The Declaration on the Elimination of Violence against Women (CEDAW) enacted by the United Nations in 1981 calls for an end to all gender-based forms of discrimination and requires that nations modify their cultural and social patterns of conduct to eliminate prejudices and practices based on gender inequality and social stereotypes.[57]

In 1984, the United Nations Convention against Torture and Other Cruel, Inhuman or Degrading Treatment or Punishment (CATCID) specifically recognized the rights of persons with disabilities by designating any form of mistreatment and discrimination of such individuals a violation of human rights. CATCID defines torture as any act by which severe pain or suffering, whether physical or mental, is intentionally inflicted on a person for purposes including any reason based on discrimination of any kind.[58] The fight for the rights of people with disabilities was motivated by United Nations treaties such as the International Convention on Civil and Political Rights and the International Covenant on Economic, Social and Cultural Rights, which established universal rights that cover all people, including persons with disabilities. As the movement to protect people with disabilities has grown, the human rights and freedoms of persons with disabilities have advanced along with it. In this charter, the United Nations proclaimed that its purpose was to "achieve international co-operation in promoting and encouraging respect for human rights and fundamental freedoms for all without distinction as to race, sex, language, or religion."[59] Under Articles 55 and 56, all signatory members pledged to take joint and separate action in cooperation with the organization for the achievement of the purpose of the United Nations.

Human rights principles, therefore, recognize that basic rights are inherent to all human beings regardless of nationality, race, gender, ability, or origin. As a political theorist, Jack Donnelly has observed, these principles are based on moral principles that set out certain standards of human behavior and are regularly protected as legal rights in national and international law.

---

57 Steiner and Alston, 244–245.
58 United Nations, *Convention against Torture and Other Cruel, Inhuman or Degrading Treatment or Punishment* (New York: United Nations, 1984).
59 Steiner and Alston, *International*, 1148.

This is because they reflect simple moral facts that all societies have cross-culturally and historically expressed in their values, even as these are interpreted in specific social contexts.[60] Human rights are embedded in significant moral positions, namely moral universalism. As a theoretical framework, moral universalism advocates for human rights.[61] It is a position that draws from four theories: (1) The natural law theory argues that human beings possess a certain degree of sovereignty regarding ideals such as freedom and honor and that all human beings possess this sovereignty equally. Therefore, imposing any restriction on human sovereignty is morally wrong.[62] (2) The theory of rationalism argues that all humans are rational and sovereign beings who are equal.[63] (3) The human capabilities theory argues that there is a need to recognize that fundamental characteristics that define what it means to be human occur across diverse societies, and that these include the basic needs for food, drink, shelter, and mobility; and the capacity for pain and pleasure.[64] (4) The doctrine of positivism argues that countries with representative forms of government should promote universal norms of behavior.[65]

The paradigm shift from the medical to the social model of disability helps to reclassify disability as a human rights issue under international law in recognition of moral universalist values. It should be noted that the introduction of the social model of disability in the 1980s led to the United Nations' acknowledgment of the rights of people with disabilities and the adoption of the convention on the rights of the child (1989), which advanced the movement that led to the establishment of major reforms, including the ADA in the 1990s. More than forty member nations adopted disability

---

60 Jack Donnelly, "The Relative Universality of Human Rights," *Human Rights Quarterly* 2, no. 9 (2007): 284–290).

61 L. Bret Billet, *Cultural Relativism in the Face of the West: The Plight of Women and Female Children* (London: Palgrave Macmillan, 2007).

62 Michael Perry, "Are Human Rights Universal? The Relativist Challenge and Related Matters," *Human Rights Quarterly* 19, no. 3 (1997): 478–481; Billet, *Cultural*, 16.

63 Elizabeth M. Zechenter, "In the Name of Cultural Relativism and the Abuse of the Individual," *Journal of Anthropology Research* 53 (1997): 321; and Billet, *Cultural*, 1.

64 Martha C. Nussbaum, *The New Religious Intolerance: Overcoming the Politics of Fear in an Anxious Age* (Cambridge, MA: Belknap, 2012).

65 Zechenter, "In the Name," 321; and Billet, *Cultural*, 6.

discrimination legislation during the 1990s.[66] In 1993 the United Nations adopted Standard Rules on the Equalization of Opportunities for Persons with Disabilities, which declared that states should recognize the principle of equal primary, secondary, and tertiary educational opportunities for youth and adults with disabilities integrated settings.[67] These rules provided the key moral imperative for change on a worldwide basis.

In 2006 the global community formally recognized the importance of advancing the human rights of persons with disabilities through the CRPD. The CRPD became the first binding UN human rights treaty to comprehensively address the equal rights of individuals with respect to disability status. By January 2015, 151 countries had ratified the CRPD, making it one of the most rapidly ratified human rights treaties in history. In recognizing the human rights of a person with disabilities, the CPRD outlined the civil, cultural, political, social, and economic rights of persons with disabilities. It declared that its purpose was to promote, protect, and ensure the full and equal enjoyment of all human rights and fundamental freedoms by people with disabilities and to promote respect for their inherent dignity. It outlines the legal duties of nations in ensuring the full enjoyment of a wide range of economic, social, civil, and political rights of individuals with disabilities. In Article 5, for instance, it commits to ensuring disability equality and nondiscrimination (Article 5). CRPD commits to ensuring that all human beings are treated equally before the law (Article 12) guarantees the right to liberty (Article 18), freedom of expression (Article 21), education (Article 24), and guarantees the highest attainable standard of health and access to medical services (Article 29) for persons with disabilities.[68] Article 2 of the Convention on the Rights of the Child calls on nations to prohibit discrimination on the grounds of disability. All nations are required to address the specific needs of children with disabilities, including the provision of special care, access to health-care services, and education. This is to be accomplished by individual countries ratifying and enforcing these conventions. Although

---

66 Frederic Megret, "The Disabilities Convention of Human Rights of Persons with Disabilities," *Human Rights Quarterly* 30 (2008): 494–516.

67 United Nations General Assembly, *Standard Rules on the Equalization of Opportunities for Persons with Disabilities: Resolution* (New York: United Nations General Assembly, 1993), http://www.refworld.org/docid/3b00f2e80.html.

68 United Nations, *Convention on the Right of Persons with Disabilities: G.A. Res. 61/106* (New York: United Nations, 2006).

the *World Report on Disabilities* recognizes these efforts, it also acknowledges challenges that continue to be faced including inadequate policies and standards, negative attitudes, lack of provision of services, problems of service delivery, inadequate funding, and lack of accessibility to services. While about 160 countries worldwide have ratified the CRPD to date and have initiated reform legislation and policies toward protecting the rights of persons with disabilities, very little is done in practice to address their rights and violations.

Africa is especially noted for partnering with the Swedish International Development Cooperation Agency (SIDA). Countries that have partnered with SIDA have also ratified the United Nations Convention on the Rights of Persons with Disabilities. These countries have also ratified the Convention on the Prohibition of the Use, Stockpiling, Production and Transfer of Anti-Personnel Mines and on their Destruction, and established to ensure that incidences of disabilities are reduced and that governments agree to clear all known areas that are contaminated by mines within ten years. In spite of this commitment by several countries in Africa that have enacted some legislative and policy steps to advance the rights of persons with disabilities, legal and policy gaps remain. For instance, of the fourteen SIDA partner countries that have ratified the United Nations' CRPD, only eight have signed the Optional Protocol to the CRPD and only six have ratified it. The Optional Protocol allows persons with disabilities whose rights have been violated to bring complaints to the Committee on the Rights of People with Disabilities.[69] In Andrew Dube's report on disability challenges in Uganda, for instance, it is clearly noted that Uganda continues to face glaring challenges with regard to complying with the national and international legal regimes and infringements on the rights of persons with disabilities. This fact is not unique to Uganda.[70]

While espousing human rights values, Africans must not forget the resource they have in the African social ethics of *ubuntu*. This ethics of the shared collective humanity rooted in the African holistic worldview emphasizes the

---

69 *SIDA*, "Disability Rights."

70 Andrew K. Dube, *Participation of Disabled People in the PRSP/PEAP Process in Uganda*, ed. Eleanor Stanley (London: KaR, 2005), https://assets.publishing. service.gov.uk/media/57a08c5ce5274a27b2001153/PolicyProject_uganda_ prsp.pdf.

interconnectedness of everything and everyone. As M. F. Murove[71] explains, *ubuntu* encompasses spiritual interdependence and respect and responsibility toward everyone including their ancestors. In emphasizing interlinked relationships, *ubuntu* promotes the ethics of care, which includes the care of all. It presents Africans with a model of social ethics that mobilizes against social injustice and toward restoring humanity and upholding individual lives and well-being as a holistic reality.[72] It locates disability within the holistic and collective understanding of humanity that acknowledges the dignity and rights of people with disabilities.

It must be recognized, however, that the growth in the movement to protect the rights of persons with disabilities in Africa has led to the establishment of various DPOs. While challenges persist, the progress that has been made is encouraging. Given that attacks such as those mentioned in this chapter are still prevalent, more work still needs to be done to promote the rights of individuals who live with disability and to ensure access to basic opportunities and services necessary for a full life. African countries need to act in recognition of their responsibilities toward this end.

Conclusion

This chapter describes the challenges that people with disabilities face in Africa. Drawing examples from a variety of African communities, the chapter highlights how people with disabilities negotiate these challenges in their day-to-day lives. It is argued that disability is a social construction of various sociocultural and religious values based on what is considered normal and abnormal and that values play a significant role in legitimizing this construction process. The chapter argues further that the persistent suffering, abuse, and mistreatment of persons with disabilities is an indicator of a deeper moral problem of socialization and discrimination. This problem requires cultural and religious confrontation through the debunking of misconceptions. While most of the negative attitudes toward people with disabilities

---

71 M. F. Murove, "An African Commitment to Ecological Conservation: The Shona Concepts of Ukama and Ubuntu," *Mankind Quarterly* 45, no. 2 (2004): 195.

72 D. J. Louw, "The African Concept of Ubuntu," in *Handbook of Restorative Justice: A Global Perspective*, ed. D. Sullivan and L. Tift (London: Routledge, 2006), 161–174; and Maria Berghs et al., *Implications for Public Health: Theories and Models of Disability* (London: NIHR, 2016).

are mere misconceptions that stem from ignorance, a change in attitude and behavior toward these people can only come through an interrogation of the social-cultural contexts within which these values exist. An examination of these values is the first necessary step toward deconstructing discriminative behavior toward people with disabilities. To promote and protect the rights of people with disabilities, the chapter describes core moral foundational values of human rights and the rise of various activist movements toward respecting the rights of people with disabilities.

There is a need for aggressive criminalization of behavior that undermines the welfare of people with disabilities. This second step should involve efforts to empower the community through education toward fostering the transformation of attitude toward embracing people with disabilities. Third, an attitude shift from a discriminative mindset to one of inclusiveness should be enforced through some form of punishment. To stand for the rights of persons with disabilities, all countries should live up to their responsibility of protecting the vulnerable. As United Nations members, all African countries must ratify the UN conventions that protect the rights of people with disabilities. Cultural and religious values that sanction the suffering of people with disabilities should be revisited through a cultural appraisal process. This process involves critical reflection on the relevance of existing values to determine whether they are discriminatory and need to be done away with or whether they protect the vulnerable and are worth upholding.

Chapter Six

Disability and Cultural Meaning Making in Africa

Kathryn Linn Geurts

Making meaning around and about disability in African contexts is a diverse, multifaceted, and often contested phenomenon. Historically, African languages rarely contained terms designating a broad category encompassing all forms of impairment. Instead, terminology reveals how communities perceived people as "without eyes" or "without ears" or when a body part was not functioning well, they were sometimes said to have "dead organs."[1] Physical disabilities caused by polio or limb amputation were perceived as wholly different than deafness and blindness, as were intellectual and cognitive disabilities. Meaning making, therefore, has evolved significantly with the influx and growth of rights-based approaches to disability. However, several enduring themes can be traced both in time and across the continent's space: misfortune and disruptions in kin groups; coalescing of "therapy managing groups" as an unresolved illness transmogrifies into disability; situating an anomalous body/mind in a continuum from normal to aberrant and a consequent shifting sense of identity with associated struggles over belonging. Long before the label of disability entered an African consciousness, concerns with misfortune, its cause, and accountability served as a powerful meaning-making practice for many families and lineage groups. Drums/cults of affliction were precursors to self-help groups. When a "therapy managing group" exhausted its quest for cure, a shift ensued into an identity replete with inadequacies and inabilities that often precipitated a crisis of belonging.

---

1   Kathryn Linn Geurts, *Culture and the Senses: Bodily Ways of Knowing in an African Community* (Berkeley: University of California Press, 2002), 209–218.

As the pace and extent of globalization increased in the opening decade of the twenty-first century, DPOs have created alternate meaning-making opportunities and spaces. But the backdrop remains, and the themes endure, resulting in a complex hybridized set of meanings surrounding disability. So while enduring African understandings of disability have combined with rights-based meanings to create more globalized orientations toward neuro and somatic human diversity, we still find that disability connotes anomalousness, peripherality, and dependency.

"Disability questions the existence and the meaning of life," wrote Africanist anthropologist Patrick Devlieger. It was not simply an assertion but rather embedded in a longer thought, a question, really: "If the why of disability in the African context can be understood existentially, in the sense that *disability questions the existence and the meaning of life*, then what does this mean in the European context?" (emphasis added)[2] Devlieger pointed to World War II as a critical moment for disability histories because an "ideology of equal chances" began to globalize in the ensuing years. He sees it stemming from the United States and the notion of handicap. At an earlier time "hand-in-cap" was a game or contest involving three people, two of whom put their hands into a cap but with an ultimate goal of producing a relatively equal exchange. It evolved, of course, into a term deployed in horse racing and golf, and it eventually was used to signify people who needed extra help from society—not unlike equalizing of chances in a horse race with weight determined according to ability. After the shock of eugenics playing such a horrific role in World War II, people began to think society was obligated to equalize chances for all sorts of people who were treated (during the war) as disposable. As Devlieger put it, "In the concept of handicap, a contract is forged between the individual and the state, containing a promise of a 'new opportunity' . . . in the United States . . . the concept of 'handicap' . . . refers to life as a lottery, in which despite your best will to participate, misfortune can happen. Society must get involved in such a case and provide you with new chances to integrate again."[3] He is quick to point out, however, that an "ideology of equal chances" (handicap) was not extended to African populations. Still in the throes of colonization, Africa was perceived as a

---

2   Patrick Devlieger, "Why Disabled? The Cultural Understanding of Physical Disability in an African Society," in Disability and Culture, ed. Benedicte Ingstad and Susan Reynolds Whyte (Berkeley: University of California Press, 1995), 94–106.
3   Devlieger, "Why Disabled?," 391.

disease-ridden place where impairment was considered "natural" given the ecological conditions of the continent. Disabled soldiers, however, did not fit into that picture. The existence and meaning of their blindness, lost limbs, deafness, and so forth were explicitly tied to experiences serving European colonial forces. And we find numerous charities for the blind, crippled, "deaf and dumb" springing up throughout the continent at this time. The period from the 1960s to the 1980s ushered in surface-level change from charity to rights-based organizing, but structural analysis suggests dependency persists in the processes of transnational NGOs and other quasi-aid/quasi-business arrangements. Neoliberalism of and from the 1990s onward has only reinforced capitalism's use of disability as a commodity, making an "ideology of equal chances" even more remote. Poverty/disability/exclusion constitutes an overwhelming reality for so many living in Africa and other Global South settings; more of humanity may be living with some variant of this condition than any other. And since we are meaning-making cultural creatures (or, in Rosi Braidotti's parlance, "intelligent, self-organizing matter,"[4] how sense gets made in such circumstances can be instructive to us all. Consequently, Devlieger's argument, in which he weaves back and forth from "African Indigenous Knowledge" to a "Posthuman Present" is particularly relevant to our explorations here of disability and cultural meaning making.

In engaging Rosi Braidotti's philosophy, Devlieger highlights how she moves beyond postmodernism by not simply dwelling on fragmentary social life, constructed identities, and the "importance of one's 'own voice' as a response to the realization that modernity is about to end" but by examining the irrelevance of dualities such as life and death, self and other, material and immaterial.[5] Invisible-immaterial realities, porosity of selves and intersubjectivity, and a continuum of living earthly beings and ancestors are core African ontological and epistemological concepts. We are coming full circle when we bring Braidotti's "posthuman knowing subject" together with so-called African indigenous knowledge. Devlieger's brilliant move, therefore, must be followed up because Africa is all too often left out of theorizing that purports to be global in scope.[6] Braidotti asserts that "the posthuman knowing subject has to be understood as a relational embodied and embedded, affective

---

4   Rosi Braidotti, "A Theoretical Framework for the Critical Posthumanities," *Theory, Culture and Society* (2018): 1.
5   Devlieger, "Why Disabled?," 394.
6   James Ferguson, *Global Shadows: Africa in the Neoliberal World Order* (Durham, NC: Duke University Press, 2006).

and accountable entity and not only as a transcendental consciousness."[7] Relational, embodied, embedded, affective, accountable: these are qualities or descriptors core to African ontologies. We will turn to accountability, first, to explore how Braidotti's "posthuman knowing subject" in Africa makes meaning around and about disability.

Disability and Misfortune

Long before a label of "disability" entered an African consciousness, concerns with misfortune, its cause, and accountability led to powerful meaning-making practices among many families and lineage groups. British anthropologist E. E. Evans-Pritchard wrote a compelling account of Azande cultural logic and explanations of unfortunate events—which no doubt captured sentiments held in many societies across the continent.[8] Witchcraft and magic, of course, were central in this important work. And while we might be tempted to think that nearly a century later Evans-Pritchard's observations would no longer be relevant, eminent health researcher Tim Allen has stated, "Surprisingly, this is by no means entirely so."[9] Allen himself examined HIV/AIDS in a specific Azande community (in the early twenty-first century) and found that "many customs and practices Evans-Pritchard analysed remain extant, although there have obviously been adaptations."[10] More to the point, as one of Allen's interviewees explained, "If someone has a disease like malaria or sleeping sickness and begins to change shape (become slim), people will suspect it to be AIDS."[11] And in fact, "An HIV positive person has characteristics that are similar to those of a witch or a sorcerer, in that he or she looks like everyone else, but is secretly killing them."[12]

Evans-Pritchard observed that *accountability* mattered deeply among Azande people from whom he learned about witchcraft, so while natural causes were clearly understood, a deeper issue was assumed to be at play, and

---

7   Braidotti, "A Theoretical Framework," 1.
8   E. E. Evans-Pritchard, *Witchcraft, Oracles and Magic Among the Azande* (Oxford: Oxford University Press, 1937).
9   Tim Allen, "Witchcraft, Sexuality and HIV/AIDS Among the Azande of Sudan," *Journal of Eastern African Studies* 1, no. 3 (2007): 364.
10 Allen, "Witchcraft," 364.
11 Allen, "Witchcraft," 366.
12 Allen, "Witchcraft," 388.

human agency was understood to be behind the misfortune. More recent analyses of witchcraft emphasize how stresses of economic scarcity lead to suspicion, resentment, and charges of being cursed so that those considered a burden are more easily discarded.[13] In part this is rooted in relational, embodied, embedded, affective, accountable ontologies (deeply African and now heralded as central to the "posthuman knowing subject") in that misfortune is understood to occur not by accident but because of the agency and power of some "intelligent self-organizing matter" (to use Braidotti's posthumanist terminology).[14] Such cultural logic was sometimes made to sound infantile or akin to magical thinking. Of course, people with cancer in certain Global North contexts who trace their illness to years of living under high-voltage power lines are also perceived by some to be imagining a causality and a human agency that does not exist. A quest for accountability for an aggrieved person is not difficult to understand if the cultural context is more familiar. The trick here is to tease out power dynamics and meaning making in ways that are grounded in cultural processes.

In Sierra Leone, in part because of witchcraft, people with amputation from the war (1991–2001) made a clear distinction between their condition of lost limbs and the circumstances of other physically disabled citizens—actually "reject[ing] any notion of themselves as disabled."[15] A worker from the French-based organization Handicap International explained to researcher Maria Berghs that "the amputees say, we are not disabled; we are different from the polio victims. And the polio victims say, the amputees are not like us because we have been suffering from birth, and we have to combat witchcraft."[16] Their misfortunes were assigned different meanings and hence they placed themselves into distinct cultural categories. In addition, people with disabilities were suspected of participation in the war in ways that angered persons with amputations: "Stories and rumors apparently circulate among local people about how the disabled were often spies.

---

13 *Witches in Exile*, directed by Allison Berg (Accra, Ghana: Newsreel, 2005); Silvia Federici, "Witch-Hunting, Globalization, and Feminist Solidarity in Africa Today," *Journal of International Women's Studies* 10, no. 1 (2008): 21–35.

14 Braidotti, "A Theoretical Framework."

15 Maria Berghs, "Disability as Embodied Memory? Questions of Identity for the Amputees of Sierra Leone," *Wagadu: A Journal of Transnational Women's and Gender Studies* 4 (2007): 86.

16 Berghs, "Disability as Embodied Memory?" 87.

Disabled people, such as people with polio, would enter into villages and then report back to the rebels allowing them to plan attacks."[17] Amputation was a war tactic used by all sides to create terror and to weaken the fighting force of enemies. Most people who had limbs amputated did not survive, but those who did ended up largely in refugee camps and eventually formed a self-help group called the War-Affected Amputee Association. There was the expectation that being identified as a "victim" (rather than embracing a "disability" identity) might enable those with amputations to access reparations after the war. Therefore, since "disability is understood as caused by witchcraft and voodoo,"[18] and people with disabilities were rumored to aid and abet perpetrators during the war, the negatives of assuming a disability identity outweighed the positives. "People with amputations initially resisted the 'disability' identity on moral grounds," Berghs explained, "in favour of identification as 'victims,' . . . until 'persons with disabilities' became linked to greater NGO resources."[19] Clearly, meanings of disability shift as material and political circumstances change. Berghs concluded, in part, that "ascribing a disability identity to amputee and war-wounded people was a means of making them invisible, avoiding giving them reparations and declaring something about their [lack of] moral worth in society."[20]

The present theme of misfortune is also followed often by disruptions in family dynamics, and this is illustrated by a case study of a Ghanaian woman called Ruth who "lived with severe uncontrolled diabetes and chronic physical impairments: loss of appetite, severe weight loss, joint pains and body sores."[21] Ruth had been a food hawker in the town of Nkoranza (in the Brong Ahafo Region) before she got sick, and she had been a robust, buxom woman. When the uncontrolled diabetes caused dramatic weight loss, people in her community speculated that she had contracted AIDS and they stopped purchasing her food. Ruth's twenty-nine-year-old daughter, Adjoa, attempted to take over her business, but this wasn't successful "because

---

17 Berghs, "Disability as Embodied Memory?," 87.
18 Berghs, "Disability as Embodied Memory?," 87.
19 Maria Berghs, "Local and Global Phantoms: Reparations National Memory and Sacrifice in Sierra Leone," in *Rethinking Disability*, ed. Patrick Devlieger et al. (Antwerp-Apeldoorn: Garant, 2016), 276.
20 Berghs, "Local and Global Phantoms," 287.
21 Ama de-Graft Aikins, "Reframing Applied Disease Stigma Research: A Multilevel Analysis of Diabetes Stigma in Ghana," *Journal of Community & Applied Social Psychology* 16 (2006): 431.

people were unwilling to buy food from an individual living in close proximity with an alleged AIDS sufferer."[22] Interviewers asked Ruth what she thought caused her diabetes, and she explained that "a certain woman came here to work. She worked with my brother. . . . One day, she and my brother had a quarrel. . . . In the course of the quarrel, she told my brother 'You have bought disease for your sister.'"[23] As the expense and stress of trying to support Ruth increased, family relationships became "fraught with emotionally charged misunderstandings" and eventually Ruth became "convinced that her family had abandoned her because they perceived her as either an AIDS sufferer or a witch."[24]

In separate interviews it was clear that her daughter, Adjoa, did not believe Ruth was a witch; however, she did experience conflicting emotions about her mother:

> Even as Adjoa recognized the extent of her mother's impairments, she glossed over her disabilities. Thus she criticized Ruth's inability to carry out her duties as a grandmother (e.g. taking on baby-sitting duties) and her culturally inappropriate response to her condition (emotional disintegration rather than stoicism at misfortune).[25]

Researcher Ama de-Graft Aiken indicated that Ruth felt despair, cried frequently during the interviews, prayed that she would die and be relieved of her suffering, and contemplated suicide (though her Christian faith contradicted that impulse).[26] So, in terms of disability and meaning making, Ruth herself seemed to associate nothing but deeply negative ideas with her predicament. She believed that her diabetes meant her brother ensorcelled her; she believed that her illness caused others to see her as a witch. In addition, while Adjoa definitely did not think that Ruth's diabetes meant she was a witch, it did mean that she was plagued with inabilities. In fact, she was no longer able to even respond in culturally appropriate ways ("stoicism at misfortune"). Disability in Africa often means strained kinship relations, broken expectations with regard to standards of mutual support among kin, and not infrequently it means completely severed ties.

---

22   Aikins, "Reframing," 432.
23   Aikins, "Reframing," 431.
24   Aikins, "Reframing," 432.
25   Aikins, "Reframing," 432.
26   Aikins, "Reframing," 433.

In Alison Berg's film *Witches in Exile* one woman states, "A witch is someone who is not wanted."[27] Typically older women who no longer bear children and may not be sexually desirable are accused of witchcraft. In his article "Peripheral Everywhere" James Charlton uses the term "double outcast" to emphasize the predicament, globally, for people with disabilities.[28] As an older woman disabled by diabetes, Ruth likely saw herself as no longer useful and thus unwanted by her kin (hence a witch). In a cultural context emphasizing relational, embedded, embodied, affective, and accountable ontologies—coupled with an economic context of insecurity—the meanings of disability are typically dire.

Disability and Therapy Managing Groups

"Medical pluralism" exists everywhere—with people sequentially as well as simultaneously consulting popular practitioners, clinical professionals, friends, family, pharmacists, and so forth in their quests to cope with debilitating episodes and chronic illnesses. Anthropologist John Janzen's groundbreaking study of this phenomenon in Zaire (now known as the Democratic Republic of the Congo; DRC) helped us understand that while outsiders (or Global North observers of African societies) often bogged down in dichotomous thinking about a seemingly incompatible schism between "traditional" African medicine and "Western" (or "cosmopolitan/biomedical") approaches, "central African clients have long been cognizant . . . that medical systems are used in combination."[29] In addition, Janzen spotlighted "therapy managing groups" rather than singling out individual sufferers, and his work helped draw attention to the dynamism of processes he identified as a "quest for therapy." Why should this matter to us here? When it comes to things African, a tendency to exoticize, demonize, simplify, and negate persists.

As an example of how this has impacted our understanding of disability and cultural meaning making in Africa, let us consider Benedicte Ingstad's critique of the idea that Africans hide their children (and other family

---

27 Berg, *Witches in Exile*.

28 James I. Charlton, "Peripheral Everywhere," *Journal of Literary and Cultural Disability Studies* 4, no. 2 (2010): 195–200.

29 John M. Janzen, *The Quest for Therapy in Lower Zaire* (Berkeley: University of California Press, 1978), xviii.

members) who have disabilities. She suggested that this notion (or "myth of the hidden disabled") developed in large part because the United Nations Decade of Disabled Persons (1983–1992) necessitated garnering sympathy to raise money; hence Global South people with disabilities were presented as "living in a state of utter misery and neglect."[30] Ingstad emphasized that these portrayals failed to account for the poverty and lack of basic health care facing the majority of the population and instead zeroed in on (and blamed) individual caretakers who confined disabled family members when lacking resources and support for effective care. In 1984–85, in Botswana, she asked district rehabilitation officers to take her to homes where they believed disabled children or family members were being hidden, neglected, or abused.[31]

One case involved a young man born with an intellectual disability whom she first met in the mid-1980s. When he was about eight years old his family was encouraged to "send him to the mental hospital in Lobatse so that he could get cured and become 'normal.'"[32] He was institutionalized for several years, treated by psychiatrists and other medical personnel, and family members went to see him on a regular basis. They witnessed a downward spiral as he became "restless and violent to the extent that his front teeth had to be pulled out so he could not bite people."[33] Against great odds his parents spent several years lobbying to have him released so they could take control of his therapy. The family was finally successful after involving a local politician, but also:

> This happened to coincide with the time (late 1970s) when it was decided to decentralize the psychiatric services and return as many as possible of the mental patients to their home communities. The young man was released to the family on the condition that they would build a special hut for him and keep him locked up so that he would not be able to harm others. They were told that they would be made personally responsible if anything happened.[34]

---

30   Benedicte Ingstad, *Community-Based Rehabilitation in Botswana: The Myth of the Hidden Disabled* (Lewiston, NY: Edwin Mellen, 1997), 246.

31   Benedicte Ingstad, "Mpho ya Modimo—A Gift from God: Perspectives on 'Attitudes' toward Disabled Persons," in *Disability and Culture*, ed. Benedicte Ingstad and Susan Reynolds Whyte (Berkeley: University of California Press, 1995), 249.

32   Ingstad, "Mpho ya Modimo," 250.

33   Ingstad, "Mpho ya Modimo," 250.

34   Ingstad, 249.

"Hidden" in a mud hut with no windows, he screamed and howled. This distressed the family terribly, and even though he was large and strong his father could physically restrain him when necessary. So now and again they let him out of the hut to walk around. Unfortunately, he would occasionally act in ways that neighbors considered violent and frightening. So after his father died, his mother kept him in the hut for fear that "the authorities" would take him away. This, of course, is the predicament that led to a rumor that his family was hiding him away out of shame. When Ingstad visited, she and some rehabilitation officers encouraged the mother to let him out to be around other people and to teach him simple tasks. Eventually he became proficient at sweeping, chopping wood, looking after goats, stamping corn, and so forth. And in the 1990s he was no longer confined but rather living outside the village at what was called "the lands"—an agricultural area where cattle were kept and where crops of vegetables and cereals were grown. Eight cases of "hidden disabled" were examined by Ingstad and only two struck her as fitting such a judgment. More often she found what I would consider a therapy managing group who was struggling to cope with dynamic and complex circumstances. A dominant (negative, exoticizing) meaning (revolving around shame, stigma, and hiding) was popularized at that time, but Ingstad revealed that the young man's kin group was, in a sense, on a quest to get him therapy. Once again, we can see a relational, embedded, embodied, affective, and accountable ontology at play and cultural meaning making around disability as highly contested.

Among Hubeer agro-pastoralists in southern Somalia, Bernhard Helander conducted ethnographic research in the 1980s and heard the saying "a sick person governs one hundred" or "a sick person orders about one hundred people."[35] Helander described a woman who had been ill for several years with what her family believed to be *dabeyl* or polio, and he invoked this aphorism in part to illustrate and generalize the socially embedded nature of health-seeking processes. "Gradually, beginning within the household, other people are introduced to the problem," Helander explained. "Even with such a widening sphere of people and resources mobilized, there is a final point beyond which further health seeking is seen as pointless, or where costs in

---

35   Bernhard Helander, "Disability as Incurable Illness: Health, Process, and Personhood in Southern Somalia," in *Disability and Culture*, ed. Benedicte Ingstad and Susan Reynolds Whyte (Berkeley: University of California Press, 1995), 82.

money, time, and relations would be too high."[36] Meaning would be made along the way, of course, and Helander referenced numerous "illness-labels" that encoded how signs and symptoms were being interpreted. Degrees of mobility were telling, in a Hubeer world, about the severity of what might have initially seemed like an illness but evolved into what they then would call *naafo*, a term that Helander explained, "suggests a finality—nothing more can be done."[37]

A more recent example of a quest for therapy is found in northern Nigeria in 2005, when a fifteen-year-old boy experienced paralysis in his leg, and the family asked anthropologist Elishe Renne for advice.[38] There to investigate polio, she recommended they go to the university teaching hospital in the area, and she inquired about whether or not the boy had received an immunization. The father said that he had been immunized against polio. At the hospital they X-rayed his leg, said they could not find a specific cause for the paralysis, gave him an injection, and sent him home. The family watched their son's condition worsen, which then prompted them to travel out of town to consult with a *malam*, or Muslim teacher, who told them "it was a spirit that was causing the problem."[39] Several days later a boil formed on the boy's ankle, and the *malam* instructed the family to have it lanced at the teaching hospital. While this situation resolved relatively quickly, Renne explained that the situation caused confusion because of "the uncertain cause of this young boy's paralysis and the apparent inability of Western medicine to cure it."[40] Indeed, pursuing perceived meanings behind why one case of paralysis would resolve and another case would lead to serious physical impairment was a conundrum African families sometimes tried to rationalize through examinations of witchcraft and notions of accountability discussed in the earlier section.

Julie Livingston more explicitly deployed the idea of a quest for therapy in her study of disability and debility in Botswana.[41] Her account of its aptness is worth quoting at length.

---

36 Helander, "Disability as Incurable Illness," 88.
37 Helander, "Disability as Incurable Illness," 82.
38 Elishe Renne, *The Politics of Polio in Northern Nigeria* (Bloomington: Indiana University Press, 2010), 1–2.
39 Renne, *Politics of Polio*, 2.
40 Renne, *Politics of Polio*, 2.
41 Julie Livingston, *Debility and the Moral Imagination in Botswana* (Bloomington: Indiana University Press, 2005).

> Disability, or *bogole*, is a status that arises out of a "quest for therapy." It signals that this search, which may have taken many different paths, is petering out. The quest varies. Often it is an arduous one, taking patients and relatives from site to site, healer to healer, draining resources, and leaving controversy and a fractured family in its wake. . . . Those who are involved may spend their time yearning for the reputed skill of healers long gone and yet lack the means or will to pursue any palpable action. A time will come when even this metaphoric quest for healing sputters and dies and a new identity sets in. The *molwetsi* (patient) of the quest shuffles from the foreground of local drama quietly to the back and becomes *segole* (disabled person).[42]

Meanings of *segole* (disability) among Batswana were wide ranging and context dependent, of course. In naming a few such meanings, Livingston provided the following list of adjectives: "brave, idle, useless, determined, unfortunate, stupid, clever, sanguine, bitter, irresponsible"; caregivers, in turn, could be described as "generous, patient, selfish, uncaring, demanding, greedy sad, martyred."[43] The contradictions are instructive because they remind us to not look for monolithic, homogenous meanings and to remember that relationality always involves negotiating power.

Mining accidents have disabled many southern African men, and Livingston recounted stories of several of these men she came to know in the late 1990s in Botswana.[44] For example, a man in his mid-forties named Kago was struck on the head and subsequently experienced a massive cerebral hemorrhage. Conflict among family members erupted immediately—first over whether or not he should receive an operation, then over what or who caused the illness, and next over who would receive and administer the $1000 lump sum of money the mine company was doling out. Kago's situation also brought on "conflict over the value of rehabilitation" that Livingston indicated she witnessed countless times.[45] This stemmed in part from cultural expectations around women and caregiving. Tswana values emphasized how wives, sisters, mothers, daughters were expected to indulge, pamper, and comfort their debilitated kin while clinical rehabilitation professionals encouraged patients to practice activities that pushed them toward greater independence.[46] While Kago's wife wanted the rehabilitation

---

42 Livingston, *Debility*, 9.
43 Livingston, *Debility*, 9–10.
44 Livingston, *Debility*, 40–47.
45 Livingston, *Debility*, 43.
46 Livingston, *Debility*, 43.

regimen to work, Kago's mother believed his wife should cater to his needs. Livingston made sure readers understood that "Kago's mother, sisters, and wife all loved him and wanted the best care for him but did not agree on what that meant."[47] Another man, Rra Molefi, had worked in the mines for twenty-seven years, supporting his family but believed that his tuberculosis was caused by the work he did.[48] At the age of fifty-six his spine collapsed from the TB. He could no longer work but did not get a pension. Rra Molefi was in a wheelchair, but unlike Kago, who could barely communicate, his mind allowed him to engage in what Livingston identified as "agricultural, pastoral, and building tasks." Despite this, for his wife the meaning of his disability was dramatically expressed when she said, "Look at him—he is useless! You will find him always seated." This example speaks volumes about contested and multiple meanings.

Each family, each case, and each therapy managing group encountered variated and complex challenges and emotional journeys. No case was held up as typical, and in fact Livingston explained that "no debilitated person whom I met had a 'typical' story to tell."[49] However, certain themes crop up again and again as people try to make sense of their debilitation. Livingston pointed out that "modes of interpretation, care, conflict, and coping are all rooted in the time before the impairment or illness started" and "case studies allow us to see how local meanings of debility are negotiated through relationships. In Botswana, debilitated individuals and their family members and caregivers alike read the meanings of debility as the product of relationships."[50] Debility as well as disability, then, is always social and intersubjective; it amplifies and intensifies already relational, embodied, embedded, affective, and accountable African ontologies.

Disability and Belonging

In the summer of 2005, I was living in Accra, the capital of Ghana, and doing ethnographic research with a range of DPOs. I had spent several days and nights baking with a group who had built their accessible bakery from the ground up. Ghanaians (especially city dwellers) had been transitioning

---

47 Livingston, *Debility*, 44.
48 Livingston, *Debility*, 46.
49 Livingston, *Debility*, 27.
50 Livingston, *Debility*, 28.

away from reliance on their staple foods made from starchy tubers (cassava and yams) to purchasing bread in record numbers. The small group of "disables" (an affectionate and respectful term in Ghanaian English) employed at the bakery were trying to compete in a cutthroat market.

It was about six o'clock in the morning and I was bleary-eyed. I had just put my seven-year-old daughter to bed as she had been up all night with us baking buns and loaves. We were making deliveries to petrol stations, convenience stores, and small grocery shops when my companion—who I'll call Abla—pointed to the label on the bags that read, in part, "Made by People with Disabilities." Abla explained that the workers had a disagreement with their European volunteer because they wanted to change the wording to: "Buying this product helps support people with disabilities." Earlier in the year they had discovered consumers avoiding their products because they believed (and openly expressed to others in the stores) the idea that since it was made by disabled people, the bread was surely "dirty" and unsafe. "Dirty" did not simply mean soiled but also referenced the idea that disability could be transferred to a person who bought, touched, and ate the product. The European volunteer working with this bakery sponsored by Hope for Life believed they should stick with the original label. I think he wanted them to use the controversy to try to raise awareness. Abla and the other employees, however, were distressed by how the stigma was hampering sales. Economic- and livelihood-related dimensions of this dilemma were easy to grasp and not even that contentious to discuss. But there were deeper semantic issues at play, and teasing them out may help set the stage for our ensuing discussion of belonging.

I opened this chapter with an assertion about how abiding African understandings of disability combine with rights-based meanings to create more globalized orientations toward neuro and somatic human diversity. I also made the observation that we still find disability connoting anomalousness, peripherality, and dependency. Being employed, receiving a paycheck, going to work on a regular basis, and having the ability to appear and feel like a contributing member of society were circumstances dreamed of by many people with disabilities I interviewed in Ghana. A pragmatic aspect of this obviously lies in the chipping away of dependency that an income (small as it may have been) enacted. But "fitting in" and being part of the flow of life (rather than on the periphery) were values that directly paralleled the relational, embodied, embedded, affective, and accountable ontologies I have suggested are deeply African. The bakers from Hope for Life were deeply hurt by suggestions that their embodied relationality (working with the dough, touching the loaves as they bagged them and prepared the bread for the public to buy) was somehow dirty, contagious, or toxic. This is not an uncommon stereotype in Ghana,[51] so it is understandable that those with a rights-based and activist orientation would want to challenge negative (and "backward") responses to "Made by People with Disability." It was a paradoxical predicament. The notion that it "helps support" disables highlights dependency; the negative ideas about contagion, however, played into relentless reminders of anomalousness and being "other."

Somali refugee women living in London at the turn of the twenty-first century also experienced othering by the general citizenry as well as medical staff.[52] Many were circumcised prior to fleeing war-torn Somalia, and since circumcision was defined differently in London than in Somalia, they suddenly acquired a "defect" or a "disability" whereas their bodies were previously "normal." "With reference to . . . discussion of disability," Aud Talle explained, "female circumcision is not a disability in the ordinary sense, as the condition of impairment is neither a consequence of 'misfortune' nor a congenital difference nor a condition caused by disease."[53] Instead, "it has been intentionally inflicted by close family members in order to create a culturally 'beautiful' and moral woman."[54] However, the gynecological problems that frequently brought Somali women to London hospitals contributed to culturally and politically redefining their circumstances as disabling. "Stories about unhappy encounters with 'rude' and 'ignorant' doctors" were "told and retold among the exiled women in London."[55] Both the initial "barbaric" genital cutting and then the cruel, demeaning treatment

---

51 Jacqueline Slikker, "Attitudes towards Persons with Disability in Ghana," *VSO, Sharing Skills, Changing Lives, Ghana Volunteer May* (2009); and Kathryn Linn Geurts and Sefakor G. M. A. Komabu-Pomeyie, "From 'Sensing Disability' to Seselelame: Non-dualistic Activist Orientations in Twenty-First-Century Accra," in *Disability in the Global South* (Cham, Switzerland: Springer, 2016), 85–98.

52 Aud Talle, "From 'Complete' to 'Impaired' Body: Female Circumcision in Somalia and London," in *Disability in Local and Global Worlds*, ed. Benedicte Ingstad and Susan Reynolds Whyte (Berkeley: University of California Press, 2007), 56–77.

53 Talle, "From 'Complete' to 'Impaired,'" 57.

54 Talle, "From 'Complete' to 'Impaired,'" 57.

55 Talle, "From 'Complete' to 'Impaired,'" 64.

by medical professionals began to be discussed as a human rights issue. The attention and othering, however, was not really welcome. As one woman expressed, "We do not like all the fuss about our circumcision."[56] They certainly wanted adequate medical care but without being subjected to stigma and shame.

A Somali gynecologist named Khadiya, whom Aud Talle knew prior to the East African woman's migration to London, had a position as an assistant and interpreter in a health clinic. In talking to Talle about the situation for patients, she "recounted how tense their bodies were when she and the British nurse examined them. This was never the case when they came to her clinic in Mogadishu."[57] The "bodily disquietude" Khadiya observed was, in her opinion, a result of "the whole situation" or a confluence of physical symptoms, social stigma, and hostility, and "their acute and often painful awakening to being [culturally] 'different.'"[58] Eventually an African Well Women's clinic was opened in northeast London, and a significant number of the women seeking treatment wanted what is called a "reversal."[59] A very tight infibulation often caused urinary and menstrual problems as well as difficulty and pain when having sexual intercourse. A "reversal" involved surgical opening of the scar. While this procedure was also performed in Somalia, usually for a married and pregnant woman, in London women were requesting reversals in much greater numbers—even young, unmarried women. Talle indicated that this was "a new situation."[60] There was a practical reason for this, according to Talle, in that the operation was "quick, painless, easy to obtain, and free of charge."[61] Beyond functionality, though, we have the semantic issues that are well illustrated by the following story Talle recounts under the subhead, "The 'Impaired' Body."

> Sagal, an attractive mother of four, attended an information course for immigrants. During one of the lectures, she heard two African men whispering behind her back: "You see this woman there [referring to Sagal]: she is very beautiful, but she is from Somalia, and Somali women do not have vaginas." Being a brave woman and secure in the knowledge that she had after all given birth to four children, Sagal turned to them and laughed at their comment. Whereupon

---

56 Talle, "From 'Complete' to 'Impaired,'" 64.
57 Talle, "From 'Complete' to 'Impaired,'" 64.
58 Talle, "From 'Complete' to 'Impaired,'" 68.
59 Talle, "From 'Complete' to 'Impaired,'" 66.
60 Talle, "From 'Complete' to 'Impaired,'" 66.
61 Talle, "From 'Complete' to 'Impaired,'" 66.

they . . . felt ashamed and apologized for their indiscrete remark. Sagal told the anecdote in order to show how life may present itself for exiled Somali women. They have to "fight" all the time, she said, not only for existence and survival, but also against prejudices, misunderstandings, and far-fetched fantasies and delusions about their bodies.[62]

The pain of being different and othered also motivated women to seek a reversal. "The growing popularity of reversals among young Somali women in London may be interpreted as a way of 'normalizing' the body by bringing it back to its 'natural' condition and thus up to standards of the encompassing community."[63] Circumcised female bodies in London were anomalous, so in an effort to fit in better and belong to their new and more "cosmopolitan" environment, many Somali women opted for this surgery.

Belonging is a theme that critical disability studies scholar Denise Nepveux dealt with directly in her study focused on women with disabilities in Ghana.[64] Nepveux was initially interested largely in issues of women's autonomy—more specifically, "how women's involvement in disabled people's organizations shaped the way that women saw themselves in relation to others" and the question of "how urban Ghanaian women with disabilities defined, valuated, and pursued personal autonomy." She was also interested in "how they might also redefine or subvert it in favor of other values."[65] As the two-year field-based study evolved, however, a question of *belonging* seemed to emerge more palpably than any deep longings for "autonomy." Women with disabilities clearly wanted skills, ways of attending to their livelihoods, and the ability to move about, but these goals took them toward belonging (in their imaginations) more than toward something we consider autonomy.

For example, a woman who Nepveux called "Elizabeth" had a strong desire to sew when she was in her teens and worked tirelessly to try to launch such a business. Her grandparents pushed her to take school more seriously, but Elizabeth was much more inclined toward entrepreneurial ventures, and she truly wanted to sew. Throughout her late teens and all through her twenties she was unable to garner enough support to invest in a machine and

---

62   Talle, "From 'Complete' to 'Impaired,'" 72.
63   Talle, "From 'Complete' to 'Impaired,'" 72.
64   Denise M. Nepveux, "'In the Same Soup': Marginality, Vulnerability, and Belonging in the Life Stories of Disabled Women in Accra, Ghana" (PhD diss., University of Illinois at Chicago, 2008).
65   Nepveux, "In the Same Soup," 66–67.

the apprentice training, so Elizabeth did not succeed in realizing that dream. She did, however, start a family, and Nepveux described her as "an unusually gifted and diligent businesswoman."[66] But in her late thirties, the glaucoma that had been troubling her for years worsened, and Elizabeth lost her vision. Neither her own nor her husband's families were forthcoming with help or support, and the relations in many ways became quite hostile. On the other hand, Elizabeth devoted herself to her children, and they in turn were loyal to their parents. So despite difficult economic circumstances they experienced a bit of security within the nuclear family unit.

In addition, Elizabeth found a sense of belonging in the Ghana Association of the Blind (GAB). She "especially found solace and solidarity in her friendships with women members," Nepveux explained. "She appreciated the culture of warmth and acceptance she felt in the group, among men and women alike. She commented that at GAB, bumping into one another was commonplace, and it led to introductions and embraces rather than the insults and reproach that one experienced on the street."[67] Hearing stories and experiences of other blind people, strategizing about how to respond to negativity from family and strangers alike, and sharing information about the rights all people with disabilities should have were ways that GAB meetings created camaraderie and community. For Elizabeth, GAB was "a place of belonging, within a larger context hostile to blind people. Elizabeth found comfort and kindness in the disability community. Her friends were unmarried blind women, and they exchanged support, they visited her, and she advised them and taught them skills."[68]

Nepveux compiled the life stories of thirteen different women with disabilities in Ghana—nine had a physical disability, one was deaf, and three women were blind. Unlike Elizabeth, the two other blind women attended a "School for the Blind." Nepveux explained that for one of the women, Lydia, "This experience represented a turning point in [her] life. Here she was delighted to meet other blind adults and children. She gained confidence in her ability to manage her life."[69] Abigail, too, who went blind at a young age, had a transformative experience at the school. She told Nepveux during an interview, "I saw that there are many [children] who are also blind like myself. So that has even comfort me a lot." And Nepveux reflected that

---

66   Nepveux, "In the Same Soup," 479.
67   Nepveux, "In the Same Soup," 490.
68   Nepveux, "In the Same Soup," 494.
69   Nepveux, "In the Same Soup," 387.

women related that they feel a sense of community with others with disabilities: "They remembered this experience of commonality and mutual support as transformative: it enabled them to begin re-envisioning themselves as productive and valuable girls and women, engaged in a process of becoming."[70] While Lydia was at the school, she learned about the Ghana Association of the Blind. "She eagerly joined and became active when she had re-established herself in Accra. She said that she felt encouraged to be in the presence of other blind people, and to chat and share problems. 'We are in the same soup,' she said, 'so we must agitate together!'"[71]

The sense of belonging captured by the phrase "We are in the same soup" is perfectly illustrative of our central concern—disability and cultural meaning making. The metaphor points to a reality that is inherently relational, embodied, embedded, affective, and accountable. Most people have emotional connections to their natal food, and soup is a mainstay in Ghana. Richly blended and embodied, the onions, spices, crabs, and spinach (for example) must relate in an appetizing way, or the cook will be held accountable for causing distress. Bad cooking can cause terrible tensions in a household. A soup that's well blended and coheres can bring people together. At the end of her study, Nepveux reflected that

> some women commented that beginning to attend disability group meetings was their first experience of feeling comfortable and welcome in a public space. Here they learned that many shared their "situation"—broadly construed—and that the impairment itself, or the identity of "deaf," "blind" or "disabled," need not be major hindrances to a flourishing life. Disability groups served as crucial resources for solidarity, relief, and positive identity to each of the women who participated in the study. As such, their affiliation with disability groups became a strong part of women's identities.[72]

In eastern Uganda, in the border town of Busia, a community of men with disabilities (largely from polio) experienced a fellowship similar to how some of the Ghanaian women described their "in the same soup" sense of belonging. Disabled men were attracted to this bustling commercial center in the early 1990s because as long as you made connections with customs authorities, you could do business: "More and more men on tricycles began crossing the border to purchase commodities on the Kenyan side, bringing them back

---

70 Nepveux, "In the Same Soup," 318.
71 Nepveux, "In the Same Soup," 387.
72 Nepveux, "In the Same Soup," 515.

for sale at a profit in Uganda."[73] In fact, friends and relatives would say to people in rural areas: "Your fellow disabled are making money at the border. You better join them instead of sitting redundant in the countryside."[74] But by 1992–93 revenue authorities began demanding tax payments from the traders, and this led to the establishment (in 1994) of the Busia Disabled Association (BDA), which advocated on behalf of the tricyclist businessmen. While Whyte and Muyinda's main goal in this piece was to show that the "realization of disability policy depends on linkages between national policy, local situations, and the efforts and resources of social actors,"[75] they also demonstrate a fellowship and sense of common identity that builds among the men involved in BDA and working the transport trade in this town. This contrasts with the social isolation they often experienced prior to their relocation to Busia: "People who came to town were mostly from rural areas where they had not had other disabled people with whom to identify."[76] In a somewhat spontaneous way, however, what emerged were "communities of people who identified with one another on the basis of having a disability."[77] Elizabeth and Lydia (in Nepveux's study) described similar sentiments about coming to know other people who were "in the same soup." The way that people with disability are continually marked as anomalous, peripheral, and dependent can set up not only disenfranchising power dynamics in social relations but also psychological stress. All this together—membership in an advocacy association, collegial relationships with other disabled tricyclist businessmen, ability to attract and marry a woman, and opportunity to have children—created "belonging." Whyte and Muyinda reflected that "again and again, as we talked with the tricyclists and visited their homes, we heard accounts of the ordinary desire for social being."[78] Social being is another way of referencing the relational, embedded, embodied, affective, and accountable values so important in African ontologies.

In Kinshasa, DR Congo, a group of people with disabilities also found a sense of belonging through creating spaces where they could produce

---

73   Susan Reynolds Whyte and Herbert Muyinda, "Wheels and New Legs: Mobilization in Uganda," in *Disability in Local and Global Worlds*, ed. Benedicte Ingstad and Susan Reynolds Whyte (Berkeley: University of California Press, 2007), 290.
74   Whyte and Muyinda, "Wheels and New Legs," 290.
75   Whyte and Muyinda, "Wheels and New Legs," 287–288.
76   Whyte and Muyinda, "Wheels and New Legs," 302.
77   Whyte and Muyinda, "Wheels and New Legs," 302.
78   Whyte and Muyinda, "Wheels and New Legs," 302.

theater that would challenge negative views of disability. "Society thinks of us as being unproductive," a participant explained to anthropologist Jori De Coster,[79] and they wanted to demonstrate their creativity, engagement, and contributions to those around them. While critiquing neoliberal emphasis on productivity, De Coster introduced two different theater groups in Kinshasa that organized largely to reclaim space, create a sense of belonging, and counter the way Congolese television represented people with disabilities. "We use theatre to sensitize society about what it means to be a person with a disability," one person explained.[80] *Mabin'a Maboko* ("Dancing Hands") was made up of "a majority of actors with an auditory impairment and four actors who have their full auditory ability."[81] In a group discussion about the purpose and goals of the theater troupe "Dancing Hands," one person expressed to De Coster that deaf people in Kinshasa were "completely closed off from communication. Often the people who know our centre [theater] come here when they feel sick and can't explain what is wrong with their family. . . . We have difficulty obtaining jobs and often do very 'low' work [such as sewer cleaning]."[82]

They considered deafness in this context to be "one of the most severe impairments one could have,"[83] so creating a sense of community and belonging was only one part of their mission. Addressing issues such as traffic safety or providing factual information about HIV/AIDS were also major goals. Doudou, the artistic director, and Freddy, a social scientist, were both founders of Dancing Hands; they were also members of Journalists for Human Rights.[84] JHR is a Canadian-based international NGO devoted to training journalists all over the globe to report on social justice issues in their own communities. They were able to facilitate connections with artists with disabilities in a variety of countries through Dancing Hands' participation in an international multiyear festival.[85] While only a few participants were able to travel to the festivals, the international attention, visitors from abroad (to Kinshasa), having films of their plays screened in other countries, and so

---

79 Jori De Coster, "A Dialogue with Society: Disability, Theatre and Being Human in Kinshasa, DR Congo," in *Rethinking Disability*, ed. Patrick Devlieger et al. (Antwerp-Apeldoorn: Garant, 2016), 184.
80 De Coster, "A Dialogue," 190.
81 De Coster, "A Dialogue," 191.
82 De Coster, "A Dialogue," 191–192.
83 De Coster, "A Dialogue," 191.
84 De Coster, "A Dialogue," 192.
85 De Coster, "A Dialogue," 193.

forth, clearly helped to create an understanding of the importance of their work. De Coster concluded that in Kinshasa "Artists with a disability use theatre to engage with society on a number of different levels."[86] It gave them a profession (even if they received a miniscule salary), it helped "call attention to their struggle with society's disabling conditions," and it countered "negative perceptions and stereotypes associated with a body with an impairment."[87] Finally, to return to the theme of belonging and a sense of being in the same soup, De Coster indicated that making theater was "about being part of and being valued by society," and it offered an "opportunity to create a (feeling of) community across borders and even frontiers."[88]

Conclusion

This chapter has examined three themes that pervade disability and cultural meaning-making activities and case studies from Africa. They include notions of misfortune and how these create disruptions in kin groups; a coalescing of therapy-managing groups focused on sickness that evolves into disability; and people with disabilities, throughout Africa and in the diaspora, seeking out spaces and communities (and even remaking their bodies) so they can feel a sense of belonging. Brief examples from Uganda, Nigeria, Botswana, Sierra Leone, and other countries brought to life certain real people and their actual predicaments, but these only scratched the surface. They point toward an array of deeper, more extensive accounts of the often-dire circumstances faced by people with disabilities who are continually marked as anomalous, peripheral, and dependent. Power and history come to bear on all of these situations. But this dominant cultural meaning (of anomalous, peripheral, dependent) gets disrupted when men on hand-cranked tricycles form an organization to advocate for their business interests, when blind women join an association devoted to the ins and outs of life without sight, or when deaf people make theatrical shows displaying their intelligence and creativity. As relational, embodied, embedded, affective, and accountable beings, the Africans with disability we have met in this chapter are at the forefront of cultural meaning making in these dynamic and precarious posthuman times.

---

86   De Coster, "A Dialogue," 194.
87   De Coster, "A Dialogue," 194–195.
88   De Coster, "A Dialogue," 195.

Part Three

Representation and Cultural Expressions

Chapter Seven

Disfiguration, Trauma, and Disability

Reclaiming the Body and the Case against Prosthetics

Ernest Cole

Introduction

The disfigured body tells a story. It is a horrific story of mutilation and amputation that creates a sense of dependency and dysfunction. It also tells a story of adjustment and overcoming of obstacles that articulates a sense of agency. The power of the disfigured body lies not in either story that it tells but in its complex ability to tell both stories at the same time. The uniqueness of the disfigured body lies not in its limitations but rather in what it potentially can achieve in spite of them.

Sorious Samura's documentary, *Cry Freetown*,[1] provided the original impetus for this chapter and was eventually the catalyst for my work on trauma and disability studies. As an amateur photojournalist, Samura documented the brutal carnage that characterized the January 6, 1999, invasion of Freetown by the RUF rebels and the resulting battle with Nigerian peacekeepers for control of the city. While seeking refuge in the Gambia,

---

1 *Cry Freetown*, directed by Ron McCullagh (Atlanta: CNN, 2000).

I watched the CNN broadcast of *Cry Freetown,* hosted by veteran CNN anchor Jim Clancy through GRTS (Gambia Radio and Television Services).

I must also state that this chapter is a continuation of my earlier work[2]. While I draw from my monograph to make critical claims on the ambivalence of the disfigured body, I also incorporate new findings from my ongoing research on body studies and semiosis, prosthetics and clinical therapy, and trauma and resilience. In addition, I explored my findings on the connections between body and body politic as a way of understanding violence and trauma within the political and social constructs of postwar Sierra Leone. This chapter, then, is a component of the larger significance of my work: to investigate the choice of the body as medium of punishment, put forward as a set of critical formations regarding that choice, and to theorize about the meanings of the mutilated body during and after the civil war. This chapter investigates the connections between injury and identity and how injury can be used to deconstruct hegemony and domination through the creation of a culture of disability that seeks to transform cultural perceptions of disability rather than disabled people.

In watching *Cry Freetown* in 2001, two major incidents in the documentary caught my attention, and since then have been the catalyst for my work on trauma and bodily disfiguration. The first is the opening scene in which a Nigerian peacekeeper summarily executed a teenage boy by shooting him in the back for allegedly being a rebel. The officer's claim was that there were marks on the boy's body that could not be convincingly explained but that clearly indicated to the officer that they were sustained in the bush, thus confirming the boy's identity as member of the Revolutionary United Front (RUF).

My interest in the body as witness or evidence of crime was ignited. I was struck by how the body could literally be read as text and marker of identity—or perhaps mis-identity. I was stunned by the fact that the teenage boy could die because his own body seemingly gave evidence against his claims of innocence. It was both alarming and fascinating to me. The image of the teenage boy as he stumbles to his death from the barrage of bullets discharged from the peacekeeper's submachine gun has never left my mind.

The second incident was the image of a young man sitting at the back of a truck whose hands seemed to have been partially amputated by the rebels.

---

2   Ernest Cole, *Theorizing the Disfigured Body: Mutilation, Amputation, and Disability Culture in Post-Conflict Sierra Leone* (Trenton, NJ: Africa World, 2014).

The flow of blood was copious, and his hands were dangling in the air, still barely attached to his body by some skin and fragile tissues. I was captivated by the phenomenon of punitive amputation: the cruel strategy of intimidation and punishment used by the rebels to control and destroy the civilian population. As I watched in horror, I was struck by this method of punishment: it seemed to defy the conventional logic of warfare. In my estimate, war is senseless and destructive, and so using guns against one another is expected. However, when combatants put aside the bullet and take up the machete, it would seem to me that a different statement is being made. Thus, the choice of the body as canvas of execution of intent was instructive.

These two incidents forced me to reflect deeply on the significance of the body in the Sierra Leone civil war. With the record of punitive amputations of hands, arms, and legs, and the scarification and mutilation of body parts as lips, ears, and noses, I wondered why the body is held to account and made to pay. I asked: what it is about the body that makes it such a powerful medium for deployment of power and of effecting communication, this time, as military strategy of fear and control? What do markings on the bodies of victims signify, and why would the mutilated or disfigured body be preferred by the RUF combatants over the bullet-ridden body? Regardless of how hard I tried to understand the choice of the body as site for punishment and control of victims, I could not grapple with its inhumane connotations and the wanton disregard it signifies in terms of human rights violations.

From these reflections, I began to theorize on a twisted but cruelly effective logic that the RUF rebels may have been pursuing in using the disfigured body as mechanism of control. I figured out that in the culture of Sierra Leone, the body is a psychosocial entity in everyday life. In Krio, the lingua franca in Sierra Leone, Sierra Leoneans greet one another by saying "Ow de bodi?" Loosely translated, this means "How is the body?" However, in the cultural context of Sierra Leone, "Ow de bodi?" goes way beyond an inquiry into the physical state of the body of the individual. It is an inquiry into the physical, mental, emotional, and spiritual state of the person. It is about "shalom," the overall state of harmony of being and the working together of body, mind, and spirit. It is about man in relation to himself, others, and his environment.

Therefore, in the context of the Sierra Leonean culture, when the body is mutilated or amputated, it is an individual destruction of mind and body, a total emasculation of self, and a rupture of kinship or community ties with the perpetrator. At the same time, punitive amputation is a destruction of the body politic. In amputating the body, the physical, spiritual, and psychological bodies of victims and the "body" of society are destroyed. Thus, it is in the context of the psychological, spiritual, and physical destruction of "bodies" that the logic of punitive amputation is to be understood. In the choice of the maimed body over the dead body, the RUF was articulating the logic of memory and permanence: since amputation is permanent, the markings on bodies and their signification would be preserved as long as the victim lives and even after the cessation of hostilities.

Another audio-visual document of crucial significance to me in developing interest in semiotics, trauma, and body studies was the Hollywood blockbuster *Blood Diamond*.[3] I was particularly struck by the cruelty of the opening scene and the significance of the body as witness to memory and trauma.

In this scene, the RUF colonel is addressing one of the innocent civilians captured in a village raid shortly before the amputation of his hands: "You are the messenger. Spread the/ word. Guv'ment say da future is in/your hands? We say RUF is da/ future. Revolution is at hand." After this monologue, the machete would then be swung and brought down with brute force on the limb of the villager after choosing either "long or short sleeves": that is, amputation below or above the elbow. After the amputation, the victim would be instructed to go to the president of the country and ask for new hands. In some instances, a message written on a piece of paper is hung around their neck for them to take to the president.

The full import of the colonel's words, "revolution is at hand," is realized in the context of the 1996 general elections. Its significance is predicated on the logic that if hands are instruments of change, as may be expressed through the ballot box, then their absence is an impediment or hindrance to that process of change. Thus, the future of that society is to be secured not by change through a democratic vote but by total dependence, physically and psychologically, on the RUF after the amputation of limbs. In this twisted logic, "RUF is da future."

These two artistic products were crucial in framing the research questions for this chapter. They provided the context to engage violence and bodily disfiguration but also provided the critical tools to rethink punitive amputation and the culture of disability in postwar Sierra Leone. As I reflected on the significance of the episodes in the documentary and movie, I recognize

---

3   *Blood Diamond*, directed by Edward Zwick (2006; Burbank, CA: Warner Home Video, 2007).

the complexity of bodily disfiguration and the ideological and theoretical constructs that will help us understand the significance of such wanton cruelty and the place of the body in the matrix of violence and human carnage. As my interest in the disfigured body grew, I was again confronted with a set of questions: what does it mean to be wounded, scarred, branded, or have a limb amputated? What message is inscribed on the body when it is subjected to these atrocities? What story does the branded, mutilated, or amputated body tell, and what is the relation between the individual, their bodies and the stories their bodies now tell? How does the victim perceive and relate to their body after it has been amputated or deformed? How does society view the mutilated or deformed body? What is the relation between body and language? Are the scars texts of memory or of amnesia? Are there areas of intersection between the body, name, and place?

These questions point to the complexity of amputation and the complicated ways in which it could be understood. In recent times, the American wars in Iraq and Afghanistan, for instance, have further complicated notions of amputation as war veterans return home without limbs to face a lifetime of prosthetic therapy. However, in my work with persons with amputations, it is clear that amputation and its symbolic representation, and at times castration, have undergone a reformulation that posits a new aesthetic of the person with amputation and the psychology behind the loss of the limb. In this chapter, I argue that in the context of the Sierra Leone civil war, the residual limb is one of ambivalence; that is, in reclaiming the use of the body, the amputation victim is asserting agency. In a sense, by reclaiming bodily function with a disfigured body, the person with an amputation is articulating a counternarrative to the master discourse that characterizes amputation as physical and psychological castration. In confronting the physical and psychological barriers associated with amputation, the survivor rejects the discourse of dependency, redefines his identity, reclaims his body, and ultimately achieves healing. It is at this point that they can forgive the victimizer and allow the process of reconciliation to begin. I argue, therefore, that reconciliation should start with the survivors and their empowerment through a process of reclaiming the disfigured body and changing the culture of disability in which person with amputations find themselves. Human agency and not prosthetics, as I argue later in this paper, is the way to healing and forgiveness.

I divide this chapter into four sections. First are the research questions where I tease out the basis of my investigation by raising a set of critical questions in order to develop a hermeneutic of disfiguration that will shed light on punitive amputation and its signification. Second, I focus on instances of bodily scarification or mutilation and amputation. I draw from eyewitness accounts published in *Human Rights Watch*, the 2004 Truth and Reconciliation Committee (TRC) Report in Sierra Leone, and a work of nonfiction by a journalist and witness to the carnage.

Third, I use these incidents to theorize the disfigured body and to articulate my argument of ambivalence: that this is a story of limitations and possibilities that are juxtaposed uniquely in the disfigured body and that to privilege one over the other is to miss the subtleties associated with the complexities of its nature and function. I bring in the social and medical models of disability as theoretical constructs to make the claim that bodily agency after disfiguration is not achieved wholly by prosthetics. One must also understand the psychosocial needs of the victims of amputation and effect a change in the culture of disability in which they live. This will allow persons with amputations the possibility of reclaiming their bodies and regain locomotion, function, and dignity. My argument rejects the medical model of disability and advocates for a reformulation of disability within social and cultural contexts.

I conclude that the nature of the amputation impacts the strategies for healing and possibilities for reconciliation. I argue that the psychosocial needs of those whose limbs were lost through punitive amputation are vastly different from those who experienced medical amputation. To conflate the two is not only to miss the power of the disfigured body to transcend its limitations and challenges but also to predicate healing entirely on mobility or locomotion, which prosthetics suggest. I argue from this conception that since the loss of limbs occurs in different ways, it would be uncritical to categorize or conflate all those with amputations as one homogeneous entity. In fact, prosthetics are in reality a small part of the process of healing. If the psychological realities of punitive amputation are not addressed before a person with amputation is fitted with prosthetics, the prosthetics achieve the opposite effect—they become a reminder of the loss of limb and are counterproductive to the healing process. I conclude that practitioners of trauma and body studies should engage in creating a counterdiscourse of amputation that will deconstruct notions of disability as handicap, and work toward reformulating negative social and cultural perceptions in order for survivors to reclaim agency and human dignity.

Disfiguring the Body: Mutilations and Amputations

In order to understand the extent of the carnage, it is important to draw from accounts of witnesses as documented in Human Rights Watch, the 2004 TRC Report on Sierra Leone, and other published materials on the war in Sierra Leone. Sebastian Junger's article is quite revealing in its depiction of the horrors of the carnage that characterized the 1999 invasion of Freetown.[4] He describes the scenario:

> Realizing that they were going to lose the city, [the RUF] started rounding up people and detaining them until special amputation squads could arrive. The squads were made up of teenagers and even children, many of whom wore bandages where incisions had been made to pack cocaine under their skin. They did their work with rusty machetes and axes and seemed to choose their victims completely at random. "You, you, and you," they would say, picking people out of a line. There were stories of hands being taken away in blood-soaked grain bags. There were stories of hands' being hung in trees. There were stories of hands being eaten.[5]

The TRC annual report of 2004 identifies wide-ranging atrocities committed by all warring factions including members of the Sierra Leone Army and the Economic Ceasefire Monitoring Group (ECOMOG), foreign peacekeepers, and mainly Nigerians. My aim is not to replicate the details of the atrocities as documented in these works (as crucial as they may be to my analysis and theorizations) but rather to analyze how particular methods of recruitment, pain, and punishment adopted by all warring factions provided a lens through which to "read" the assumptions and objectives of the insurgency, and to understand the implications to both victim and perpetrator. And through this understanding, we can collectively come to grips with the horrible lessons learned and forge a new identity and future.

The brutal civil war in Sierra Leone was perhaps most remarkable in its techniques of forced conscription of young men and women as fighters of the infamous RUF. The violence of the atrocities committed by the warring factions has been well documented. Lansana Gberie points out the connections, historical and political, between the RUF and the destruction of Sierra

---

4 Sebastian Junger, "The Terror of Sierra Leone," *Vanity Fair*, August 2001, http://www.vanityfair.com/politics/features/2000/08.
5 Junger, "Terror."

Leone.⁶ Greg Campbell, a journalist, presents a comprehensive statement of the violence perpetrated on civilians by the RUF.⁷ He writes:

> Composed of mostly uneducated . . . the RUF was quickly revealed as an army of murderous thugs rather than justice-seeking rebels. RUF fighters fueled this inspiration at every opportunity. . . . Their "tactics" of warfare were unbelievably brutal. Sometimes after capturing a village, RUF fighters would gather civilian prisoners in the town square and make them choose small strips of paper from the ground that described different forms of torture and death, such as "chop off hands," "chop off head," or simply "be killed." Soldiers would bet with one another about the sex of pregnant women's unborn children. Winners are determined after the baby had been removed from the womb with a bayonet. In one instance, a young boy was beaten and roasted nearly to death on a spit in front of his mother for refusing to kill her.⁸

The Truth and Reconciliation Report of 2004 also provides details about the violence of the civil war and the mutilation of victims. In the 2004 report, for instance, one child testified to the commission of the violence and carnage: "Before I was captured, the rebels shot my father and mother in front of me, and having killed them, one of the Commandants grabbed me by the throat, tied both of my hands, cut parts of my body with a blade and placed cocaine in it."⁹ In this and other techniques, the forced conscription and retention of child combatants was ensured mostly by the RUF rebels. In the testimonies of child soldiers, scores of abductees testified to the use of branding as technique of forced conscription and retention of captives. Thus, throughout the civil war, it was common for captives to be branded across the forehead, chest, and back with the acronym of the movement, RUF.

In the events leading up to the 1996 General Elections, the rebel movement called in vain for a national boycott of the polls. When it became clear that the SLPP intended to go ahead with elections, it resorted to

---

6   Lansana Gberie, *A Dirty War in West Africa: RUF and the Destruction of Sierra Leone* (Bloomington: Indiana University Press, 2005).

7   Greg Campbell, *Blood Diamonds: Tracing the Deadly Path of the World's Most Precious Stones* (Boulder, CO: Westview, 2002).

8   Campbell, *Blood Diamonds*, 71–72.

9   United Nations, *Final Report on Ten-Year Sierra Leone Conflict Published; Seeks to Set Out Historical Record, Offer Guidance for Future* (2004), https://www.un.org/press/en/2004/ecosoc6140.doc.htm.

indiscriminate mutilations and amputations. A worker for International Crisis Group who monitored the situation reported the following:

> Hundreds of Sierra Leoneans had their fingers, hands, arms, noses, or lips chopped off with machete in the cause of democracy. They were being punished either for voting in, or for the mere fact of, the first round of the country's first multi-party elections in more than twenty-five years. . . . Among those I met in Bo . . . was a man who had had his right ear and his lips slashed off. Someone had carved with a knife the word TERROR on his chest and on his back AGAINST THE ELECTION FEBRUARY 26. Some men and women had had their arms hacked off above the elbow; some had lost their hands at the wrist.[10]

The use of the body as site of punishment was rampant during the civil war. Bodily mutilation by rebels of the RUF was intended to deter voting; however, in many ways, as this chapter will explore, these acts of violence on the body reveal the complex conception and operation of a dynamic of power and control that goes far beyond disenfranchisement of the population.

Apart from bodily mutilation, there was rampant amputation of limbs. *Human Rights Watch* further documents several cases of punitive amputation during the January 1999 RUF offensive in Freetown. The report states that

> during the month of January, Freetown's three main hospitals Connaught, Brookfield, and Netland Hospital treated ninety-seven victims of amputations resulting from attacks with axes and machetes. The majority of amputations were of the hands and arms, including thirty-six double amputations. One hospital treated over forty cases of attempted amputations, serious lacerations to the arms and legs, where medical staff were able to save the extremity or extremities.[11]

In interviews conducted with persons with amputations during this period, *Human Rights Watch* records the story of Lansana who, together with his two brothers, had their hands hacked off by rebels on January 18, 1999. He describes the incident:

> They told us to lie down in the road, face down; they had their guns to our heads. The first to be cut was Brima; they cut his left hand with an axe. Then my

---

10   William Shawcross, *Deliver Us from Evil: Peacekeepers, Warlords and a World of Endless Conflict* (New York: Simon and Schuster, 2002), 193.

11   Human Rights Watch, "Getting Away with Murder, Mutilation, and Rape: New Testimony from Sierra Leone," *Human Rights Watch* 3, no. A (1999), https://www.hrw.org/reports/1999/sierra/.

left hand was hacked off and then Amara's right hand . . . we were all bleeding so much. Brima tried to get us a few times, but he stumbled and fell. The last time he only made it a few yards and stumbled and collapsed. . . . We had to leave our brother right there on the street. After we got out of the hospital we went back to the place where it happened. The people told us Brima had been buried later that day in a common grave, right near where he fell.[12]

Similarly, Ramatu and five of her neighbors had their arms or hands amputated by rebels during the January invasion of Freetown. She describes the incident:

They then marched us at gunpoint to the hill near Kissy mental Hospital. . . . When we arrived they ordered us to lay face down and started cutting us. They dragged us, they had us get down on our knees and put our arms on a concrete slab. They had others standing over us and holding us from behind. One rebel did all the cutting. A few had both hands cut off; others just one. And then they walked away.[13]

Finally, Tejan's description of the brutal amputation of his two hands on January 20, 1999, completes the picture of wanton cruelty and reckless abandonment:

After they set fire to my house they caught me trying to escape out the back door. Then they brought me to the compound next door where I saw they'd captured two of my neighbors. They started arguing whether to kill me or cut my two hands. Then the one who seemed to be in-charge gave the order to amputate both my hands and called forward a fifteen-year-old boy they called "Commander Cut Hands." I refused to lie down. They beat me and it took several of them to hold me. They tripped me and when I fell to the ground three of them had to sit on my legs and back and a few had to hold my arms. Then they took out that axe. I was crying and after they had hacked off both of my hands, I screamed, "just kill me, kill me." They also cut off the hands of my two neighbors.[14]

The brutal hacking of limbs and the frequency of its occurrence has been documented in Lansana Gberie's (2005) groundbreaking work in which he discussed the January 6, 1999, invasion of Freetown by the RUF and the

---

12   Human Rights Watch, "Murder."
13   Human Rights Watch, "Murder."
14   Human Rights Watch, "Murder."

amputation of limbs that followed. He points out in "Operation No Living Thing" and "Terror as Warfare" the chilling irony that excited the warped mentality of the rebels and galvanized them into mass amputation of their victims' limbs. Gberie writes:

> It was during this period, while the rebels were terrorizing eastern Freetown and the Nigerians were advancing from the West, that a cruel twist of fate allowed the rebels to open up a new phase of horror in the city: a group of them raided a World Food Programme (WFP) warehouse at Kissy looking for food, but instead discovered hundreds of brand new machetes which had been brought in by the UN agency to be given to peasant farmers. Intended to be used for the cultivation of food, the machetes were now used by the rebels crudely and methodically to cut off the hands of people, including hundreds of people who could have used them to grow food. The perversion was complete: the tragedy was brutally surreal.[15]

The enactment of this perverse and brutal tragedy on the population forms part of the public testimonies of April 15, 2003, conducted and documented by the Truth and Reconciliation Commission in Sierra Leone. In one of the testimonies, Witness 007, Morlai Bizo Conteh, explains:

> I was going to visit my mother in Kono. On my way going, we fell into an ambush . . . when the rebels saw that I was trembling, they thought I was going to put up some resistance. He got hold of my throat and held on tightly to it. One of the rebels who was in military fatigue and who was also having a cutlass hit my hand seriously and chopped off the right arm. The arm did not fall off completely but hanged dangling. I bled profusely and fell unconscious . . . I was taken to the Makeni (Arab) Hospital for a surgical operation where they cut off my hand.[16]

Another witness, Isatu Kamara, who testified to the commission notes:

> My mother had gone sell her wares on the day the village was attacked. She escaped. They gathered us together and locked us in a room, and they started taking us out one after the other. Some had their ears cut off; some had their

---

15 Lansana Gberie, *A Dirty War in West Africa: The RUF and the Destruction of Sierra Leone* (Bloomington: Indiana University Press, 2005), 129.
16 Morlai Bizo Conteh, "Appendix 3, Part 1: Memorials and Transitional Justice," The Sierra Leone Truth and Reconciliation Commission (website), 2003, https://www.sierraleonetrc.org/index.php/appendices/item/appendix.

arms cut off. . . . They came to me; they took me, outstretched my foot and cut it off with a cutlass. I fainted.[17]

Further instances of amputation by the RUF were documented in the child-friendly version of the TRC's report of 2004. As recorded, one twelve-year-old girl told the commission during the closed hearings in Makeni: "At about 2 am, the rebels attacked our town. . . .They lined up a number of people, sent for a mortar and asked each of us to put our hand and they cut them off. . . . I placed my right hand and it was chopped off."[18]

Mutilation and amputation are indicative of psychological control of victims and are closely linked to the discourse of silence and the resulting subjugation of survivors to their situations. Human branding in war produces a culture of silence emanating from fear and intimidation. The marks on the body create a submissive and compliant prisoner imprisoned by and his own body. Practically entrapped in his body, the victim is made to be complicit in his own abuse. The inscription RUF across the chest, forehead, arms, and back of child combatants announces their culpability in the mayhem. The scarred body further implies that their survival depends on the signification of the inscription to the "reader" or interpreter. Given the atrocities committed by the RUF, it is clear that the branded body signifies destruction, rape, decapitation, and summary execution. The individual with the branded body would then be made to pay for its signification. As in the opening scene in *Cry Freetown*, the young boy loses his life because of the marks on his body. In other cases, young men with marks on their bodies face mob justice, vigilante execution, and death at the hands of government soldiers and peacekeepers.

Importantly, it stands to reason that the signification of the branded body may constitute ambivalence because it has the tendency to disclose as much as it conceals. In many ways, the "reading" given to the body would depend on the perspective of the body's "reader" , and interpretations could range from complicity to innocence. The scarred body is a mask that both designates and disguises: while the scar may be "read" as identification and belonging, the circumstances in which the branding is done may allow for

---

17 Isatu Kamara, "Appendix 3, Part 1: Memorials and Transitional Justice," The Sierra Leone Truth and Reconciliation Commission (website), 2003, https://www.sierraleonetrc.org/index.php/appendices/item/appendix.

18 Quoted in Marc Pilisuk, *Peace Movements Worldwide* (Santa Barbara: ABC-CLIO, 2011), 24.

a reading of the same scar as forced conscription, loss of innocence, and domination rather than guilt and complicity. Thus, there is tension between what it signifies or designates (child combatant) and what it conceals (forced conscription) or that which remains undisclosed or unknown. The failure of warring factions to work out this gap between revelation and concealment resulted in the deaths of thousands of people, some in the most gruesome or horrifying of circumstances.

At the same time, human branding accentuates the theory of the body as signifier in the sense that the branded body creates a new identity for the victim that is incriminating and produces guilt and shame. The scars are permanent designations of complicity and participation in the atrocities of the civil war and imply the need for some form of punishment and justice on the part of the afflicted in society. In addition, and with the scar on his body, the victim internalizes its signifiers: anger, hate, self-recrimination, and violence. In their internalization, the psychological control of the victim is complete. The situation is one of acute mental agony for the victim in realizing that his marked body, in its visual representation, is a betrayal of his humanity and, in the context of the Sierra Leone civil war, a betrayal of the political ideology of resistance to armed insurgency and the promotion of civil disobedience. The victim has to confront the signification of his marked body as traitor and executioner for the rest of his life. The weight of shame, guilt, and self-hate on child combatants accounts for the refusal of scores of former child soldiers to return to their communities and to reintegrate into society.

Branding of the body is also a physical marking of the body politic. The marked body becomes the geographical space where the boundaries of power and control intersect to reconstruct a new space on the body of the victim that illustrates both bodily and territorial possession. The marking of RUF on the body of the captive ensures the geographical boundary or physical space that the individual can safely inhabit. Since RUF is inscribed on his body, the continued existence of the captive is henceforth circumscribed, defined, and regulated within the terrain or physical space under the control of the RUF. Hence, the marked body is the space where bodily contours or "mappings" reflect or are equal to the geographical boundaries the captive lives within. Since the boundary is "drawn" by the RUF inscriber, the branded captive has no alternative but to submit to his control and exist within the space he operates in.

Further, branding is an attempt by the inscriber to impose a new national identity on the body of the victim. It is almost as if the victim's body offers the perpetrator a new geographical canvas to redraw the map of Sierra Leone.

Accordingly, the inscription of RUF on the victim's body signifies possession of the state by the rebels. In short, bodily possession is indicative of territorial or state possession. Hence, possession of the body of the victim is metonymically possession of the body politic. Within this construct, the body of the victim is akin to the "body" of Sierra Leone where possession of the scarred body is indicative of territorial possession and where the traumatized condition of the branded victim is reflective of the physical state of the country both in terms of destruction of infrastructure and of the national psyche of Sierra Leoneans. The branded body is the physical and psychological text of violence and trauma that defines Sierra Leone during the civil war and threatens to destabilize reconstruction and reconciliation in postconflict Sierra Leone. Accordingly, the RUF pursues human branding to demonstrate possession of both body of individuals and the body politic.

Theoretical Constructs: The Disfigured Body and Disability Theory

In articulating a theoretical construct for analysis, I develop a phenomenology of the body that establishes a point of connection between bodily wound and the name given to it. I theorize that at the moment the body is wounded or disfigured, it is given a new name and that the name is reflective of the type or nature of the bodily wound and becomes the label attached to the victim or his identity. Thus, the label "amputee" becomes the name of both the bodily disfigurement ("amputation") and the carrier of that body. Since the disfigured body is the locus of intersection of both the name of wound and the name of carrier of the wound, those who experience amputation develop a new sense of self in relation to his or her label. Therefore, part of the objective of this chapter is to develop an ontology of the body by which we would begin to understand the ways in which the amputated body is conceptualized by both victim and society.

It is important to make a distinction between punitive and surgical forms of amputation and hence emphasize the difference between the victims of amputation and the patient. In medical amputation, the loss of the limb is a remedy to a bodily ailment. In some cases, it is prescribed as a deterrent to the spread of an ailment. Therefore, the person who loses his leg, for instance, to avoid gangrene occasioned by diabetes confronts a different psychological reality about himself and his situation. Further, as a result of this realization, he relates to his residual limb and the surgeon who performed the operation in a different way than the person who had a limb hacked off with a machete by a combatant in war. Thus, even though the patient could be described as "disabled," the circumstances surrounding his "disability," the psychological effect it produces, and his relation to and understanding of himself and society are of a different form than the survivor of punitive amputation.

On the other hand, punitive amputation is neither intended as cure nor remedy to a medical situation. It is a deliberate, calculated, and cruel decision of a perpetrator to inflict bodily harm as punishment on another person. In its epistemologies of power, control, domination, abuse, and cruelty, punitive amputation proffers a different psychological reality to the individual and his relationship to his body and his society is anchored in feelings of resentment to the perpetrator and pain from the loss of the limb.

The literature of Sierra Leone reflects the horrors of punitive amputation. And for purpose of analysis, I will cite a few. Eugene Harkins's *Where Witch Birds Fly*, Ian Stewart's *Freetown Ambush: A Reporter's Year in Africa*, Von Doen's *How di Body?*, Greg Campbell's *Blood Diamonds: Tracing the Path of the World's Precious Stones*, Ishmael Beah's *A Long Way Gone*, and Mariatu Kamara's *The Bite of the Mango*, are examples of such works of literature. The psychological realities of punitive amputation in the brutal civil war in Sierra Leone are glaringly captured in Greg Campbell's work:

> Dalramy was shoved to his knees in the red dirt, and as one of the young rebels tossed the amputated hands of the pervious victim into the thick bush—twirling them in a spray of blood toward a solid wall of green leaves, where they disappeared like food into the mouth of a giant beast. . . . An AK-47 barrel was pressed to his left temple. Dalramy looked at the indentation around his thick finger where he'd just removed his son's ring. There was a quick glint of sunlight on the blade of the homemade ax, and Dalramy squeezed his eyes tight against the blow. The blade slammed through the bones of his arm above the wrist. The hand came off with one clean chop, a blessing considering many such crude amputations required more than a dozen blows to sever a limb. He saw his hand bounced off the edge of the stump, gleaming white ulna bone seeing the sun for the first time.[19]

Campbell's diction is particularly effective in conveying the excruciating pain, the trauma of the incident, and the inhumanity of the perpetrator. As Dalramy "squeezed his eyes tight" to psychologically block or detach himself from the impending amputation, the unspoken discourse of cruelty and

---

19   Campbell, *Blood Diamonds*, xvii.

indifference of the axe-wielding rebel in the background sharply heightens the cruelty and human rights abuse contained in the incident. He suffers the crushing "blow" of the axe; the blade "slammed through the bones" and the hand "came off" in one clean "chop." In the immediate aftermath of the amputation, Dalramy through the gaze confronts the horror of the situation as he "saw" his hand "bounced off the edge of the stump," and he sees the white ulna, which is also "seeing" the sun for the first time. Invariably, his residual limb, like the stump on which it was placed before it was chopped off, takes on the meaning of the "stump."

It is clear from Campbell's narrative that punitive amputation involves a much more complex relationship between perpetrator and victim and that in view of these complexities the victim of amputation's injury shapes both a sense of self and his relation to society. Thus, in postconflict societies like Sierra Leone, where punitive amputation was rife, theories of disability and of the disabled should consider the peculiar circumstance of the situation: intentionality, psychological trauma, perception of the disfigured body, and the ambiguities and ambivalences characterizing the disfigured body when the disabled body is analyzed and theoretical assumptions about it are constructed. Furthermore, it is crucial to make a brief remark on the difference between the person who undergoes punitive amputation and the veteran who returns home after losing a limb, for instance, to a landmine. In spite of the fact that both have lost limbs in the context of war, the circumstances are clearly different, and the individual and society respond to and interpret the residual limb in different ways. To the veteran, his residual stump carries much sentiment—associated with courage, honor, patriotism, bravery, sacrifice, and resilience. On the other hand, the amputation victim's residual limb carries feelings of stigma, humiliation, and resentment.

Victims of amputation in postconflict Sierra Leone face a crucial problem of image and function. With the loss of limbs, the survivor assumes a new label (amputee) that gives him a new identity, one predicated not only on visual image (physical appearance) but also on bodily function (mobility and physical function). I emphasize that crucial to healing, forgiveness, and reconciliation is how a victim of amputation addresses this new image in order to negotiate a new sense of self and function.

In June of 2009 I interviewed a person with a double amputation at the Jui amputee camp in the east of Freetown, Sierra Leone. The interview focused on the issue of body image or physical function. The amputation victim, Mr. Sesay, pointed out to me the conflicting perspectives of the individual person with an amputation and society with regard to the limitations and possibilities of the amputated body. He demonstrated ingenious ways he has developed to cope with the physical challenges he encountered in the camp in order to maintain his independence and reassert his dignity. During our dialogue, it became clear to me that he was essentially advocating for a conceptual shift from the amputation victim as helpless to being accepted as functional and independent. He reiterated the point that a continued perception of persons with amputations in the light of dependency and dysfunction inhibits autonomy and promotes self-hate and revenge. This sense of the amputated body's ambivalence and its ability to reverse conventional cultural perceptions of the body is crucial to understanding my position in this chapter.

However, I am well aware that such an analysis or ontology of the body requires a theorization of the relationship between name and wound. In his work on the poetics of the wounded body, Dennis P. Slattery asked the following questions:

> What is this phenomenal body, this poetic body of markings? What is the wound in its relation to language, to identity, and to being named? Does being wounded, marked, scarred, tattooed, violated in some bodily way change our relation to the way we express ourselves incarnationally through body gesture or in language? Does it change the way we are placed, or in place in the world?[20]

Using Slattery's questions, I hypothesize the following: that there is a point of connection between bodily wound or scar and the name or label given to it. What this means is that at the moment the body is wounded or damaged, it is given a new name. Thus, the word "amputee" becomes the name of both the nature of the wound (amputation) and the identity of the carrier of the wound (amputee). At this intersection, the person with an amputation develops a new sense of self in relation to language, an identity that is circumscribed around the word or label that is now used to describe him. In this circumstance, the body becomes both the sites for deployment of power (as the process of amputation occasions), and for resistance and recalibration of that notion of domination (as a theory of transcendence depicts). It is both, as Slattery asserts, a "location and a field for experience as well as for interpretation," for as he further emphasizes "our wounds name us and give the trajectory of our destiny. They identify and mark us. Our name, along

---

20 Dennis P. Slattery, *The Wounded Body: Remembering the Markings of Flesh* (Albany: State University of New York Press, 2000), 7.

with our wound, records us in the world. And in our identity rests our vulnerable moral limits."²¹

Another influential article in understanding punitive amputation in the context of the civil war in Sierra Leone provides a deeper insight into the nature and impact of amputations on the survivor. In his conversation with Eric Duret, a French psychologist treating persons with amputations in Freetown, George Parker writes:

> Sierra Leoneans seldom say, "My hand was amputated." They say, "I was amputated" [Duret] told me that when he sees his patients they continue to show him the stump. "Sometimes it's so present, so painful, that they are no longer anything but that," he said. "The amputated part takes the place of the whole." The arm has lost its face and voice; especially in the case of a double amputee, it's as if he had been gagged as well as bound. When I first met Sierra Leoneans, I kept imagining that the tongue had been cut off along with the hands.²²

George Parker's article is crucial in this regard, as it depicts the cultural context in which amputation and its resulting disability are perceived in Sierra Leone. Parker's article is influential not only in articulating the culture of disability in Sierra Leone but also in calling attention to the need for a reformulation of disability and its cultural significations.

Parker explores a metonymy of amputation that substitutes the residual limb for the whole body, both individually and nationally. In conflating the amputated limb with the amputated body, "the amputated body not only takes the place of the whole," but dehumanizes, silences, emasculates, and incapacitates the individual and hinders society's transformation. Here, the amputation of the limb is metaphorically the cutting off of the tongue, and so he postulates that in amputation "the tongue has been cut off along with the hand." Such a representation achieves a double effect: it unveils the violence but also (and unfortunately) conflates that violence with identity. In this way, it disempowers survivors and takes away their agency. As I discuss later, such a conception of amputation articulates the medical model of disability.

In this chapter, therefore, I focus on intervention strategy aimed at such forms of representation that will explore possibilities of reformulation of ideas pertaining to image and function of victims of amputation. I argue in favor of engaging disability through the theory of "complex embodiment,"

---

21   Slattery, *Wounded*.
22   George Parker, "The Children of Freetown," *New Yorker*, January 13, 2003, 6.

a phrase I borrow from Tobin Siebers, and stress the point that disability is ideologically constructed: through a complex reformulation of amputation, survivors can reclaim their bodies and reassert dignity. I argue that the amputated body is a site of resistance rather than domination and that with cultural transformation it can deconstruct notions of physical challenges and psychological trauma associated with it. Hence, the amputated body should be "read" both in terms of its impairment as well as its potentials. As I theorize, the disfigured body is not constructed entirely from its place in the environment. Rather, it acknowledges the social construction while also embracing the physical impairment. It is in this state of complex embodiment that the survivor achieves liberation and autonomy.

The medical model of disability constitutes a deficit model that characterizes impairments as problems that have to be corrected. Pfeiffer illustrates three variations of the deficit model: medical, rehabilitation, and special education.[23] Mitchell and Snyder suggest that "disabled subjectivities are constituted in a struggle with the able-bodied public's projections and investments in maintaining disability as alterity."[24] Similarly, Hughes maintains that the medical model of disability leads to the creation of a culture of paternalism and a theory of ableism whereby the disabled are constructed as dependent and in need of charitable assistance. Hughes notes that this invokes the gaze of pity and sympathy for the disabled from those considered nondisabled: an act anchored in social responses as almsgiving and segregation, as well as in "charitable paternalism and exclusion."[25] Therefore, the conceptualization of disability as "abnormality" and essentially as personal tragedy is limiting.[26] As Hughes succinctly puts it: "The ontological essence of disability [as] physical or mental impairment or a biological "deficit" or "flaw" . . . limits what disabled people can do."[27]

---

23   David Pfeiffer, "Disability Studies and the Disability Perspective," *Disability Studies Quarterly*, no.1 (2003): 142–148.

24   David Mitchell and Sharon Snyder, "Introduction: Disability Studies and the Double Bind of Representation," *The Body and Physical Difference*, ed. Mitchell and Snyder (Ann Arbor: University of Michigan Press, 1997), 23.

25   Bill Hughes, "Disability and the Body," in *Disability Studies Today*, ed. Colin Barnes, Mike Oliver, and Len Barton (Cambridge: Polity, 2002), 62.

26   Michael Oliver, *The Politics of Disablement: A Sociological Approach* (New York: St. Martin's Press, 1990).

27   Hughes, "Disability," 60.

Elaborating on the theme of deficit in the medical model, Siebers notes that this model "defines disability as an individual defect lodged in the person's defect that must be cured or eliminated if the person is to achieve full capacity as a human being."[28] Siebers affirms what to the individuals who have gone through punitive amputation is at the core of their reality or existence: amputation of limbs is not equivalent to "sub-standard" or "incomplete" humanity and that human potential, its manifestation and accomplishment, is a fundamental function of will, the implementation of which has little to do with "ableism" or bodily ability.

Ability intricately linked to identity in this way implies that the identity of the victim of amputation is in part socially constructed. And that identity contains and reflects complex assumptions and theorizations about the body and the social realities it is located in. Accordingly, based on the paradigms and critical formations embedded in these theories or models, some bodies like the disfigured or amputated body stand to be excluded, stigmatized, labeled, discriminated against, and undervalued by a dominant social ideology or master narrative of "ableism" or "normality." As Siebers contend, these bodies are ideologically constructed as they "display the workings of ideology and expose it to critique and the demand for political change."[29]

The core of my argument is that since loss of limbs occurs in different ways, it would be uncritical to categorize or conflate all persons with amputations into one homogeneous entity. Because loss of limbs may occur either accidentally, as in landmine explosions or in other violent accidents, or deliberately, as in punitive amputation, the psychological and social realities that characterize these situations vary widely. If persons with amputations from medical or surgical treatment are included, the picture is further complicated. And because the psychosocial realities of those with amputations are predicated on the circumstances surrounding the amputation, persons with amputations have different needs and would require different rehabilitation strategies and procedures. Use of prosthetics alone may not be as effective a method of rehabilitation to the person with an amputation who has gone through punitive amputation as it may be for the victim of a landmine explosion or a patient recovering from a surgical operation to prevent the progress of a malignant tumor.

---

28   Tobin Siebers, *Disability Theory* (Ann Arbor: University of Michigan Press, 2008), 3.
29   Siebers, *Disability Theory*, 13.

While the need for physical mobility may be desired by all people with amputations, their psychosocial needs differ. In a situation where all persons with amputations are identified and categorized under the medical model of disability, the objective of the rehabilitation process is to "fix" the deformity or malfunction, and mobility is perceived as the first step toward rebuilding their lives, transforming a life of dependency on others into a life of dignity and independence. However, the needs of victims who have experienced punitive amputation go well beyond being fitted with prosthetics as guarantee of locomotion. There also needs to be not only an understanding and engagement with the social dimension of disability but also the reconstruction of a new identity and creation of a culture of disability.

Conclusion

I recognize that such a view of prosthetics and their use is bound to stir up controversy, and I must again state that while this chapter would critique and theorize prosthetics, it does not seek to vilify or devalue them. On the contrary, this chapter's intention was to advance the following theoretical assumptions: that prosthetics imply the construction of impairment as a deficit from which the person with an amputation is relegated to a state of incompletion, inferiority, and inadequacy; they signify a condition where the person with an amputation is cast as coping with a disabled identity rather than confronting, challenging, and deconstructing that identity. Prosthetics must engage the psychosocial dimensions of amputation, address the use of language as a construct of identity and the power dynamics it engenders, and amplify or lend credence to a state of brokenness or something that requires fixing.

From these assumptions, it is evident that prosthetics seek to create a "before" and "'after" image; an extreme "make-over" prosthetics edition, where the prosthetics restore normalcy to the abnormal. In this way, the prosthetics, albeit unintentionally, overlook or downplay the significance of the message inscribed on the body of the amputation victim, which, in fact, is the reason why the amputation was conducted in the first place. Thus, the prosthetics avoid the core of the issue—the deconstruction of the message on the body of the person with an amputated limb—and unwittingly promote locomotion or function over psychological trauma. In this case, then, prosthetics function as reminders of the loss and pain encountered during the atrocity that led to the amputation. Instead of the transformation they strive to achieve, prosthetics could potentially accomplish exactly the opposite. In fitting prosthetics onto individuals who have internalized the narrative of dependency and dysfunction that come with punitive amputation, there is the danger that the prosthetics will amplify this message while assuming that the victims of amputation have been liberated and rendered "whole." In this context, rather than emancipation, prosthetics could promote depression, grief, sorrow, and disillusionment.

Therefore, there is need for a counterdiscourse to the master narrative of deficiency in order for prosthetics to accomplish their goal. Victims of amputation must realize that their identity as dependents is not physical but rather socially constructed. It is critical then to postulate that it is the medical model of disability (and the extreme social model that eliminates impairment from disability) that makes it difficult or impossible for impairment to be embraced.

Consequently, the individual who has gone through punitive amputation comes to recognize that his condition should not relegate them to the status of second-class citizen abandoned and isolated in some remote camp for persons with amputations.[30] He or she comes to see that amputation should not constitute barriers, impediment, segregation, and discrimination and should neither be articulated in disabling terms (grief, guilt, bitterness) nor in heroic terms (courage, nobility, transcendence) that would indicate either the deficit model or the compensation model. Rather, it would be more productive for amputation victims to examine and reconstruct their own personal ontology and social reality in order to reverse the stereotypes associated with amputation and recast them into liberation contingent on the creation of a new value system.

My view of prosthetics centers on the fact that full restoration of bodily function in cases of punitive amputation has to engage the mental and psychological processes of the individual for the prosthetics to be meaningful and for psychological liberation to be achieved. In this regard, I make the claim that bodily function is to be conceptualized in both locomotive and

---

30 One such foundation is the Prosthetic Outreach Foundation (POF) and because of its pivotal work in Sierra Leone, some attention is devoted to its operation, especially with the setting up of the prosthetic clinic (Makeni Government Hospital Rehabilitation Center) at the Makeni Government Hospital in the northern part of Sierra Leone. See ISSUU, *Prosthetics Outreach Foundation: 2009 Annual Report* (Copenhagen: ISSUU, 2009), 3, https://issuu.com/pofsea/docs/2009_annual_report.

psychological terms and that for liberation to be achieved, there should be a counterdiscourse to engage and reverse the negative connotations, cultural and otherwise, associated with punitive bodily amputation. While prosthetics afford persons with amputations the opportunity for physical mobility, they do little to transform the mind, a crucial aspect of the healing process. However, it is in the transforming and renewal of the mind that the amputation victim reverses the socially constructed notions of handicap, dismisses humiliation, and embraces functionality. Psychological liberation anchored on both the limitations and possibilities of the disfigured body is the linchpin for agency, as it is through this process that survivors reverse domains of power and assert agency.

Since persons with amputations have to face the fact that the prosthesis is an "artificial limb," a foreign body (and so must come to terms with the fact that the "natural limb has been lost irrevocably"), it is essential to articulate a phenomenology of the disfigured body that would promote acceptance of it but also rework its negative signifiers to fully comprehend the dynamics of the amputated body and promote agency.

In reclaiming the disfigured body, the individual is articulating the possibility of imagining the body as something other than what the perpetrator had in mind when he amputated or disfigured it. Thus, accepting the residual limb is the first step toward reclaiming agency and establishing a sense of subjectivity. Conceptualizing the disfigured body as agency rather than disability illustrates, in Carol Henderson's phrase, "the paradoxical nature of remembering."[31] This way, the body becomes a site of objection and resistance, a means of empowerment and defiance against the insanity that led to its disfigurement in the first place and confronts the mentality behind the action.

Finally, my critical formations regarding the disfigured body as agency rest on a number of theoretical principles. First, disfiguration is not the end of meaningful existence. For the person with an amputation, the question is not whether the prosthesis has replaced the natural limb but rather how by virtue of the difference amputation and prosthesis make to the individual and society, the person with an amputation can use that difference to his or her advantage. Second, those with amputations must be provided with the

---

31   In 2009 and 2010, I interviewed amputation victims of the Sierra Leone civil war in two resettlement camps, Jui and Newton camps, in the outskirts of Freetown. It was evident that the camps were in dire need of medical facilities and social support.

psychological tools that empower them to redefine the cultural norms that interpret disfigurement as deformity and dysfunction. Third, prosthetics do not guarantee that the psychological problems associated with loss of limbs have been engaged. While they offer and restore some degree of mobility and function, they do not provide the tools for handling the negative feelings and behaviors that persons with amputations would have to deal with. The availability of prosthetics is in reality a small part of the process of healing.

My contention, therefore, is that the amputated body is to be perceived through images that interrogate, contest, and rework the notion of dependency and helplessness. My conception of the amputated body provides a framework to rethink it as a site where the master discourse of domination and dependency is resisted, transformed, and transcended. This framework reimagines the amputated body as an ambivalent entity: one that denies, challenges, and subverts conventional notions of disability.

Chapter Eight

Paradoxical Dramaturgies

Disability, Ritual, and Resistance in the Plays of Wole Soyinka

Nic Hamel

The dramas of Nigerian dramatist, poet, novelist, and essayist (as well as Africa's first Nobel Laureate in literature) Wole Soyinka often combine seemingly disparate elements of West African subjects, cosmologies, and performance traditions with European tragedy and absurdism. He is acclaimed, and indeed canonized, by literary and theatrical critics, primarily for what Biodun Jeyifo describes as "a convergence of the *aesthetic* and *political* radicalism which, apart from Soyinka, we encounter only in a few other African writers."[1] However, alongside the copious praise he has received over the last several decades, Soyinka has also developed a reputation as an often difficult writer, or even an obscurantist. Critics like Bernth Lindfors and others lament that Soyinka's dramaturgically and culturally complex works too often contain "enigmatic obfuscations," which are "perverse and irresponsible" for an artist who ostensibly values ethical social commitments.[2] To interpret the political content of Wole Soyinka's dramas requires a focused consideration of context and nuance, particularly when approaching as overdetermined and ambiguous a concept as disability. Many of the literary tools

---

1   Biodun Jeyifo, *Wole Soyinka: Politics, Poetics, and Postcolonialism* (Cambridge: Cambridge University Press, 2004), 14.
2   Bernth Lindfors, "Wole Soyinka, When Are You Coming Home?" *Yale French Studies*, no. 53 (1976): 197.

developed by critical disability studies cannot easily be applied to Soyinka's dramatic creations and the readings demanded by their particular Yoruban contexts.

Disability and disabled characters are ubiquitous in Soyinka's plays, and fulfill a multiplicity of dramaturgical functions, operating variously as metaphor or metonym for vulnerability, mysticism, and postcolonial debilitation. Yet disability in Soyinka is not easily articulated in the terms developed by traditional disability studies. As articulated by Afro-Caribbean poet, playwright, and fellow Nobel Laureate, Derek Walcott:

> One does not need to look very far for the usual location of such characters in Soyinka's writings . . . in the spaces between worlds—the worlds of the living, the dead and the unborn . . . here reside the dwarfs, cripples, and idiots in Soyinka's plays—all of the usual candidates for grotesque status. No particular stigma attaches to any of these figures . . . they all partake of the special dangerous energy of transition that lies in the space between worlds . . . they have the capacity to explode contradiction into power and energy.[3]

Enmeshed both in Soyinka's intricate social commentary and in his engagement with traditional Yoruba cultural practices, disability is important to the dramatic and symbolic logic of his theatre. In his landmark study of disability in Soyinka's plays, Ato Quayson indicates that "the combination of the ritualistic with the political is something for which Soyinka has become notably famous . . . disability acts as a marker of both ritual and the political, but in ways that interrupt the two domains and force us to rethink the conceptual movement between the two."[4] Through the combination and juxtaposition of indigenous Yoruba beliefs and practices with the anxieties of postcolonial Nigeria, Soyinka uses disability to both suture and disrupt his audiences' cultural identity.

Certain critics downplay the centrality of the indigenous African context on Soyinka's dramaturgy, arguing particularly that interpretations that privilege Yoruban cosmology serve more to distract than inform. Derek Wright claims: "The mythographic lore of deities dismembered in chthonic gulfs and its ritual embodiments have had a loud voice—perhaps too loud, disproportionate to their true importance—in Soyinka's criticism, and reassessment of

---

3   Derek Walcott, "Transition and the Grotesque: Soyinka's *Madmen and Specialists*," *Commonwealth (Dijon)* 18, no. 2 (1996): 21–22.

4   Ato Quayson, *Aesthetic Nervousness: Disability and the Crisis of Representation* (Bloomington: Indiana University Press, 1997), 29.

their proper place in his work is long overdue."[5] This criticism is due largely to the emphasis that Soyinka himself has placed on mythic aspects of his work, particularly when addressing non-African audiences.[6] Henry Louis Gates suggests that "the fact of Soyinka's Africanness only makes visible an estranged relation which always stands between any text and its audience. As Shakespeare used Denmark, as Brecht used Chicago, Soyinka uses the Yoruba world as a setting for cosmic conflict, and never as an argument for the existence of African culture."[7] Indeed, any interpretation of Soyinka that flattens African or Yoruba cosmologies into a mere trope of his work ignores a great deal of the dynamism both of Soyinka's writings and of Yoruba culture itself. As Quayson argues:

> The limitations of criticism of Soyinka's work derives from implicit assumptions informing the critical enterprise in the first place. Traditional Yoruba culture is seen as a stabilized entity articulable in its rituals and myths. What Soyinka is seen as doing is to have captured the essence of Yoruba culture in his theorizing and to have dramatized it in his plays. Since he speaks on behalf of his own culture, the assumption is that his theorizing coalesces the essence of the culture with a highly sophisticated mode of articulation.[8]

To evaluate Soyinka's plays, and the functions of disability within them, it is important to adequately contextualize their Yoruba settings and influences without essentializing either their forms or functions.

While Soyinka's dramaturgical deployment of disability may be partially described within disability studies' frames of stigma, metaphor, and prosthesis, I contend that attention to the specific cultural and material conditions of Soyinka's plays will produce a substantially more nuanced reading. Critical disability methodologies, developed almost exclusively in the Global North, often prove inadequate tools for examining postcolonial literature and performance, and this is certainly the case with Soyinka's multivalent metaphysical

---

5   Derek Wright, "Ritual and Revolution: Soyinka's Dramatic Theory," *ARIEL: A Review of International English Literature* 23, no. 1 (1992): 57.

6   Wole Soyinka, *Myth, Literature, and the African World* (Cambridge: Cambridge University Press, 1976), 151.

7   Henry Louis Gates Jr., "Being, the Will, and the Semantics of Death," in *Perspectives on Wole Soyinka: Freedom and Complexity*, ed. Biodun Jeyifo (Jackson: University Press of Mississippi, 2001), 74.

8   Ato Quayson, *Strategic Transformations in Nigerian Writing* (Bloomington: Indiana University Press, 1997), 66.

significations. Soyinka's "predisposition toward enigma, open-endedness, and dramaturgic experimentation"[9] forces any serious consideration of his work to engage beyond established theories and disciplinary distinctions, particularly with regard to such hotly contested issues as the position of the fictionalized disabled body. I explore in this chapter the functions of disability what Awam Amkpa terms Soyinka's "metaphysical dramas";[10] that is, those plays written largely between 1958 and 1970 that reflect a complex engagement with traditional Yoruban cultural and religious practices, as well as a keen postcolonial critique. I read the signification of disability specifically here through the plays *The Swamp Dwellers* (1958), *The Strong Breed* (1964), *The Road* (1965), and *Madmen and Specialists* (1970). In these texts I deal with historical and cultural narratives of the Yoruban deity, Obàtálá, traditional Yoruban masquerade performances, and postcolonial debilitation and resistance.

I will argue that critical attention must be paid not only to the metaphorical significance of the characters with disabilities but also to the specificities of Yoruban ritual and seemingly paradoxical modes of postcolonial resistance. By attending to each of these valences, I argue that Soyinka's theatrical approach to disability is not reducible to any ready formula, whether it be from postcolonialism, Africanism, or critical disability studies but instead that his work simultaneously offers provocative challenges to each of these disciplines. In approaching Soyinka's plays from multiple methodological directions, I hope to both reiterate the importance of disability to his work and also to revise and expand the consideration of the ritualistic, performative, and postcolonial valences of disability as a concept.

Aesthetic Nervousness and Postcolonial Representation

Quayson's evaluation of disability in Soyinka frames his approach within the larger literary stance that he terms "aesthetic nervousness," briefly: "when the dominant protocols of representation within the literary text are short circuited in relation to disability."[11] This short-circuiting, Quayson claims, arises from the discomfort related to the social encounter with disability, which relies on "the implicit assumption that disability is an 'excessive'

---

9   Quayson, *Aesthetic Nervousness*, 145.
10 Awam Ankpa, *Theatre and Postcolonial Desires* (London: Routledge, 2004), 24.
11 Quayson, *Aesthetic Nervousness*, 16.

sign that invites interpretation. . . . Following from this first point is the issue of subliminal fear and moral panic."[12] The crisis produced by a real-world encounter with disability then destabilizes the traditional functions of representation when utilized in writing but immediately places aesthetic concerns in an ethical context so that "the representation of disability oscillates uneasily between the aesthetic and ethical domains, in such a way as to force a reading of the aesthetic fields in which the disabled are represented as always having an ethical dimension that cannot be easily subsumed under the aesthetic structure."[13] This always-incomplete effort to represent disability engenders an aesthetic nervousness for both the writer and the reader that places them in an unstable relationship with the ethics of oppressed and stigmatized bodies.

Quayson's aesthetic nervousness functions largely as a revision and expansion of David T. Mitchell and Sharon L. Snyder's earlier theorizations of disability metaphor and "narrative prosthesis." Mitchell and Snyder castigate literary metaphorizations of disability that deny actual disabled bodies and replace them with "a shorthand method of securing emotional responses from audiences because pathos, pity, and abhorrence have proved to be an integral part of the historical baggage of our understandings of disability."[14] For Mitchell and Snyder, representations of disability evoke patronizing patterns of responses in their viewers: "Once narrative mobilizes the question of disability's ambiguous relationship to morality a duality is established, and the point is not whether the connection is forged or broken but rather that the two perpetually coexist and define each other."[15] Further refining this process, Mitchell and Snyder coin the term "narrative prosthesis" to indicate a literary device that foregrounds a disorienting encounter with disability: "Making comprehensible that which appears to be inherently unknowable situates narrative in the powerful position of mediator between two separate worlds."[16] In a manner more forceful than Quayson's, Mitchell and Snyder

---

12   Quayson, *Aesthetic Nervousness*, 14.
13   Quayson, *Aesthetic Nervousness*, 19.
14   David T. Mitchell and Sharon L. Snyder, "Introduction: Disability Studies and the Double Bind of Representation," in *The Body and Physical Difference: Discourses of Disability*, ed. David T. Mitchell and Sharon L. Snyder (Ann Arbor: University of Michigan Press, 1997), 17.
15   Mitchell and Snyder, "Introduction," 17.
16   David T. Mitchell and Sharon L. Snyder, *Narrative Prosthesis: Disability and the Dependencies of Discourse* (Ann Arbor: University of Michigan Press, 2000), 6.

portray narrativization as an always-impossible endeavor to exert control over the unruly concept of disability. The assumption that Mitchell and Snyder make is that because of the social erasures of disability as an embodied and material reality, writers employ a tactic of narrative prosthesis that "seeks to accomplish an erasure of difference all together; yet, failing that, as is always the case with prosthesis, the minimal goal is to return one to an acceptable degree of difference."[17] Mitchell and Snyder imply that the ethical valence of disability narratives is nearly always a harmful reiteration of the status quo's efforts to normalize, control, or discard disabled people who do not follow their standards of acceptability.

Aesthetic nervousness, for Quayson, revises narrative prosthesis and operates in two significant directions: (1) it reconfigures the primary relationship of disability representation away from the tension between a textual signifier and an embodied referent toward an interplay of signifiers that complicate aesthetic and ethical considerations, and (2) it radically expands the possible functions that disability may serve in a literary work. Quayson rejects Mitchell and Snyder's assumption that the relationship between disabled characters and their narrative function is stable, but rather contends that "even if programmatic roles were originally assigned, these roles can shift quite suddenly, thus leading to the 'stumbling' they [Mitchell and Snyder] speak of."[18] The "short-circuiting" of aesthetic nervousness, while closely related to the "stumbling" of narrative prosthesis, manifests in a wider variety of forms. Quayson outlines what he takes to be the predominant forms of aesthetic nervousness in his—admittedly incomplete and formalistic—typology of nine disability categories, of which three are relevant to Soyinka's work:

> Disability as bearer of moral deficit/evil . . .
> Disability as signifier of ritual insight . . .
> Disability as hermeneutical impasse[19]

Quayson thus suggests that it is necessary to move beyond mere frames of narrative prosthesis toward a consideration of "disability's resonance on a

---

17   Mitchell and Snyder, *Narrative*, 7.
18   Quayson, *Aesthetic Nervousness*, 25.
19   Quayson, *Aesthetic Nervousness*, 52.

multiplicity of levels simultaneously,"[20] while retaining Mitchell and Snyder's basic framework of disability as an unsettling moral encounter.

While aesthetic nervousness softens somewhat the vitriolic implications associated with narrative prosthesis, it nevertheless maintains Mitchell and Snyder's fundamental criticism that narrativized disability engages in a troubling instrumentality that consequently flattens the concept and, by extension, devalues the lived experiences of disabled people. Taking issue with this aspect of Quayson's (along with Mitchell and Snyder's) approach, Michael Bérubé cautions against exclusively negative readings, claiming that disability should retain critical meanings in literature.[21]

Bérubé's assertion is that disability in narrative necessarily functions literarily and that to require, as Mitchell and Snyder do explicitly and Quayson does obliquely, that representations of disability should not be interpretive is to deny their inherent literary qualities. He advocates instead a continuously hermeneutic approach, which has extra resonances for theatrical texts in the sense that not only will the reader (and audience) be in a different interpretive orientation each time they encounter the work but also the text will be continuously reinterpreted from production to production (and even from performance to performance) by the actors who perform the play. Bérubé, who attributes the initial suggestion to performance and disability scholar Leon Hilton, argues for a rereading of Quayson's aesthetic nervousness in which the "short-circuiting" that occurs is free of value judgments:

> It remains to us, in other words, to do more with Quayson's metaphor than he does. For when electrical current is diverted through an areas of lower resistance, some functions that the current is supposed to serve may very well be "disabled," ... "Disabling" an aspect of narrative by way of a short circuit, therefore, implies no normative judgments about what a narrative ought to be.[22]

Bérubé's project involves an extension of this nonnormative sense of aesthetic nervousness to a variety of texts that engage, both directly and indirectly, with intellectual disabilities and so extends Quayson's complications of narrativized disability.

---

20   Quayson, *Aesthetic Nervousness*, 28.
21   Michael Bérubé, *The Secret Life of Stories: From Don Quixote to Harry Potter, How Understanding Intellectual Disability Transforms the Way We Read* (New York: New York University Press, 2016), 48.
22   Bérubé, *Secret Life*, 56.

In the context of specifically postcolonial literature occupied by Soyinka, Clare Barker articulates the central tension between postcolonial and disability scholarship: "Put starkly, postcolonial critical readers often valorize metaphor for its capacity to establish connections between divergent experiences and to draw attention to oppressive social and political practices, whereas the disability community accentuates the alienating or stigmatizing effects of metaphorical representation."[23] Quayson, as an adept postcolonial and disability scholar, attempts to navigate this contradiction in his evaluation of Wole Soyinka, arguing that "what emerges as aesthetic nervousness in this work is underscored by an apparently irresolvable paradox tied to the peculiar relationship that is established between ritual dispositions and the process for the production of subjectivity and agency, a process that is in the last instance political."[24] Soyinka's emphasis on disability as ritual, for Quayson, "acts as a marker of both ritual and political, but in ways that interrupt the two domains and force us to rethink the conceptual movement between the two."[25] Extending the ritual function into the realm of theatrical signification, Soyinka himself argues that the shared space of performer and audience "is threatening because, unlike a similar parable on canvas, its fragility is experienced both at the level of its symbolism and in terms of sympathetic concern for the well-being of that immediate human medium."[26]

The instability of disability representation intersects with the instability of theatrical representation in ways that hypostasize Soyinka's open-ended projects that "pursue diverse, even conflicting objectives, sometimes simultaneously."[27] Indeed, very little in Soyinka is subject to straightforward interpretive models, and Quayson's comparatively complex ones are an admirable engagement with an author who is notorious for resisting interpretation. However, by relying on the assumptions of traditional (western and northern) disability studies that frame disability as always already a crisis that requires a regressively prosthetic solution from normative authors and readers, Quayson risks eliding the particular postcolonial (southern) context of Soyinka's writings. Barker contends that the definition of "normal" as used

---

23   Clare Barker, *Postcolonial Fiction and Disability: Exceptional Children, Metaphor, and Materiality* (London: Palgrave Macmillan, 2011), 15.
24   Quayson, *Aesthetic Nervousness*, 117.
25   Quayson, *Aesthetic Nervousness*, 29.
26   Soyinka, *Myth*, 41.
27   Jeyifo, *Wole*, 88.

in traditional disability studies is not directly applicable to postcolonial literature, since "normalcy is culturally contingent rather than universal—what is considered to be a 'normal' or 'disabled' form of embodiment in one location does not necessarily hold true elsewhere."[28] As I will show, Soyinka's location of his plays in a hybridized postcolonial Yoruba cultural context provides an environment that may not be directly mapped onto other social configurations of disabled or "normal" bodies.

Barker also takes issue with the "crisis" model of disability that undergirds both narrative prosthesis and aesthetic nervousness, arguing that "many postcolonial disability narratives do not present this sense of 'crisis' but are flexible in their narrative strategies, empathetic towards their disabled characters, and explore disability as a matter-of-fact and quotidian aspect of complex sociocultural formations."[29] Echoing Bérubé's call for a less value-laden approach to metaphorical treatments of disability, Barker emphasizes the positive possibilities for disability representation in postcolonial writing that reflects an alternative conception of both normality and abnormality. In contrast to Quayson, Barker argues that

> "prosthetic" readings of texts . . . may signal a scarcity of critical methodologies with which to analyze disability representations more holistically, rather than any innate "crisis" in the image or narrative itself. It is through developing the analytical tools to read for disability in material terms—rather than accepting literature's prosthetic analogies at face value—that we can access the more positive disability narratives that are present in fiction and that suggest alternative, enabling trajectories for disability in postcolonial cultural locations.[30]

I would contend that Quayson's theorization of aesthetic nervousness is an important, if unfinished, stage in the development of exactly the sort of holistic analytical tools that Barker calls for. By extending aesthetic nervousness, pace Bérubé, to literary (and dramatic) texts without ascribing inherently negative values to them—and attending, pace Barker, to cultural specificities and alternative conceptions of postcolonial subjectivity—a broader and more inclusive analysis of disability may be possible.

The theater of Wole Soyinka serves as a particularly apt case study for this methodological orientation due to his simultaneous engagements with paradoxical and open-ended ideological orientations that challenge any simplistic

---

28 Barker, *Postcolonial*, 4.
29 Barker, *Postcolonial*, 20.
30 Barker, *Postcolonial*, 21.

political commitments and his devotion to specifically Yoruban cultural signifiers that offer unique orientations toward disability. As Julie Nack Ngue suggests in her review of Quayson,[31] a consideration of Achille Mbembe's concept of postcolonial vulgarity adds more nuance to Quayson's analysis of Soyinka's disabled characters. Further, a consideration of the postcolonial implications of debility, informed by the work of Julie Livingston[32] and Jasbir Puar,[33] offers a globalized political context for the specifically African settings of Soyinka's plays. In my subsequent readings of disability in three of Soyinka's plays, I will utilize this extended conception of aesthetic nervousness to explore the specific political and cultural implications for disability in his work and also to suggest that traditional postcolonial and disability readings (alone) are insufficient for a nuanced interpretation of Soyinka's theater.

"People of Obàtálá"

In a 1992 interview with the German Africanist Ulli Beier, Soyinka drew an explicit distinction among cultural treatments of disability, remarking that "Europeans tend to hide such people, whereas Yoruba religion actually accounts for them."[34] He refers here to the treatment in Yoruba cosmology of the *orisa,* Obàtálá, Yoruban deity of creation, described by Soyinka as the "god of soul purity . . . to him belongs the function of molding human beings . . . . One day, however, Obatala allowed himself to take a little too much of that potent draught, palm wine. His craftsman's fingers slipped badly and he moulded cripples, albinos and the blind."[35] As Adegbindin explains:

> The Yorùbá language and oral tradition are replete with sayings that establish these individuals as companions of Òrìṣà-ńlá. This, by implication, shows that it is not out of place to categorize the hunchback, the cripple, the albino, and the

---

31   Julie Nack Ngue, "Aesthetic Nervousness: Disability and the Crisis of Representation (Review)," *Journal of Literary & Cultural Disability Studies* 4, no. 3 (2010): 333–335.
32   Livingston, *Debility and the Moral Imagination in Botswana* (Bloomington: Indiana University Press, 2005).
33   Jasbir Puar, *The Right to Maim: Debility, Capacity, Disability* (Durham, NC: Duke University Press, 2017).
34   Wole Soyinka, *Orisha Liberates the Mind: Wole Soyinka on Yoruba Religion: A Conversation with Ulli Beier* (Beyreuth, Germany: Iwalewa, 1992).
35   Soyinka, *Myth*, 15.

dwarf as the major *eni-oòsà* and others—the blind, the dumb, persons with 'invisible disabilities', and so on—as the minor *eni-oòsà*.[36]

The special treatment that Yoruba religion requires for the disabled is reflected in *The Swamp Dwellers*, where a blind beggar finds his way to the home of the old man, Makuri, who is puzzled by the beggar's desire to work and exclaims, "But you're blind. Why don't you beg like others? There is no true worshipper that would deny you this charity!"[37] The blind beggar in *The Swamp Dwellers* reflects some of the characteristics of the divinity—in his ritual insight, patience, and healing. Patrick Colm Hogan notes how he "is scrupulously penitent, worrying over the purity of his blessings and over the alms he has accepted . . . like the sins of Obatala, minor crimes in the larger scheme of things. Indeed, Obatala forever eschews palm wine because of his errors in making, which resulted from inebriation—a point stressed by Soyinka. The Beggar too, alone among those in the play, refuses liquor."[38] *The Swamp Dwellers* concludes with an act of sanctification: the beggar grants a blessing to the house—one that he has withheld throughout the play despite the requests of multiple characters for the bestowal of his ritual power as a disabled person.

The charitable treatment of *eni-oòsà* by the Yoruba is not exclusively positive, however. Adegbindin acknowledges how among the Yoruba disabled people are subject to "institutional exclusion, enfeebling sense of shame, socio-economic limitations associated with disability."[39] Aspects of this treatment are reflected in *The Swamp Dwellers*, particularly in other characters' dismissive responses to the beggar's desire to work. However, the ritual function he serves in the play more directly recalls Soyinka's characterization of Obàtálá: "His beauty is enigmatic, expressive only of the resolution of plastic healing through the wisdom of acceptance. Obatala's patient suffering is the well-known aesthetics of the saint."[40] This near-saintliness that the beggar reflects might strike some disability scholars as reminiscent of the trope of

---

36   Omotade Adegbindin, "Disability and Human Diversity: A Reinterpretation of Eni-Òòsà Philosophy in Yorùbá Belief," *Yoruba Studies Review* 3, no. 1 (2018): 78.

37   Wole Soyinka, *Wole Soyinka: Collected Plays 1* (Oxford: Oxford University Press, 1983), 89.

38   Patrick Colm Hogan, "Particular Myths, Universal Ethics: Wole Soyinka's *The Swamp Dwellers* in the New Nigeria," *Modern Drama* 41, no. 4 (1998): 591

39   Adegbindin, "Disability," 92.

40   Soyinka, *Myth*, 143.

the innocently angelic sufferer, particularly common in sentimental Western literature and cultural production of the past few centuries.[41] However, while the portrayal of the beggar in *The Swamp Dwellers* seems to grant him some features of ritual insight, patience, and healing, the characterization, taken in its appropriate cultural context, is far more nuanced and recognizably human than a straightforwardly prosthetic reading might suggest.

A similar dynamic of ritual and godly reflection may be found in *The Strong Breed*'s character of Ifada, the "idiot" boy, who the protagonist, Eman, saves from sacrificial murder by substituting himself as the target of the village's ritual festival. The play reflects the tension between Soyinka's conception of the disabled as created and thus protected by Obàtálá and the actual treatment of disabled people among the Yoruba (and other West Africans), which is often anything but charitable. Indeed, the association with Obàtálá, and the category of *eni-oòsà*, is often used as a pretext for discrimination and a justification for stigma. In *The Strong Breed*, Soyinka portrays Ifada as an innocent, marked for victimhood and ritual purgation by the village in a way that forces Eman to sacrifice his own life in exchange. As Quayson contends, "At a very basic level, the play suggests that Ifada is 'naturally' contaminated, and yet, at another, it makes us recoil from the ultimate implication of that naturalization, that is, that he could be seized upon violently and against his will as a sacrificial carrier by the sheer fact of his disability."[42]

Wright somewhat dismissively suggests that "the imprisonment of Obatala may form a distant backdrop to the abduction of Ifada and its subsequent energizing of Eman, as Ogun-surrogate . . . but nothing is made in the text, beyond the perverse notion that he has been sent to suffer, of the idiot's sacred link with Obatala and the play operates perfectly well on a level that makes no reference to mythic archetypes."[43] Such an evaluation assumes that disability functions in the play solely as an indicator of suffering, abjection, and lack, which certainly would be consistent with the way most European writers have approached the subject. By disregarding Ifada and Eman's ritualized connections to the deities, Wright reduces both characters to stock

---

41   See Howard Margolis and Arthur Shapiro, "Countering Negative Images of Disability in Classical Literature," *English Journal* 76, no. 3 (1987): 18–22; Ann Dowker, "The Treatment of Disability in 19th and Early 20th Century Children's Literature," *Disability Studies Quarterly* 24, no. 1 (2004); and Paul K. Longmore, "The Cultural Framing of Disability: Telethons as a Case Study," *PMLA* 120, no. 2 (2005): 502–508.
42   Quayson, *Aesthetic Nervousness*, 122.
43   Wright, "Ritual," 55.

heroes and victims. Joel Adedeji's interpretation engages more directly with the dramatic action for a more dynamic reading of the character relationship:

> Eman feels towards Ifada and as he discovers him, he identifies with his spirituality. Seing beyond the latter's visible appearance, he recognises him as 'eni orisa' (the one who belongs to Obatala, the divinity). He thus assimilates the profound reality of Obatala through a cognitive process. Eman is driven to challenge a basic flaw in a society which exploits humans of the nature of Ifada as a sacrificial lamb.[44]

Eman's attitude here is consistent with Adegbindin's argument that it is a mistake to view disabled people as marked for exclusion by Òbàtálá: "Contrary to the conventional thought that Òrìsà-ńlá molds "deformed" or "abnormal" human forms as a way of punishing certain individuals, the deity molds *aesthetically* differing human forms according to his own fancy and to communicate his idea of normalcy in material terms."[45] There is nothing "naturally contaminated" about Ifada, unless we as audience members assume that the protagonist of the play is completely mistaken in his resistance to the village's persecution. A radical disability reading might rather suggest that *The Strong Breed*, like *The Swamp Dwellers*, utilizes the mythic dimensions of the *eni-oòsà* to demonstrate a condemnation of the prejudices and inhuman treatment that Yoruba culture expresses toward disabled people.

Egungun and *Adema* Masquerades

Murano, the character of the limping and (presumably) deaf servant in Soyinka's *The Road* is a far less humanized figure than *The Swamp Dweller*'s beggar, or *The Strong Breed*'s Ifada, but this is not least due to the fact that *The Road* is a substantially less humanistic play. In *The Road*, a variety of characters converge at a roadside auto parts store run by a pompous and enigmatic forger and thief, Professor, along with Murano, his henchman. Early in the play, there is an offstage accident where an *egungun* masquerader disappears and may or may not have been killed. Throughout the play's series of absurdist and tragicomic interactions it becomes clear that what has disappeared is only the *egungun* mask, which is now in the possession of the professor and Murano. *The Road* culminates with Murano's

---

44 Joel Adedeji, "Aesthetics of Soyinka's Theatre," in *Before Our Very Eyes: Tribute to Wole Soyinka*, ed. Dapo Adelugba (Ibadan: Spectrum, 1987), 110.
45 Adegbindin, "Disability," 93.

performance of a feverish *egungun* masquerade dance that so panics the other characters that the professor is stabbed, while the stage directions indicate that "[*The mask still spinning, has continued to sink slowly until it appears to be nothing beyond a heap of cloth and raffia. Still upright in his chair, Professor's head falls forward. Welling fully from the darkness falling around him, the dirge*]."[46] Murano's disabled body literally disappears through the performance of an *egungun* masquerade dance, putatively enacted to discover the truth, while ultimately capping the semiotic confusions present throughout the play.

Murano's most undeniable quality is his mysterious symbolic unintelligibility, which becomes increasingly disorienting and violent throughout the play. However, as Jeyifo contends, "if 'meaning' in this play is elusive and its articulations shrouded in esoteric discourses and symbols, nobody, reader or stage audience, could possibly miss what the play, phenomenologically, is about, what it powerfully evokes through its dramatic action: the carnage of human lives on the roads and highways of the coastal strip of West Africa."[47] Murano, through the ambiguity and discomfort related to his disability, signifies on both the material implications for precarious bodies, as well as a multiplicity of metaphysical and spiritual identities. Further, Murano, much as the villagers in *The Strong Breed*, is consistently bound up with the masquerade practices of the *egungun* ancestor cult, portrayed as a haunting, threatening, and ritualistic presence in both plays.

Murano tends to be interpreted by critics as a cipher, a divinity, or pure symbol, but considerations of the functions that he fulfills in *The Road* ought to take into account the specific contexts of Yoruba ritual, particularly with regard to the relationship between disability and the *egungun* and *alarinjo* masquerades. The origin of *alarinjo*, as a dance-drama masquerade performance associated with the *egungun* cult of ancestor worship, is connected with theatricalized representations of disability, as related by historians of Nigerian theater Dapo Adelugba and Olu Obafemi:

> Customarily, emissaries would be sent to the old site of the capital city for reconnaissance, but the Oyo Mesi sent, ahead of the king's emissaries, six ghost-mummers to frighten them off the site. . . . The ghost-mummers sent by the Oyo Mesi each represented a councilor—the albino (Alapinni), the leper (Asipa), the hunchback (Basorun), the prognathous (Samu), the cripple (Akiniku) and the

---

46   Soyinka, *Collected Plays 1*, 229.
47   Jeyifo, *Wole*, 145.

dwarf (Laguna) . . . hunters captured the ghost-mummers, who were brought to the palace where they became entertainers under Ologbin Ologbojo.[48]

The original *egungun* masqueraders then were closely associated, as in *The Road*, with both fictionalized representations of disability and a sense of spiritual intimidation and threat based on subterfuge. John Thabiti Willis, emphasizes the explicitly political dimensions of early *egungun* performance, "Egungun and Gelede emerged as institutionalized practices that harnessed the collaborative and often conflicted interests of royals, producers of material goods, and ritual specialists."[49] The political dimensions of *The Road* are external to most of the play's action and characters; however, the play's politics are implicated through the presence of *egungun*, which is suggested by Particulars Joe's generally inexplicable interest in the disappeared masquerader. Contemporary *egungun* is frequently explicitly political, particularly when utilizing the characters of "a moron (*dindinrin*), one with mumps (*eleekedindi*) one with the oversized teeth (*eleyin wambo*), one with oversized ears (*eleti ehoro*), the Hausa man (*gambari*), the Nupe man (*Tapa*), and the Whiteman (*oyinbo*)."[50] Interestingly, both the *egungun* masquerade and the palm wine that Murano taps daily for Professor in *The Road*, are considered taboo to Obàtálá, producing another culturally specific tension for Soyinka's Yoruba audiences.

An additional layer of ritualistic significance is added by the reference in the play's prologue to *agemo*, a masquerading practice similar to *egungun*, although with some important distinctions. As Indian postcolonial theater and dance scholar Ketu H. Katrak explains,

> The agemo masqueraders, like the Egungun, parade through Ijeu towns during festival times. . . . One is apprenticed to be an agemo masquerader from childhood and is initiated through chants, certain sacrifices, and two forms of puri-

---

48   Dapo Adelugba and Olu Obafemi, "Anglophone West Africa: Nigeria," *A History of Theatre in Africa*, ed. Martin Banham (Cambridge: Cambridge University Press, 2004), 141.
49   John Thabiti Willis, *Masquerading Politics: Kinship, Gender, and Ethnicity in a Yoruba Town* (Bloomington: Indiana University Press, 2018): 42–43.
50   Jubril Adesegun Dosumu, "Masks and Masques in Yoruba Ritual Festivals: Unmasking the Past for the Present and the Future," *Orisa: Yoruba Gods and Spiritual Identity in Africa and the Diaspora*, ed. Toyin Falola and Ann Genova (Trenton, NJ: Africa World, 2005), 118.

fication. Only then is one allowed to enter the agemo shrine in the forest where the costumes are always kept. The Yoruba believe that one enters the shrine as flesh and emerges as "the spirit of the dead.[51]

The most relevant distinction between the *agemo* and the *egungun* masquerades has to do with the distinctions between how they are perceived by the audience as engaging in greater or lesser degrees of theatrical illusion. Soyinka himself, as quoted by Katrak, describes the relationship thusly:

> Some agemo are just like any other egungun masquerade. There are certain others who dance within mats rolled around their bodies. The human being, the form is there [inside the mats]. After a while, this form dances, dances into a terrific whirl and then it just collapses. There is absolutely nothing inside the mat. . . . So I use agemo in this sense as illusion. It's different from the egungun in that sense, i.e., there is no attempt at illusion in the egungun masquerade as there is in the agemo. But when the parade of the agemo begins, you don't distinguish them from the main egungun.[52]

This process of the disappearance of the body in the paroxysm of masquerade dance is precisely what happens to Murano at the end of *The Road*, which reveals that what was perceived as an *egungun* masquerade was actually an *agemo* one and thus directly concerned with the disappearance (or "dissolution") of the flesh.

Katrak argues that the characters of Professor, Kotonu (a traumatized and depressed driver), and Murano are implicated by the *agemo* ritual as occupying positions on a continuum between pure flesh and pure divine, where "Professor is the farthest from experiencing the divine, Murano is the closest, and Kotonu is in between."[53] Although Katrak does not mark it, from a disability perspective the characters she identifies as experiencing some measure of divinity are all at least marginally disabled. Murano has clearly identifiable physical disabilities and is taken to be closest to the divine, while Kotonu is indirectly identified as mentally disabled. Like the Obàtálá parallels in *The Swamp Dwellers* and *The Strong Breed*, the representations of disabled characters in *The Road* exist in complex relationships to divinity, politics, and ritual traditions. The context of the masquerade in which they are presented renders these characters less immediately intelligible but certainly no less nuanced.

---

51 Ketu H. Katrak, *Wole Soyinka and Modern Tragedy: A Study of Dramatic Theory and Practice* (Westport, CT: Greenwood, 1986), 103.
52 Katrak, *Wole*, 68.
53 Katrak, *Wole*, 69.

Debility and Postcolonial Vulgarity

Written following Soyinka's imprisonment in the Biafran civil war, *Madmen and Specialists* may appear uncharacteristically materialist and bleak. The portrayal of disability in the play is even more prominent than in his other works, involving a choral quartet of Mendicants with a variety of impairments, alongside Old Man, a former "specialist" in treating war victims, whose own mental condition appears to swing considerably throughout the play. The plot, insofar as the play has one, has to do with the Mendicants' employment by Dr. Bero, an erstwhile surgeon-turned-intelligence investigator and son to Old Man, to kidnap and detain Old Man, who had previously operated the rehabilitation center where the Mendicants had been housed. Old Man espouses a cryptically subversive philosophy of "As" with which he has indoctrinated the Mendicants in order to undermine the military establishment.

The play culminates with the attempted murder of Cripple, one of the Mendicants, by Old Man along with the other Mendicants, after Cripple tries to ask a question concerning "As." However, the murder is prevented by Dr. Bero, who shoots and kills Old Man as he is about to cut open Cripple's chest. The Mendicants, presumably including the almost-murdered Cripple, end the play "gleefully" singing the song in praise of "As" that they have sung periodically throughout the play, except this time, "*The song stops in mid-word and the lights snap out simultaneously.*"[54]

Femi Osofisan, the Nigerian playwright who also happened to be an actor in the premiere of *Madmen and Specialists*, contends that the play is radically unconventional:

> It does not narrate a story as such; its main purpose, instead, is to narrate a historical *situation*, one that is macabre, and immensely frightening, by animating it with graphic and telling illustrations. Its goal is not catharsis therefore, but rather shock and psychic wounding: an attempt to confront the audience with its own mirror of horror, to immerse it in the excretions of its own prevailing brutalities, the sanious nightmare of its *condition humaine*. Hence you could not say what the play was *about*, only what it did to your psyche and to your mind.[55]

---

54 Katrak, *Wole*, 276.
55 Femi Osofisan, "A Playwright's Encounter with the Drama of Soyinka," in *Wole Soyinka: An Appraisal*, ed. Adewale Maja-Pearce (Portsmouth, NH: Heinemann, 1985), 179–180.

The disabled characters in *Madmen and Specialists*, particularly the Mendicants, do not follow Soyinka's tendencies in other works to associate disability with ritual or mysticism. Frances Harding suggests that the donning of a surgical mask by Old Man invokes a connection to *egungun* masquerade that "transforms his living self into an ancestor, anticipating and inviting his own death."[56] More thematically, Barney McCartney illustrates that the Mendicants perform parodic functions in the play analogous to *egungun* performers:

> They not only act as a chorus in the play and satirize the actions of others, but they are also satirists satirized—as all tricksters are. We laugh both with them and at them. They provide, as masks do, a distancing device, a method of indirection allowing us to look rather closely at realities we would otherwise not face. Also, our own laughter becomes a physiognomic mask for us so we can participate in what comes close, at times, to a satirical ritual.[57]

However, such connections are oblique in comparison with Soyinka's earlier works, even as the literal presence of disability in the play is much more ubiquitous.

In *Madmen and Specialists*, Quayson argues, "The representation of ritual as organically deriving from a coherent context, whether real or imagined, is no longer considered possible."[58] Quayson, following Jeyifo, attributes this shift to Soyinka's experience in the Biafran war that rendered him "no longer able to stand at any point outside the system to manufacture an artistic critique of it. He has been too emotionally affected by the chaos to be entirely free from it."[59] This view leads Quayson to consider the relationship between Dr. Bero and Old Man as a dialectic that would otherwise be either resolved or confounded by the Mendicants in their quasi-choric role, but instead "the mendicants end up providing an assimilable spectacle rather than a stubborn singularity."[60] Indeed, for Quayson, the Mendicants' mutable assimilability,

---

56 Frances Harding, "Soyinka and Power: Language and Imagery in *Madmen and Specialists*," in *African Theatre in Performance: A Festschrift in Honour of Martin Banham*, ed. Dele Layiwola (Charlotte, NC: Harwood, 2000), 113.
57 Barney McCartney, "Traditional Satire in Wole Soyinka's Madmen and Specialists," *Journal of Postcolonial Writing* 14, no. 2 (1975): 506–513.
58 Quayson, *Aesthetic Nervousness*, 129.
59 Quayson, *Aesthetic Nervousness*, 145.
60 Quayson, *Aesthetic Nervousness*, 141.

"simultaneously *within* and *without, for* and *against* the system,"[61] suggests an aesthetic nervousness because "they are capable of questioning the system, reminding its operatives of their shared humanity."[62] Moreover, Quayson contends that the Mendicants, despite their capabilities, are only assimilated by each side in turn, and ultimately portray a "lack of self-reflexivity" whereby "they are really only docile subjects."[63] Quayson laments the missed opportunities whereby the Mendicants could have become "the heroic protagonists for a way out of the impasse produced by the war mentality,"[64] thereby fulfilling the role occupied by the Ogunian figures in Soyinka's earlier plays. I contend that Quayson's ascription of docility to these characters, along with his implication of their simplistically metaphorical significations, fails to take full account of the Mendicants' performative self-awareness, histories of debilitation, or their status as complexly postcolonial subjects.

In the first scene in *Madmen and Specialists*, the Mendicants are discovered playing dice and gambling their body parts in a darkly comic and carnivalesque display that they indicate has become something of a regular practice:

CRIPPLE:	When do I get my eye, Aafaa?
AAFAA:	Was it the right or the left?
GOYI:	Does it matter?
AAFAA:	Sure it does. If it's the right one he can take it out now. The left is my evil eye and I need it a while longer.
CRIPPLE:	It was the right.
AAFAA:	I've just remembered the right is my evil eye.
CRIPPLE:	I'll make you an offer. Let me throw against both of you for Goyi's stumps. I'll stake the eye Aafaa lost to me.
GOYI:	Why leave me out? I still want to try my luck.
BLINDMAN:	You have nothing left to stake.
CRIPPLE:	You're just a rubber ball, Goyi. You need a hand to throw with, anyway.
GOYI:	I can use my mouth.
AAFAA:	To throw dice? You'll eat sand my friend.
BLINDMAN:	Sooner or later we all eat sand."[65]

---

61 Quayson, *Aesthetic Nervousness*, 137.
62 Quayson, *Aesthetic Nervousness*, 136.
63 Quayson, *Aesthetic Nervousness*, 140.
64 Quayson, *Aesthetic Nervousness*, 144.
65 Wole Soyinka, *Wole Soyinka: Collected Plays 2* (Oxford: Oxford University Press, 1974), 217–218.

The Mendicants thus begin the play with an expression of acute self-awareness, recognizing their impairments and capacities of their bodily states, cheerfully and anarchically signifying on the rituals of their military past. As Walcott describes the characters' behavior, "In their improvised satiric sketches, taught to them by the mad father at the rehabilitation centre, they parody the activities of war and totalitarian military regimes which have reduced them to this state: namely, mutilation by torture, castration or amputation (in the course of the play this grim burlesque gets out of hand and becomes increasingly hard to distinguish from reality)."[66] Throughout the play, the Mendicants engage in episodes of ribald singing alongside parodic enactments of biopower in the form of interrogations, surgeries, and sermons. This leads Walcott to the conclusion that "the Mendicants are in fact self-consciously theatrical and therefore self-determining creatures who are always, in some measure, performing. They exaggerate and control their disabilities in the service of their trade and in their various vaudeville sketches they present themselves, by turns, as victims and persecutors, alternatively mocking and identifying with official sadism."[67] While these acts of self-awareness are often in the supposed service of either Dr. Bero or the Old Man, their continued repetition and resignification indicates a complexity in function that undermines simple metaphoric or prosthetic interpretations.

In *Madmen and Specialists*, the Mendicants, along with Old Man, are disabled by the social treatment of their particular impairments; but equally, if not more importantly, they are also debilitated by their experience in the war that serves as the play's background. The sense that Julie Livingston proposes for debility in the context of Botswana is apropos to the condition experienced by the play's characters whose "impairment and disfigurement arise out of particular junctures ... and thus it gives us insight into a people's historical experience and changing assumptions about personhood and self."[68] In her Botswana case study, Livingston found that the impairments experienced by her subjects existed in a complex relationship between social stigma and postcolonial animus, so that questions of care involved both the negotiation of everyday barriers and a resentment of the colonizing forces that helped contribute to the need for care. All of the male characters in *Madmen and Specialists* have been profoundly affected and debilitated by their experiences in the war and its continued impact on their lives. The Mendicants

---

66   Walcott, "Transition," 21.
67   Walcott, "Transition," 22–23.
68   Livingston, *Debility*, 2.

are traumatized and have lost limbs or senses, Old Man has lost capacity for rational thought, and even Dr. Bero appears to have lost any appreciable moral sense. While a critic like Quayson views this aspect of the drama as serving to flatten the stories of disabled bodies into a comment on the barbarity of war, queer theorist Jasbir Puar suggests that an acknowledgment and exploration of debility, particularly in the Global South, offers a keener sense of the extent of disability's insidiousness in such contexts: "Rethinking disability through the precarity of populations not only acknowledges that there is more disability within disenfranchised and precarious populations, but also insists that debilitation is a tactical practice deployed in order to create and precaritize populations and maintain them as such."[69] Indeed, some sense of this is found in Dr. Bero's frustration at the seeming failure, under Old Man's care, of the Mendicants to remain docile in their debilitation:

> BERO: [*heatedly.*] It's not his charitable propensities I am concerned with. Father's assignment was to help the wounded readjust to the pieces and remnants of their bodies. Physically. Teach them to make baskets if they still had fingers. To use their mouths and ply needles if they had none, or use it to sing if their vocal chords had not been shot away. Teach them to amuse themselves, make something of themselves. Instead he began to teach them to think, think, THINK! Can you picture a more treacherous deed than to place a working mind a mangled body?[70]

Arising from his position as a specialist in both medicine and the military, Dr. Bero clearly views the Mendicants as invalids whose time needs to be occupied and made productive rather than personally satisfying. Dr. Bero does not see them as a threat to the biopolitical power structures that he represents.

Dr. Bero envies Old Man's capacity to manipulate and control, rather than any ritualistic or metaphysical truth that might conceivably exist in his philosophy of As. What matters to Bero is the capability to utilize the illogical language of traditional spirituality to affect and persuade those who have experienced the misfortune of debility. Both of the play's specialists are engaged in coercively biopolitical manipulations of the Mendicants, and the broader implication is that the war has turned all of the men into immoral or sadistic specialists and debilitated madmen. The implications for disability are not merely at the level of collateral (and certainly not only metaphorical)

---

69   Puar, *Right to Maim*, 72–73.
70   Soyinka, *Collected Plays 2*, 242.

damage but rather the very means by which the processes of biopower in the Global South are consciously carried out on and through debilitated bodies and minds. Barker suggests that in postcolonial contexts, "To tell a story about colonialism or its aftermath, it is often necessary to tell a story about disability. . . . 'Broken' bodies may signify partitioned countries, troubled minds represent a nation's collective trauma, and blindness might stand in for a refusal of leaders to 'see' the lives and circumstances of their subjects."[71] While such representations are undoubtedly metaphorical, at least in part, they need not be flattening, particularly in so complex a piece as *Madmen and Specialists*.

The most curious criticisms lodged by Quayson with regard to this play is that compared to the socially inquisitive characters in Soyinka's other plays, "The mendicants in *Madmen and Specialists* do not produce any such questioning outside the framework that is established for them by others."[72] This observation is central to Quayson's characterization of the Mendicants as "docile," and the consequently prosthetic function he attributes to them in the play. However, to make such a claim seems to ignore a number of events, not least among them the climactic moment of the play when Cripple dares to question Old Man about the doctrine of As. As described by Harding:

> He (the Old Man) is interrupted by the Cripple who wants to do the very thing which Old Man's lessons in thinking must lead him to do—ask a question . . . At no point is the perverted authority of either of the Beros threatened or challenged. Only when Cripple tries to ask a question which may be the very one that those in power fear the most (we never find out the question), does Old man realise the danger and shouts out.[73]

It is precisely Cripple's stepping outside the awe and worship demanded by Old Man before the metaphysical power of "As" that instigates the violent reaction from Old Man and the other Mendicants, leading both to the threat of violence and also to the actual murder at the play's climax.

Moreover, the Mendicants choric and carnivalesque behavior, following Old Man's death as well as throughout the play, indicate the particular expression of postcolonial agency that Achille Mbembe associates with vulgarity. For Mbembe, the grotesquerie of official power in the postcolonial state is reflected not necessarily by condemnation or judgment but through

---

71 Barker, *Postcolonial*, 106.
72 Quayson, *Aesthetic Nervousness*, 140.
73 Harding, "Soyinka and Power," 113.

a complex operation of vulgar ridicule where "the body of the despot, his frowns and his smiles, decrees and commands, the public notices and communiques repeat over and over: these are the primary signifiers, it is these that have force, that get interpreted and reinterpreted, and feed further significance back into the system."[74] While such repetitions do not necessarily appear critical of hegemonic forces, Mbembe argues that "by dancing publicly for the benefit of power, the 'postcolonized subject' is providing his or her loyalty, and by compromising with the corrupting control that state power tends to exercise at all levels of everyday life, the subject is reaffirming that this power is incontestable—*precisely the better to play with it and modify it whenever possible.*"[75]

This game of repetition and reconfiguration is visible throughout the Mendicants' various interruptions of the dramatic action, from the very beginning of the play when they roll dice for body parts, through to their foreshadowing parody of Dr. Bero's interrogation ("Truth hurts. I am a lover of truth. Do you find you also love truth? Then let's have the truth,"[76]) and also their exposure of Old Man's manipulative quasi-religiosity. Even as the Mendicants may appear to be submitting to the will of either Dr. Bero or Old Man throughout the course of the play, their status as demonstrably self-aware, purposefully debilitated, and vulgarly acquiescent suggests that while their submissions may not be entirely voluntary, they are also not the actions of docilely disabled functionaries. *Madmen and Specialists* is a play that is very much about the chaos of war, the insidiousness of biopolitics, and the condition of socially inflicted disabilities. It should not undermine the importance of disability in the play that it bears a complex and shifting relationship to the piece's other central themes.

Conclusion

Through an exploration of Soyinka's dramaturgical use of Yoruban cosmology, West African ritual performances, and postcolonial debilitation and resistance, I have attempted to show that Soyinka's treatment of disability is enmeshed in a social context that although not exclusively liberatory,

---

74 Achille Mbembe, *On the Postcolony* (Berkeley: University of California Press, 2001), 108.
75 Mbembe, *Postcolony*, 129.
76 Soyinka, *Collected Plays 2*, 223.

nonetheless offers a generous and multivalent engagement with disability representation. While the Global North has developed an abundant spate of tropes that marginalize, demonize, and/or instrumentalize disability, it is inappropriate to judge the role of postcolonial literature by exclusively Eurocentric standards. With a playwright such as Wole Soyinka, whose aesthetic and political techniques can be "supremely ambiguous, to the point sometimes of nihilism,"[77] it might be tempting to view his treatment of disability as problematically obscurantist or insufficiently liberating. However, to do so would be to miss the central role that disability plays in Soyinka's occasionally absurd but always penetrating dramaturgical practice. Rather than utilizing disability only as a metaphor to illustrate political concerns, Soyinka employs disability to navigate the paradoxical elements of the postcolonial condition, for both people with and without disabilities.

---

77 Jeyifo, *Wole*, 286.

Chapter Nine

Demonizing Madness

Mental Disorders as *Deus Ex Machina* in Nollywood Movies

Kolawole Olaiya

Although discrimination in different guises is a common worldwide phenomenon, people with developmental disabilities and mental health conditions are frequently discriminated against and stereotyped in many societies. Many even go so far as to argue that mentally challenged people are more discriminated against than any other group.[1] Stories about the mentally challenged in different situations of conflict feature prominently in Nollywood movies. Most of these movies rehash the discrimination against the mentally challenged and uphold the social construction of mental illness as the consequence of moral blemish and spiritual wickedness. Rather than seeing mental impairment as medical and social problems that can be treated and managed, some Nollywood movies depict mental impairments as resulting from spiritual attacks. The situation of the mentally disabled is compounded by negative responses to the impaired person's situation—responses that are largely determined by stereotypical traditional beliefs. Such discriminatory practices contribute to "the perpetuation of discriminatory and stigmatizing attitudes towards persons with mental illness," and form "a barrier to

---

1   Patrick W. Corrigan and David L. Penn, "Lessons from Social Psychology on Discrediting Psychiatric Stigma," *American Psychologist* 54, no. 9 (1999): 765–776.

accessing treatment," which can dissuade the mentally disabled from seeking medical attention where it is needed, thereby worsening their condition.[2]

The demonization of mental health challenges and the labeling of individuals with mental disability as "dangerous, dirty, and a nuisance to society" is common in Nollywood movies.[3] In some cases, the individual with cognitive development challenges becomes the butt of jokes, while in other cases, mental illness is deployed as a subplot and a deus ex machina, as in *Abela Ojomeje*.[4] There is usually a collocation between plot structure and the representations of mental illness, and there is a tendency to use mental illness as a handy resolution device. In such instances, the subplots of madness that are grafted onto the main plots as a resolution device become a very infinitesimal part of the story. The effect of this small part of the story on its overall structure is usually disproportional because it provides the missing link to the loose and sometimes unwieldy melodramatic plot.

Furthermore, while most of the motivations for the conflicts in movies about the mentally challenged are evidently secular, the sudden introduction of supernatural elements at the climax of many stories, like in *Ìwògbè Mirror*, to explain away the actions of certain characters in the movies, helps Nollywood producers to suddenly resolve the central conflict.[5] This sudden resolution is reminiscent of deus ex machina, the device employed by

---

2   Magnus Mfoafo-M'Carthy, Cynthia A. Sottie, and Charles Gyan, "Mental Illness and Stigma: a 10-Year Review of Portrayal through Print Media in Ghana (2003–2012)," *International Journal of Culture and Mental Health* 9, no. 2 (2016): 197–207.

3   O. F. Aina, "Mental Illness and Cultural Issues in West African Films: Implications for Orthodox Psychiatric Practice," *Medical Humanities* (2004): 23–26, 30; V. E. Ampadu, "The Depiction of Mental Illness in Nigerian and Ghanaian Movies: A Negative or Positive Impact on Mental Health Awareness in Ghana" (PhD diss., University of Leeds, 2012); Olayinka Atilola and Funmilayo Olayiwola, "Frames of Mental Illness in the Yoruba Genre of Nigerian Movies: Implications for Orthodox Mental Health Care," *Transcultural Psychiatry* 50, no. 3 (2013): 442–454; Saheed Aderinto, "Representing 'Tradition,' Confusing 'Modernity': Love, Sexuality and Mental Illness in Yoruba (Nigerian) Video Films," in *Mental Illness in Popular Media: Essays on the Representation of Disorders*, ed. Lawrence C. Rubin (Jefferson, NC: McFarland, 2012), 256–269.

4   *Abela Ojomeje*, directed by Sunday Alabi (Lagos: Soars Films Nigeria, 2016).

5   *Ìwògbè Mirror*, directed by Yemi Amodu and Mayor Gbenga Adewusi (Lagos: Bayowa Films and Music International, 2011).

playwrights in the fifth century "especially Euripides, to resolve his plots."⁶ When madness is used as a deus ex machina, it pushes disability as a social status to the periphery. The decentering of mental disability removes emphasis from the cause of the illness, presents the mentally ill as spectacle, and diverts attention from the illness. This chapter explores the representations of mental disorders, especially the relationship between mental illness, religion, morality, and karma, in two Nigerian movies, *Oruka Ijosi* and *Ayo Ni Mo Fe*, which socially construct mental illness as the consequence of moral deficit and spiritual wickedness. These movies also demonize the mentally challenged and use them as deus ex machina to resolve knotty and implausible story features.⁷

The social construction of madness as a consequence of moral ineptitude and spiritual wickedness is a recurrent theme in Nollywood movies. A common trend in movies that focus on popular topics like money-making rituals (the belief that some acquire wealth through rituals that involve the sacrifice of human beings or certain body parts of a living human being), jealous wives, and wicked mothers-in-law is that at the end of the movie, the main culprit (usually the jealous stepmother or aggrieved sibling) confesses to being responsible for the problems of the afflicted and then suddenly loses her mental faculties. The culprit usually ends up as the village idiot or dies. This is common in movies in indigenous languages—especially Yoruba and Ibo languages—and English-language movies that depict madness as the by-product of past infractions of the mentally ill or a family member. Most Yoruba movies perceive mental illness, especially full-blown madness, as a physical manifestation of some spiritual anomaly. As in the proverb about the person who sold sand in place of salt and so was paid in stones, mental impairment becomes the pebbles received as a reward for being dubious.

The understanding of mental illness as the consequence of metaphysical conflicts or the reward for past sins in Yoruba movies reflects the classic good-versus-evil plot. The Yoruba people live mostly in the western part of Nigeria. Adagbada describes them as very religious, and a group to whom

---

6   Oscar Brockett and Franklin Hildy, *History of the Theatre*, 8th ed. (Boston: Allyn and Bacon, 1999), 34.

7   *Oruka Ijosi*, directed by Abiodun Olanrewaju (Lagos: Cabal Production and Toyin Ogungbe Films, 2010); and *Ayo Ni Mo Fe*, directed by Tunde Kelani (Lagos: Mainframe Films and Television Productions, 1994).

"religion is life and life is religion."[8] Aderinto acknowledges the liberal attitude of the Yorubas and argues that they still cling to traditional ways of thinking in some areas. He suggests that the "21st-century Yoruba society showcases a tripartite identity of the traditional/pre-colonial, the modern, and traditional."[9] The way the Yorubas traditionally understand the causes of mental disability can be largely explained by their cosmology. Traditionally, the Yorubas see human beings as the "combination of material (biological/physical) material (spiritual) substances."[10] They see the presence of the spiritual in everything that happens in the physical realm and believe that man can deploy spiritual forces for good and evil purposes. They believe that the forces of good and the forces of evil constantly jostle for the soul of the individual; in order to succeed, the individual must overcome the forces of evil. Aderinto posits that sickness and wellness are attributed to good and evil forces. He explains that to the Yoruba, the "causation of sickness, including mental illness, is mainly coded spiritually, not scientifically. In addition, mental illness is perceived as a state of metaphysical existence controlled by *anjonnu were* or 'the spirit of madness.'"[11] Since the cause of mental illness is attributed to "*anjonnu were*," it is not usually understood as a purely medical problem.[12] Most Yoruba movie producers exploit the idea that mental illness can result from spiritual inflictions as a common trope in their plot.

The way mental illness is presented in Nollywood can affect the way mental illness is understood in Nigeria, because film, television, and newspapers play important roles in educating and shaping the opinions of society. In a ten-year review of the media portrayal of mental illness in Ghana, Mfoafo-M'Carthy, Sottie, and Gyan acknowledge that " the media plays a significant role in the dissemination of information and entertainment and sheds light on issues pertaining to current society."[13] Their study looks at the roles played by the print media in stigmatizing the mentally challenged in Ghana. It examines the influence of the media and concludes that it is in a prime position to affect the beliefs and opinions of Africans. Coverdale, Nairn, and

---

8   Oluwafadekemi Adagbada, "Sociological Analysis of Money Rituals as a Recurrent Theme in Yoruba Films," *New Media and Mass Communication* 32 (2014): 13–20.
9   Aderinto, "Representing," 257.
10 Adagbada, "Sociological," 13.
11 Aderinto, "Representing," 259.
12 Aderinto, "Representing," 259.
13 Mfoafo-M'Carthy, Sottie, and Gyan, "Mental Illness," 197–207.

Claasen aver that "in reporting, the media has the ability to use language, inference or image to either perpetuate society's perception of an issue or transform society's perception through education."[14]

Other studies have also shown that the media can play important roles in the social perception of mental illness. Peter Byrne argues that "television, radio and newspapers play an essential role in public perception of mental illness."[15] Byrne further contends that while "the media often perpetuate unhelpful stereotypes of mental illness, if properly harnessed, they may be used to challenge prejudice, inform and initiate debate and so help combat the stigma experiences by people with mental illness and their careers." Klin describes the media as prominent agents of "socialization that fuels public perceptions about mental illness," among its other functions.[16] Most of the research done in Ghana and Nigeria finds that the portrayal of mental illness in the media has been largely stereotypical and has affirmed traditional myths about mental disabilities.[17]

The discrimination against individuals with mental illness has been practiced worldwide from time immemorial. According to Wallcraft, "Madness has been stigmatized for centuries."[18] But as Salter and Byrne found out in a survey, "Various mental illnesses attracted different types of prejudice."[19] While attempts have always been made to solve the problem of mental illness, such attempts have largely been discriminatory because they rarely consider the interest of the mentally disabled. For example, toward the end of the seventeenth century, madhouses and asylums were intended to remove the mentally disabled from society because they were considered undesirable

---

14 John Coverdale, Raymond Nairn, and Donna Claasen, "Depictions of Mental Illness in Print Media: A Prospective National Sample," *Australian & New Zealand Journal of Psychiatry* 36, no. 5 (2002): 697–700.

15 Peter Byrne, "Psychiatric Stigma: Past, Passing and to Come," *Journal of the Royal Society of Medicine* 90, no. 11 (1997): 618–621.

16 Anat Klin, "Crime and Punishment? The AIDS Narrative in the Daily Press in Israel, 1981–1995 as a Cultural Construction of a Disease" (PhD diss., Hebrew University, 2001).

17 Aina, "Mental Illness"; Ampadu, "Depiction"; Aderinto, "Representing"; Atilola and Olayiwola, "Frames."

18 Jan Wallcraft, "Psychiatrists Fighting Stigma: Doing More Harm Than Good?" *Cross Currents, The Journal of Addiction and Mental Health* 13, no 3. 2010.

19 Mark Salter and Peter Byrne, "The Stigma of Mental Illness: How You Can Use the Media to Reduce It," *Psychiatric Bulletin* 24, no. 8 (2000): 281.

people that should be separated from the rest of society. Foucault has argued that the emergence of psychiatry at the end of the eighteenth century silenced the voices of the mentally disabled and led to the end of the dialogue between "reason" and "madness."[20] This was ultimately part of the impulse to separate those considered socially unfit from society at large. Even with the closure of the asylum in the mid-twentieth century, the stigma against mental illness and the mentally ill has remained rife throughout society.[21]

The pervasive social stigmatization of madness has consequences for the mentally disabled. The stigma attached to mental health conditions often deprives individuals of their agency. Because mental illness is concerned with and relates to problems in the brain, it is often viewed as malaise that affects a person's total being, and therefore the bodies of the mentally ill are seen as diseased. Unlike most illnesses, society often blames the mentally disabled for their illness, instead of focusing on the illness and characterizing adverse mental health conditions as treatable. Moreover, it is generally assumed that mental illness is permanent and incurable and that the mentally challenged, even if cured, are not capable of taking charge of their lives. Mental illness is believed to have a permanent effect on the life of the mentally challenged. The sweeping assumption that they are incapable of making rational decisions, even after their situations have changed, incapacitates them and denies them certain privileges. The myth that the mentally disabled person is abnormal exposes such persons to discrimination that increases their marginalization.[22] The stigma attached to the illness forces the mentally disabled to resort to self-denial. They often become overwhelmed by the illness, since they are ashamed to "seek treatment."[23] In addition, the social rejection and shame attached to mental disability increases their vulnerability to exploitation on many fronts. For example, caregivers, including medical doctors and traditional healers, exploit the mentally disabled, who are at their mercy. Studies have shown that the individuals with mental health challenges are

---

20 Michel Foucault, *Madness and Civilization: A History of Insanity in the Age of Reason* (New York: Vintage, 1988).
21 Corrigan and Penn, "Lessons."
22 Greg Wolbring, "Ability Privilege: A Needed Addition to Privilege Studies," *Journal for Critical Animal Studies* 12, no. 2 (2014): 118–141.
23 Lisa Barney et al., "Stigma about Depression and Its Impact on Help-Seeking Intentions," *Australian & New Zealand Journal of Psychiatry* 40, no. 1 (2006): 51–54.

violently and sexually abused more than any other persons with disabilities.[24] An Ekiti proverb states that "madness is not one of the illnesses one can own up to—while one can admit to having had a flu or a headache in the past, no one will easily admit that he or she was once mad" (my translation). This proverb illustrates the way the Ekitis perceive mental illness. It normalizes the negative social attitude to the mentally challenged.

Normalizing bias against the mentally challenged promotes distrust of individuals suffering from any form of mental illness and is common in many traditional cultures. The effects of social attitudes on disability and the disabled are one of the major concerns of scholars who have developed the social model for studying disabilities. The scholars in this field define "disabilities as being an interaction between physical impairment and the social and cultural environment."[25] They contend that disabilities entail both the "physical struggles with the physical body" and "the larger and more inchoate struggle with the negative and intransigent attitudes toward people with impairments."[26] Scholars in this field are looking beyond the medical and suggest that positive social attitudes toward the disabled can go a long way to help them live a healthy, fulfilling life.

The problems of mentally disabled individuals are compounded by the spiritual dimension to the understanding of mental illness in most African cultures. As Aina contends, in most parts of Africa there still exist "strong beliefs in the existence and the activities of witches, ancestral spirits, sorcerers, diviners."[27] In those societies, it is strongly believed that mental illness can result from harnessing and misusing supernatural forces. The myth that mental illness results from spiritual attacks is the foundation of most Nollywood movies. In some of these movies, the mental challenge occurs when the secret of the "evil" person who causes problems for the victim-hero is revealed. While the victim-hero is magically cured, the problem is resolved, and the audience learns from it. This misapprehension of the ailment turns

---

24 Eileen M. Furey, "Sexual Abuse of Adults with Mental Retardation: Who and Where," *Mental Retardation* 32, no. 3 (1994): 173-180; Dick Sobsey, *Violence and Abuse in the Lives of People with Disabilities: The End of Silent Acceptance?* (Baltimore: Paul H. Brookes, 1994); and Dick Sobsey and Tanis Doe, "Patterns of Sexual Abuse and Assault," *Sexuality and Disability* 9, no. 3 (1991): 243–259.

25 Ato Quayson, *Aesthetic Nervousness: Disability and the Crisis of Representations* (New York: Columbia University Press, 2007), 101.

26 Quayson, *Aesthetic Nervousness*, 101.

27 Aina, "Mental Illness," 23.

a solvable mental health problem into an unfathomable spiritual matter. Attributing mental disability to metaphysical reasons, rather than to social or medical ones, reinforces a myth that disability is the result of individual failures. Ultimately, in a society that believes that mental impairment is incurable because its source is metaphysical, the opportunity to correct the negative social attitudes against the disabled is missed. Instead, these movies reinforce prejudices against mentally impaired individuals and increase their suffering.

Madness as Deus ex Machina in Òrùka Ìjọsí

Oruka Ijosi is a two-part movie produced by Cabal Production and Toyin Ogungbe Films and directed by Abiodun Olanrewaju. The film's underlying philosophy is that poverty is a curse that, figuratively speaking, turns its victim into a doormat. Moyo (Kikelomo Adeyemi) is a victim of poverty in a society where women are coerced into sacrificing their self-esteem in order to survive. The movie uses different scenarios to show Moyo's travails and her vulnerability but also emphasizes the inhumanity of the rich. Like most Yoruba Nollywood movies, the morality of the story is based on the underlying Yoruba philosophy of "reaping whatever one sows." Hence, Moyo, the central female character, can only become financially stable if she does one good deed.

Oruka Ijosi has a fairly complex and unwieldy plot. Kayode, a mean and unruly high school dropout and thug, impregnates Moyo, who is a friend of his stepsister. He tries unsuccessfully to persuade her to abort the pregnancy. Moyo disagrees and has the baby anyway, much to the disappointment of Kayode. Through series of flashbacks, which are a common motif in Nollywood movies, the viewer is taken through Mayo's various sufferings. The exaggeratedly pathetic depiction of Moyo's circumstances makes for poignant commentary on contemporary Nigerian society, where few opportunities are available to the poor, including orphans. It also dramatizes how poverty can intensify the vulnerability of young women and expose them to different kinds of temptations.

In contrast to Kayode, Moyo is kind, considerate, humane, and hospitable. Her kindness pays off when she offers shelter to Adebayo, a man in search of refuge from the rampaging traditional *oro* cultists. The grateful Adebayo (Taiwo Hassan) decides to help Moyo, his benefactor. In the process, they fall in love and start a relationship. Adebayo chooses the path of peace and pays off Kayode and his gang, a costly mistake that results in almost turning Adebayo into their "Automated Banking Machine."

Adebayo decides to fight back when he is no longer able to meet the monetary demands of Kayode and his friends. He calls the bluff of Kayode and his friends, fights with them, and in the process knocks Kayode down with a magical ring given to him by an old man he helped in the past, hence the title, Òrùka Ìjosí (the ring from the past). Adebayo, who does not have the heart to kill a fellow human being, is confused and troubled because he has forgotten the antidote and cannot revive Kayode. In desperation, Adebayo runs to his brother, Alade, for help.

This revelation of the familial relationship between Adebayo and Alade introduces a major subplot that becomes pivotal to the resolution of the movie's conflicts. While the first part of the movie concentrates largely on the dysfunctional relationship between Moyo and Kayode, the second part tells the story of a homeless young man suffering from amnesia who is almost lynched by hostile neighbors. Through a melodramatic set of coincidences, the hapless man meets Alade (Yinka Quadri), who eventually adopts him. A combination of medical and personal care gradually restores his speech but not his memory. His adopted parents rename him, monitor his progress, and encourage him to socialize with their only daughter.

The sudden introduction of Gbenga, the disoriented, traumatized, homeless young man with memory loss, who happens to be the younger brother of Kayode, performs two major plot functions in the movie. First, the response of the mob to Gbenga provides critical commentary on "jungle justice" in Nigeria that has led many to untimely deaths. One of the many effects of Nigeria's stifling economic problems is the increase in burglaries and armed brigandage. In the absence of effective policing, citizens act—and in most cases, hastily—to defend themselves. But this sometimes leads to the death of innocents. For example, if the crowd chose to attack Gbenga, the innocent young man could have died. Second, this subplot suggests that the producers are aware of the need for a positive attitude toward those suffering from this form of mental impairment. But the poor handling of the situation shows the family's condescending attitude to Gbenga in a way that affirms the stereotypical attitude to the mentally disabled. The story of the traumatized young man adds to the catalogue of atrocities perpetrated by Kayode's stepmother. It is an important but hidden factor in the story design that becomes the plot resolution device: the deus ex machina.

Alade, the benefactor of the nameless young man, is kind, humane, and considerate. He starts by giving the young man a name—and thus, an identity. But Alade treats him with condescension. In spite of the diagnosis of Gbenga's ailment, Alade and his family treat him as an intellectually disabled young man, one with the mentality of a five-year-old. He is shown as a man who prefers to play with children's toys. This portrayal reflects the traditional way in which the mentally disabled are framed in the movie. This falsely frames a person suffering from memory loss, incorrectly suggests the way they should be treated, and showcases the mentally disabled as objects of pity.

The incidents involving the wicked stepmother, who suddenly becomes afflicted with mental illness, and the young man with amnesia, are important dramatic devices in the story design of *Oruka Ijosi*. The movie begins with the story of Moyo and her travails at the hands of the ruthless thug, Kayode. The interactions between these coincidental lovers appear to be the main focus, until the middle and near the end of the story, when the incidents of Gbenga and revelations about their stepmother's wicked acts are introduced. The absence of any hint about the possibility of connections between the major plot and these subplots makes the resolution of the story appear contrived. The revelations of the familial relationship between Gbenga and Kayode, on the one hand, and the relationship between Gbenga and the stepmother on the other, are melodramatic devices used to explain away the initial erratic behavior of Kayode. This structural shift changes his status from a villain to a victim.

The last scene of the movie is reminiscent of a scene in Henrik Ibsen's famous play *A Doll's House*. This dramatic style allows the characters to review past events in order to learn a lesson. The principal characters in the movie gather to revive the comatose Kayode in the herbalist's house, and through flashbacks, viewers know how Adebayo acquired the magic ring that put Kayode into a coma. Gbenga, who is with his benefactor, Alade, sets eyes on his stepmother and miraculously regains his lost senses, and the stepmother loses her sanity. Almost simultaneously, Adebayo remembers the remedy to the charm and wakes up the comatose Kayode, while the wicked stepmother now confesses that she has been responsible for all the calamities that befell the family and begs for forgiveness. While twists and turns in plots are expected to introduce unexpected outcomes, it is assumed the outcomes must be something plausible or likely to happen given the chain of events surrounding a story, but this is not the case in *Oruka Ijosi*. The misunderstanding and crisis between Kayode and the stepmother are not unusual in a polygamous family, especially where the stepmother despises her adult stepson. In the Yoruba cultural system, Kayode's behavior would not be acceptable and neither would the stepmother's actions toward Kayode. However, the introduction of the supernatural and the revelation that she is responsible for Kayode's actions exonerates Kayode and lays the blame on the wicked stepmother.

This movie demonstrates the problems associated with the representation of mental illness in Nollywood movies. The plot of *Oruka Ijosi* illustrates the reasons why the issue of mental health, introduced toward the end of the film, is an important story element. It helps to contextualize and explain away the actions of the main actor. The film uses the activities of the stepmother that result in her mental disability as the remote causative factor and the invisible hands responsible for myriad problems in the lives of two major characters in the movie. At first it seems like the film will focus solely on the socioeconomic factors that underlie the sufferings and afflictions of a poor family, a common theme in Nollywood movies. However, the emphasis shifts to dysfunctional families (Kayode's being a central focus) and serves to decenter madness as an important factor in the movie. The narrative structure of *Oruka Ijosi* follows the recurrent pattern of Nollywood movies: a nonlinear plot, in which the majority of issues from the present originate in the past and are caused by a wicked stepmother, who later confesses her sins and then goes mad. When the audience witnesses the jealous mother admitting guilt and taking responsibility for harming Kayode, any lingering questions about Kayode's actions are answered. These revelations also resolve all of the conflicts in the movie. The now-demonized madwoman serves as a kind of deus ex machina used to resolve implausible conflicts in the movie.[28]

When madness is used as a deus ex machina, it pushes disability as a social status to the periphery. The problem with this kind of story design is that it decenters the complex realities of the life of the mentally disabled person. The representations of able persons in *Oruka Ijosi*— including the purportedly wicked stepmother before her affliction—reflect different aspects of their lives. The focus on these different aspects humanizes them, while the mentally disabled character is used to teach moral lessons. Ato Quayson categorizes this kind of representation as "disability as articulation of disjuncture between thematic and narrative vectors"[29] It is quite common for Nollywood films to deploy for didactic purposes supernatural explanations for what appear to be ordinary realities. This is prevalent in movies based on traditional sources. In *Oruka Ijosi*, the sudden mental affliction of the

---

28 Brockett and Hildy, *History*, 34.
29 Quayson, *Aesthetic Nervousness*, 40–41.

wicked stepmother is not a major concern for the people who inhabit the world of the movie and the target audience; rather, it becomes a visible warning to those who might want to choose the path of evil. In that sense, only a handful of people—usually the biological children of the mentally challenged—are concerned about the health of their parents. But they cannot do anything to help because of the stigma and moral deficit associated with the sins that earned their parents the anger of the gods, which the movie presents as the cause of their mother's mental health problems. They cannot get help from the community precisely because their mother's mental disability is self-inflicted and because of the accompanying shame that comes with being the offspring of a wicked woman who has justly been rewarded.

The cause of most of the problems in the movie—even quotidian happenings whose origins appear obvious—are spiritual in nature. For example, the conflicts between Kayode and his stepmother, a common feature in polygamous families, are given unorthodox explanations. The overt spiritualization of the mundane is one way the producers explain the friction between Kayode and the wicked stepmother. It is a subtle means of introducing the element of the Yoruba concept of destiny. In Yoruba cosmology, the head is highly valued. It is seen as the source of everything that happens to a human being. Writing on "Ori and Man's Choice of Destiny," Wande Abimbola, the revered professor of Yoruba culture and an expert on Ifa, states that "a man's destiny, that is to say his success or failure in life, depends to a large extent on the type of head he chose in heaven."[30] Ifa configures the head as the most important determinant of a person's future, fate, and destiny. The Ifa corpus tells many stories about how the fortune of any individual depends on his *ayanmo* or *kadara* (destiny). But predestination is a complex phenomenon. According to the Yorubas, with some appropriate sacrifices, destiny can be modified for good or bad. This is what Kayode's stepmother attempts to do with him and his brother, Gbenga. But she did not succeed and is punished with mental derangement for her wickedness.

Gbenga's illness presents another telling instance of how the producers smuggled in a spiritual explanation for what appears to be a basic medical problem. For instance, Alade suddenly (and implausibly) sees a connection between the sudden upsurge in his wealth and the presence of the young man. The spiritualization and framing of the response to amnesia, a medical challenge, as a moral imperative with rewards promote the Yoruba idea

---

30   Wande Abimbola, *Ifa: An Exposition of Ifa Literary Corpus* (Ibadan, Nigeria: Oxford University Press, 1976), 126.

that being nice to the disabled attracts spiritual blessings. This idea that being charitable to the disabled is profitable suggests that it is the religious and moral obligation of the normate to help those shaped by the "error of Obatala."[31]

Like most melodramatic stories, a rash of contrivances and coincidences lead to the unconvincing conflict resolution, which leaves more questions than answers. The unanswered questions did not result from the open-ended nature of the conclusion: rather, there is a sense of forced realignment of consciousness about the culpability of Kayode and the decentering of Moyo; there is also no practical explanation for the sudden mental illness of the stepmother. The stepmother suddenly begins losing her senses and starts to misbehave. Her body language suggests someone who is uncomfortable and embarrassed that she has been exposed, but her discomfort and paranoia exhibit signs of the onset of madness. The herbalist erases all signs of doubt when he says: "What she sows is what she is reaping. Her madness is self induced."[32] Everybody concurs, except her daughter, who will likely have to live with the stigma of madness. The situation of the daughter is particularly bad because she is single. In Yoruba traditional culture, where mental illness is believed to be hereditary, most families would not approve of their son marrying the daughter of a mentally disabled person. The movie ends with little attention paid to the situation of the stepmother, since she is merely a catalyst to resolve the story and convey a moral message. This deliberate consignment of the mentally ill to the margins of the story sums up the fate of most mentally ill characters in Nollywood movies.

Tunde Kelani: The Normalization of Sexist Myths in *Ayo Ni Mofe*

Tunde Kelani, an accomplished Nigerian scriptwriter, producer, and director, is the director of *Ayo Ni Mo Fe*. One of the earliest producers in the Nigerian movie industry to seek social change through film, Kelani wants

---

31 Wole Soyinka, "Morality and Aesthetics in the Ritual Archetype," in *Myth, Literature and the African World* (Cambridge: Cambridge University Press, 1976), 15.
32 *Oruka Ijosi*.

his movies to promote what he considers the positive aspects of African culture.³³ Described as one of the "most sought after" Nigerian filmmakers, Kelani has produced Yoruba- and English-language movies that have garnered worldwide critical acclaim.³⁴ Kelani's works reveal his deliberate attempt to bridge the gulf between Yoruba culture and Western ideas while simultaneously promoting his Yoruba heritage. He self-consciously utilizes Yoruba cultural resources to address contemporary social ills, and this deliberate attention to relevant social issues made him a darling of the masses. Akin Adesokan described this as Kelani's proclivity to "thematize . . . social issues" as something that "encourages us to think of aesthetic populism as approaching opportunism."³⁵ The insertion of snippets from different aspects of society in Kelani's movies dealing with traditional themes is one of the most common illustration of his "aesthetic populism."³⁶

In *Ayo Ni Mo Fe,* Tunde Kelani adopts a radically different approach to the representation of mental illness. The movie addresses the illness and the personality of the mentally disabled, provides a plausible and practical cause for the illness, exposes the charlatans, deceivers, and fake spiritualists that exploit the mentally disabled, explodes Yoruba myths about the mentally disabled and suggests orthodox medical cures for the illness. His dramatization also includes the motiveless spectacle that emanates from the mentally disabled gestures and antics and the different ways they are exploited by their family and caregivers. Kelani uses this film to debunk the myth that mental illness is a spiritual problem that can only be cured by traditional herbalists; however, he takes an ambivalent stance on some fundamental questions concerning the attitudes and myths about madness. Unlike *Oruka Ijosi,* where madness is a minor subplot that nevertheless controls the central plot, *Ayo Ni Mo Fe* pays more attention to the causes, management, and social issues surrounding mentally disabled women. The movie draws attention to the stigmatization and exploitation of the mentally disabled and suggests medical and social interventions are desperately needed.

---

33 See Jonathan Haynes, ed., "Nigerian Video Films," in *Africa Series* 73 (Athens: Ohio University Press, 2000); and Onookome Okome and Jonathan Haynes, *Cinema and Social Change in West Africa* (Jos: Nigerian Film Institute, 1997).
34 Akin Adesokan, *Postcolonial Artists and Global Aesthetics* (Bloomington: Indiana University Press, 2011), 81.
35 Adesokan, *Postcolonial*, 81.
36 Adesokan, *Postcolonial*, 81.

The plot of *Ayo Ni Mo Fe* revolves around the lives of two lovers, Jumoke and Ayo, who planned to marry but ultimately could not because of Ayo's unfaithfulness. Their plan to marry was going well up until Ayo (who has been cheating on Jumoke) impregnates Adunni, the teenage daughter of the tough, no-nonsense police commissioner, Dabiri. To save face, the police commissioner and his wife force Ayo to marry their teenage daughter. Upon hearing the news of Ayo and Adunni's marriage, Jumoke has a mental breakdown. As is customary under such circumstances in Yoruba culture, Jumoke's elderly mother takes her to the local herbalist for treatment. However, the herbalist is a charlatan who specializes in exploiting vulnerable individuals with mental health conditions. The herbalist brutalizes the male clients under his care and uses the females as sex objects. He subjects Jumoke to sexual advances and immediately sets out to rape her. Jumoke escapes the rape only to be left living on the street, where Chief Tomobi, who has been told that his wife could only become pregnant after he sleeps with and impregnates a mentally challenged person, meets Jumoke and lures her into having sexual intercourse with him.

Meanwhile, Adeleke, the rich polygamist—and one of her suitors—offers to help Jumoke. He takes Jumoke for medical treatment in an orthodox hospital where she gets the right diagnosis and appropriate medical attention. The combination of good medical attention, loving care, and positive attitudes from her family and friends appears to cure Jumoke. Contrary to the Yoruba popular traditional belief that mental health problems are incurable, she regains full use of her mental faculties. This has tremendously positive consequences. She happily marries Adeleke and moves in with him as the youngest of his wives. Favored by Adeleke and helped by her educational qualifications and business acumen, she becomes the head of Chief Adeleke's business and ends up doing well. Not surprisingly, the other wives become jealous of Jumoke. In one of Kelani's critical comments on the evils of polygamy, the wives conspire against Jumoke and remind her of her mental illness. The condescending treatment and the negative attitude toward Jumoke lead to depression and mental breakdown, a clear case of how negative social attitudes can exacerbate disability. But with the help of the caring husband and a competent doctor, Jumoke bounces back and continues to lead a normal life.

Unlike *Oruka Ijosi*, Kelani's *Ayo Ni Mo Fe* has a more practical, thoughtful, and realistic treatment of madness in contemporary Nigerian society, it nonetheless endorses another way of thinking about how copulating with a mentally challenged person can spiritually ameliorate their illness. The travails of Chief Tomori, an important subplot of the main story, is significant to the representation of the mentally challenged in Yoruba culture as a cure for some forms of illness. This claim is consistent with the Yoruba myths about the mentally challenged, especially the belief in the healing powers Olodumare, the Yoruba God of creation, deposited in the body of the disabled to compensate them for the mistakes that led to their inadequacies. In Yoruba mythology, the disabled were created by an inebriated Obatala. To show remorse for his drunkenness, Obatala became a teetotaler. In order to compensate the disabled, Olodumare gave them the gift of spiritual insight that is denied the normate.[37] This ties into the Yoruba belief that having sex with and (if possible) impregnating a mentally challenged woman can spiritually solve a variety of problems.

Kelani uses the affair between the mentally disabled Jumoke and Chief Tomori to illustrate this myth in *Ayo Ni Mo Fe*. For instance, Chief Tomori has three wives, none of whom has been pregnant. In one of his searches for a cure, a female priest told him that his inability to impregnate a woman is not a medical problem but a spiritual one. It is understood that the cause of Chief Tomori's spiritual problem stems from his mother once humiliating a man caught having sex with a mentally challenged woman in the past. She exposed the man despite his pleas. The man then placed a curse on her children. Thus, the curse will only allow Chief Tomori to be cured of his infertility after impregnating a mentally challenged woman.

In a society where infertility is stigmatized and procreation is the main reason for marriage, Chief Tomori, determined to have children, lures the mad Jumoke into his bed and impregnates her. His intentions are not to cure Jumoke of her "madness" since he had to rape her to solve his problem. The rape of Jumoke that later results in pregnancy furthers the movie's tendency to exploit the mentally challenged. It is pertinent to note that Chief Tomori's rape of Jumoke is one of several attempts by different men to sexually exploit her. This is not surprising, since research has shown that "people with intellectual disabilities experience more violence in general when compared with those without disabilities" and are more likely to be sexually abused than those without disabilities.[38] However, unlike the case of the fake herbalist

---

[37] Kolawole Olaiya, "Commodifying the 'Sacred,' Beatifying the 'Abnormal': Nollywood and the Representation of Disability," *Global South* 7, no. 1 (2013): 137–156.

[38] Leigh Ann Davis, "People with Intellectual Disabilities and Sexual Violence," *The Arc* (2011): 1–3; Furey, "Sexual Abuse"; Sobsey, "Violence"; and Sobsey and Doe, "Patterns."

who uses the madwomen in his care as sex objects, the filmmaker did not condemn the objectification of the mentally disabled woman or Jumoke by Chief Tomori. Instead, the subplot focuses on the moral lessons of restraint and understanding. This authorial silence on the crime against Jumoke normalizes the injustice committed against her.

It can be argued that the punishment given to Chief Tomori by Karma is intended to serve as a lesson to mothers and warn them to be careful, lest their offspring bear the consequences of their actions. This opportunity to show the painful price of overcoming the punishment of inherited sins is illustrated with the pregnancy of Chief Tomori's wives. This occurs after he performed the disgraceful act of sleeping with a mentally disabled woman, for which his mother disgraced another man. But portraying the pregnancy as the consequence of Chief Tomori's disgraceful exploitation of Jumoke is tantamount to rewarding Chief Tomori for raping Jumoke, and this should not be the case. The focus on the didactic lesson inherent in the unguarded actions of Chief Tomori's mother at the expense of the consequences for Jumoke also confirms the myth that copulating with a mentally challenged woman is a spiritual cure for his infertility. Ultimately, this sends the wrong message: one that can appear to endorse the Yoruba traditional sexist myth that sleeping with a mentally disabled woman will cure complicated medical problems and solve other troubles in life.

Tunde Kelani's *Ayo Ni Mo Fe* has mental disability as its thematic center and advocates the adoption of orthodox medicine and social acceptance in the treatment of mental health problems. Aderinto argues that the movie "offers some counter-narratives to established ideas about the superiority of African over Western psychiatry."[39] *Ayo Ni Mo Fe* reveals some of the weaknesses of Yoruba traditional medicine in the treatment of mental health problems and exposes the fraudulent antics of some fake practitioners who exploit the mentally challenged. But the film does not stop there; Kelani also beams his creative searchlight on the way social attitudes compound the problems that trigger the illness of Jumoke, the movie's heroine. His claim that the causes of mental illness are medical and social can help in refocusing the attention of doctors and society in the right direction. This is a radical step at a period when most people attribute the cause of mental illness to spiritual attacks.

Kelani's *Ayo ni Mo Fe* makes a brave attempt to debunk the myth that mental illness is caused by spiritual forces and can only be cured by herbalists

---

39   Aderinto, "Representing," 262.

who know how to appease the gods. The movie exposes those herbalists who treated Jumoke as "fake, violent, and retrogressive."[40] The upheavals and triumph of Jumoke illustrate how the combination of social acceptance and Western medicine can help reduce the challenges faced by the mentally disabled. This important departure from the formulaic representation of mental disability is commendable. Despite these accomplishments, Kelani seems to use the left hand to rescind what he offers to the discourse on mental disability with the right hand. While the main plot of the movie suggests that his society should embrace orthodox Western psychiatric treatment and accept the mentally challenged as normal human beings, he uses the subplot of the Jumoke-Adeleke encounters to reinforce a retrogressive myth. The plot suggests that Chief Tomori's wives became pregnant because he slept with the mentally ill Jumoke, which is an unethical message to send to viewers. This subplot is the deus ex machina that helps to end the story in a positive, "live-happily-forever" manner that often ends comedies. But this sudden introduction of a spiritual solution to what appears to be an intrinsically medical problem is retrogressive and unhelpful in a movie that boldly charts a different narrative of madness and cure.

Conclusion: Humanizing Mental Illness and Centering the Mentally Disabled

This chapter demonstrates how two Nigerian movie producers treat mental disabilities in *Oruka Ijosi* and *Ayo Ni Mo Fe*. A critical look at the way they represent mental disorders in these movies shows that the content and form of both movies were shaped by traditional beliefs and social attitudes. *Oruka Ijosi* starts as a story about Kayode's rascality and moral turpitude as well as his problematic relationship with Moyo, which showcases the adverse effects of poverty on young Nigerian girls. But it ends in a melodramatic and improbable way that reveals Kayode's stepmother as the witch responsible for his past actions and all the family's problems. Her sudden confession—sudden because it is extraneous to the plot—magically revives Kayode, restores his brother's sanity, and results in her madness and death. More importantly, it redeems Kayode, who the audience now sees in a new light and casts him as the victim of his wicked stepmother. Consequently, instead of condemnation, the audience pities Kayode. *Ayo Ni Mo Fe* starts on a radical, hopeful,

---

40   Aderinto, "Representing," 262.

note that proves that with appropriate medical attention and family support, mental illness can be cured. The use of a credible story that debunks the commonsense myths that have normalized unproven traditional practices to cure mental illness radically departs from most representations of mental illness in Nigerian movies. But the raised hopes of proper education of the populace on mental illness are dashed by questionable resolutions of some conflicts in *Ayo Ni Mo Fe*.

Oruka Ijosi portrays mental illness as resulting from spiritual actions that are extraneous to the human body. The spiritualization of the causes and cures for madness performs major functions for Nollywood producers, portraying the mentally disabled as either objects of pity or derision—and both of these reactions derive from traditional myths about mental disabilities. When the source of madness is adduced to spiritual affliction by a third party—which, in Nollywood movies, is usually the wicked mother-in-law or rival wife, like the case of Kayode in *Oruka Ijosi*—the mentally disabled person automatically becomes an object of pity. But in a situation where the mentally disabled are seen as wicked people, he or she is automatically condemned as guilty and deserving of their ailment. The disability is often seen as a "reward" for personal or familial sins. It is a distortion to portray mental illness as a spiritual affliction instead of an ailment that requires medical and social attention.

Movies can profoundly shape and produce meanings. As de Lauretis, suggests, cinema technology is "directly implicated in the production and reproduction of meanings, values, and ideology."[41] Hence, the power of film and the technology that enables it to combine sound and image to make powerful social statements cannot be overemphasized. Given the popularity of Nollywood movies in Nigeria, it is important that movies send the right message to viewers. Producers must be self-conscious and pay attention to details in movies that deal with the disabled. Scriptwriters and movie producers need to do more to give an accurate portrayal of the causes of mental health problems and suggest solutions that can empower those with mental disabilities. Nollywood movies can and should educate society about mental illness and can play an important role in treating the mentally challenged as important members of society.

---

41   Teresa de Lauretis, *Alice Doesn't: Feminism, Semiotics, Cinema* (Bloomington: Indiana University Press, 1984), 37.

Chapter Ten

Masculinity, Disability, and Empire in J. M. Coetzee's *Waiting for the Barbarians*

Saloua Ali Ben Zahra

In James Clifford's article "On Ethnographic Allegory," allegory is defined as "a story in which people, things and happenings have another meaning, as in a fable or a parable: allegories are used for teaching or explaining."[1] Read as such, the allegorical claims of the magistrate in *Waiting for the Barbarians* backfire. In the magistrate's writing and teaching, as will be discussed in this chapter, events are "not themselves but stand for other things."[2] This chapter offers a reading of *Waiting for the Barbarians* that serves as a remodeling of imperialist masculinity and relations for the sake of redeeming empire. This definition of allegory and my reading of the disabled woman's character in Coetzee's novel are inspired by Ato Quayson's concept of "aesthetic nervousness." As Quayson advances, "Because disability in the real world already incites interpretation, literary representations of disability are not merely reflecting disability."[3] Accordingly, I read the disability of the female char-

---

1   James Clifford, "On Ethnographic Allegory," in *Writing Culture: The Poetics and Politics of Ethnography*, ed. James Clifford and George E. Marcus (Berkeley: University of California Press, 1986), 98.
2   J. M. Coetzee, *Waiting for the Barbarians* (London: Secker and Warburg, 1980), 40.
3   Ato Quayson, *Aesthetic Nervousness: Disability and the Crisis of Representation* (New York: Columbia University Press, 2007), 32.

acter in question within Coetzee's narrative as allegorical and conducive to thought-provoking interpretations.

The magistrate's ethnographic project is merely an autoethnography in progress. His goal is the production of the knowledge and meaning that would allow him to relate to the new young men of empire and construct an appropriate model of masculinity to serve empire. The magistrate in the narrative tries to forge a masculine bond through explaining his ideas to the young officer. This endeavor stands in contrast to the magistrate's relations with the old colonel and the barbarian woman, with whom no dialogues are attempted. The colonel and the barbarian woman are representative of old colonial models and relations. Accordingly, the magistrate does some ethnographic work on them. As he studies these two, he explores his reactions. The underlying autoethnography voices a rejection of what the colonel and the woman stand for and what he shares with them. He rejects old age, feminization, and open brutality as inadequate for the purpose of continuing occupation and distant nonviolent coexistence. His autoethnography could also mean self-rejection; however, the magistrate seems to regard his ability to see these aforementioned shortcomings and his ideas about them as a redeeming act.

This chapter presents a textual reading of the novel's narrative starting with the magistrate's ethnographic project. In this analysis, Colonel Joll and the barbarian woman are brought together because this connection stands for a model of relations between masculinity and femininity. Colonel Joll stands for the brutal-yet-effeminate type whose methods the magistrate disapproves of, mainly because these traits threaten the future of empire. Inadequate and incorrect methods are described as effeminate, just as women are seen as unfeminine if they give the impression of understanding their situation in terms of colonial and male domination instead of dutifully performing their roles. The magistrate says that Colonel Joll "walks with his hands clasped before him like a woman."[4]

The principal punitive methods of Colonel Joll are captivity and torture. They provoke violence and ignore the distance that should be maintained between the races. For these reasons, the magistrate is against open warfare and the opening of the occupiers' world to the natives. He does not want the barriers to collapse or the different bodies and cultures to violently interrelate in a way that involves negative consequences for empire. He wants to leave the old culture of empire in the past. Both the colonel's methods and

---

4   Coetzee, *Waiting*, 4.

the barbarian woman's body/land culture are treated as objects of study from which to learn how to conduct the ongoing colonial project.

In the field of the barbarian body and land, the magistrate portrays the barbarian culture as an "ethnographic present (which is always in fact a past)."[5] The findings from his excavations are always ruins that are hard to decipher. The magistrate's claim amounts to writing the history (and the future) of the barbarians. He says, "I hope that the history of their captivity enters their legends, passed on from grandfather to grandson" (the mothers and daughters are not included). The magistrate continues: "But l hope too that memories of the town, with its easy life and its exotic foods, are not strong enough to lure them back. I do not want a race of beggars on my hands."[6] The natives' culture is merely a site for excavations of ruins and a world to be kept separate. The natives' future cultural life is also planned for them by the magistrate. The magistrate's desire to be studied, his legacy preserved and glorified, is expressed in the following: "If we were to disappear would the barbarians spend their afternoons excavating our ruins? Would they preserve our census rolls and our gain-merchants' ledgers in glass cases, or devote themselves to deciphering the script of our letters?"[7]

Quayson interprets Benita Parry as saying, "Inarticulateness is distributed in [Coetzee's] work in such a way as to imply a hierarchy among various Others. . . . This implied hierarchy rehearses the ways in which the power to (self-)represent is dispersed with the colonial archive."[8] The colonials are to know their place and study their colonial past and the historical exploits of their old teachers and masters. They are not to master indigenous technologies and should spend their youth and life studying the letters and romantic literature of the dominant culture. The prospects of employment for those who want to specialize in the study of their own language and letters will be discouragingly few. Colonials should rely on what remains of their natural resources or face a beggarly future if they go to the cities of their rulers.

The masculinity and femininity of empire as modeled by the magistrate are mutually defining. Whereas homosocial and homoerotic bonds are appreciated, women are cast to believe and perform within the framework of limited models and patterns. Out of commitment to empire, the magistrate finds it important to reactivate his own awareness of how the genealogy of

---

5   Clifford, "Ethnographic," 111.
6   Coetzee, *Waiting*, 19.
7   Coetzee, *Waiting*, 52.
8   Quayson, *Aesthetic Nervousness*, 154.

masculinity works in the process of colonial relations. When he proposes to visit the barbarians, he rewrites and validates the original version of the benevolent claims. He says, "To repair some of the damage wrought by the forays of the Third Bureau, I write and to restore some of the goodwill that previously existed, I am undertaking a brief visit to the barbarians."[9] The magistrate believes in the original good intentions of empire that have been corrupted by the extremist and ill-informed agents of the Third Bureau. His sense of identity and masculinity is contingent on this historicizing move back to the ostensibly benevolent origins and intentions of empire. He opposes those who harm the interests of empire: "My alliance with the guardians of the Empire is over, I have set myself in opposition, the bond is broken."[10] However, the bonds between the men of empire should prevail against all odds and, if broken, they should be reconstructed on a healthier basis.

The woman's body is modeled to serve as a ground for homosocial and homoerotic continuities: "And here I am patching up relations between the men of the future and the men of the past, returning, with apologies, a body we have sucked dry." Whereas the barbarian history is reduced to obscure underground ruins from the past, the magistrate tries to situate himself within a history and relate to other men of empire. Even in his fall from grace and his trial for mixing with a street woman and for watching a girl flog a barbarian man, he is still busy figuring out and expressing what he stands for. He asks, "What after all do I stand for besides an archaic code of gentlemanly behavior towards captured foes, and what do I stand against except the new science of degradation that kills people on their knees, confused and disgraced in their own eyes?"[11] He aims at fashioning a middle ground between masculinity and colonial relations, something beyond the archaic, politically amateurish old class but that does not resemble the brutal present one. Empire needs officers who can control the natives in a reasonably innocuous manner that falls just short of provoking them into embracing technologically advanced weaponry: such a scenario would lead to the kind of carnage that would make the world too unsafe to accommodate long-term imperialist masculinity.

In fact, the barbarians, or the colonized people in general—men, women, and cultures—are a common reference point for the new men of empire to relate to each other and their shared history, as well as understand themselves

---

9   Coetzee, *Waiting*, 57.
10   Coetzee, 78.
11   Coetzee, 108.

and each other better so as to promote the interests of their institutions worldwide. The magistrate assumes that the apologies should suffice and that the barbarian men—who are thought of like animals in their desire to remain outdoors in their own space—will accept them. Even though he disapproves of brutality—mainly because it bothers his conscience and threatens the empire that makes his livelihood possible—the magistrate manages to make excuses for the torturers in that they are simply fallible men. The magistrate focuses on the construction of a more appropriate model of masculinity among the young men of empire. The magistrate says, "I am sure that among these men . . . are some that who have slept with the girl. It is not that I imagine them sniggering behind their hands. On the contrary, never have I seen them stand more stoically. . . . Never has their bearing been more respectful."[12] Like a good teacher, the magistrate instructs his disciples to bury the bodies of deserters because "it is good for the morale of their comrades."[13]

This is the model of masculinity that the magistrate tries to construct: young, healthy, hardy, and honest males willing to lose their lives for the sake of safeguarding the empire. Later, he says, "I picked these men because they were hardy and honest and willing."[14] Before engaging in his teachings and explanations with the new officer, the magistrate says, "I like this young man's energy."[15] And this is the kind of man the magistrate tries to share knowledge and dialogue with. He molds these youths in military styles of dress and conduct and is certain that an encounter with the barbarians should not affect the masculinity of the men, especially such an outward model of masculinity. On the way back from the visit, the magistrate describes their state: "We are exhausted, but we walk like men . . . it would have been better if I had told the men to put on their armor for these last few miles."[16]

In terms of the mutual definition dynamic at work in the masculine/feminine encounter, the woman's body is not only a site for such interactions but is also representative of what happens to the model of femininity in the process. The desirable model of femininity is that of the informant and sympathetic silent listener: "I discover that I am not without friends, particularly among women, who can barely conceal their eagerness to hear my side of the

---

12   Coetzee, *Waiting*, 54.
13   Coetzee, *Waiting*, 54.
14   Coetzee, *Waiting*, 61.
15   Coetzee, *Waiting*, 49.
16   Coetzee, *Waiting*, 76.

story."[17] The magistrate says earlier about the barbarian woman, "It occurs to me that whatever I want to say to her will be heard with sympathy, with kindness."[18] Women are excluded from the privileging dialogues of the magistrate. They are objects of study in the magistrate's pursuit of information, knowledge, and pleasure. The magistrate's fascination with how the barbarian woman deals with her people[19] casts the woman in the role of a native informant. In this guise, the magistrate could observe the workings of an untapped potential that he belatedly and vainly tries to harness. His appreciation of her banter with male companions redeems her in his eyes for a brief moment: he no longer sees the barbarian woman as a worthless being. Her fluency and intelligence flatters and affirms his masculine self-esteem. The notion of belatedness is important in understanding the consequences of the lack of substantive male/female dialogue in that particular colonial historical period.

The concept of forced birth control works at the heart of the model of femininity. The feminine model in question is rendered sterile, and a culture of death is imposed on the former colonies. The woman in the novel who lost a child was shunned by the other prisoners.[20] They seem to reject her because of the loss of her child and fear that the same will befall them. The people seem to have a myopic vision of the crippled woman's predicament, a destiny shaped by the men of empire for colonial women. Colonial masculinity is complicit in this shunning, and this is one of few contexts where the latter is allowed to have an existence, albeit an effaced one. It seems that this complicity in shunning marked colonial women is what imperialist masculinity demands from colonial masculinity; that is, marking those women more deeply and sterilizing them more irrevocably. Children die in the colonial encounter. Women and cultures lose valuable years trying to reason with imperialist men and hoping they will make good on their promises. From the start, the barbarian woman tells the magistrate in no uncertain terms that he would not want someone like her.[21] He stays with her and gives her false hope, and her initial misgivings about the relationship are proven valid. Meanwhile, the magistrate had been indulging in his private fantasies and using her body for his selfish pleasure. It was as if he subconsciously wanted

---

17   Coetzee, *Waiting*, 126.
18   Coetzee, *Waiting*, 22.
19   Coetzee, *Waiting*, 63.
20   Coetzee, *Waiting*, 20.
21   Coetzee, *Waiting*, 27.

to mark her to the point at which marriage and childbearing, her birthright, were unattainable: "However kindly she may be treated by her own people, she will never be courted and married in the normal way."[22] He seems to forgive himself for this because he sees a prestigious role for her within the empire.

The successor to the barbarian woman was another lonely woman, this one living with her mother. The magistrate listens to her while she plays the role of informant.[23] When it comes to her need to understand what happened to the barbarian woman, the magistrate tells her: "You don't understand.... There is a whole side to the story you don 't know, that she could not have told you because she did not know it herself. Which I don't want to talk about now."[24] The magistrate does not want to share his knowledge with women as he thinks that they do not understand (although they do on many occasions). The ironic response of the barbarian woman to the magistrate's pleas for her to tell her people the truth betrays a deeper knowledge than he imagines. But she apparently tells her people nothing that would complicate the relations between the magistrates and colonial men and, consequently, the relations among men of empire. This is a model of the role the magistrate would like colonial femininity to perform in the service of future imperialist masculine interests. Regarding the barbarian woman, the magistrate goes on to say, "I imagine her trotting through the open gateway at the head of a troop of horsemen, erect in the saddle, her eyes shining, a forerunner, a guide, pointing out to her comrades the lay of this foreign town where she once lived. Then everything will be on a new footing."[25] The magistrate does not want barbarian men to come to the town, but his fears tell him that it may happen someday. In such a case, he hopes the "brutal" and "feminized" barbarians will come led by a woman, probably because she would be more manageable than a male. He also counts on her indirect education in the colonizers' ways to bear fruit in the form of an expression of gratitude. The imagined new footing is one of easy commercial exchange and exploitation of the natural resources of the former colonies. The magistrate's wishful idealizing of the disabled woman's new or "neo" role can be read as an attempt on his part to erase colonial and neocolonial violence. In dialogue with Gorman and Udegbe's interpretation of such a trope in African literary

---

22 Coetzee, *Waiting*, 135.
23 Coetzee, *Waiting*, 128.
24 Coetzee, *Waiting*, 152.
25 Coetzee, *Waiting*, 152.

representations of disability,[26] the magistrate's strategy is another instance of such suppression and erasure.

Thus, in one of his dreams, the magistrate sees the child building a clay oven and holding out a loaf of bread to him.[27] There also comes a point when the magistrate is fed by the fisher folk and admitted among them without suspicion. It could be for this reason that he was against cheating them in town at the beginning. He seems to have a long-term vision about the ethics of business as promoting trust among people for the sake of future economic relations and ethnic diversity. The magistrate plans to marry one of the prettiest girls of the fisher folk. This vision of future interdependence and cooperation is better articulated in the following statement: "But when the barbarians taste bread . . . and gooseberry jam, they will be won over to our ways. They will find that they are unable to live without the skills of men who know how to rear the pacific grains, without the arts of women who know how to use the benign fruits."[28] According to this model, it is the men and women of empire who have the know-how and power. The postcolonials are dependent, underskilled, and destined to be kept in servitude.

The model of femininity that the men of empire construct for the women of empire is shaped by imperialist masculinity and relations. The mothers are expected to be meticulous and care about the honor of the men. The magistrate's new lover lives with an "exacting mother"[29] and partly because of this, the model of relationships outside marriage fails. A guard reads the charges against the magistrate:

> Despite being principal administrative officer . . . he contracted a liaison with a street woman who occupied most of his energies to the detriment of his official duties. The liaison had a demoralizing effect on the prestige of imperial administration because the woman in question had been patronized by the common soldiers.[30]

---

26   Rachel Gorman and Onyinyechukwu Udegbe, "Disabled Woman/Nation: Re-narrating the Erasure of (Neo)colonial Violence in Ondjaki's *Good Morning Comrades* and Tsitsi Dangarembga's *Nervous Conditions*," *Journal of Literary & Cultural Disability Studies* 4, no. 3 (2010): 310.
27   Coetzee, *Waiting*, 109.
28   Coetzee, *Waiting*, 155.
29   Coetzee, *Waiting*, 128.
30   Coetzee, *Waiting*, 83.

It is meaningful that the general term "woman" is used here instead of "barbarian woman," which is used elsewhere. This could be because the model of proper feminine behavior is meant to cover the women of empire as well and stigmatize prostitution as an unproductive alternative that expends energy better deployed within a productive heterosexual, matrimonial, and labor contract. Accordingly, the relationship with the magistrate's favorite does not continue. Nonetheless, there is redemption for the girl but not for the barbarian woman. The former finds a young man with whom she may still have children and have a beautiful, healthy, and productive family. Her relationship with the magistrate would have been sexually uneventful and unproductive because of his old age. Her race is meant to multiply. The barbarian women are to be rendered effectively sterile through writings on their bodies and left to age alone. Forgiveness and repair are for the women and men of empire.

Expressions of unease and guilt abound in this narrative. The final and dominant note, however, is one of self-forgiveness, and there is a commitment to the idea that empire should carry on successfully. What redeems the magistrate's participation in the work of empire is his wish not to be part of it. He says: "I wanted to live outside the history that Empire imposes on its subjects, even its lost subjects. I never wished for the barbarians that they should have the history of Empire laid upon them. How can I believe that this cause for shame."[31] The magistrate's view of the barbarian culture does not change. He nostalgically continues to see the desert relics as its only valuable manifestation. He claims the work of writing history: "It seems right that as a gesture to the people who inhabited the ruins in the desert, we too ought to set down a record of settlement . . . and to write such a history no one would seem to be better fitted than our last magistrate."[32] The magistrate ends up writing a nostalgic plea to continue living in that "paradise on earth."[33] Though he feels uneasy about such a message of his, he thinks that his words will not be held against him and that what will endure is the security of the ruins of the barbarians: "When one day people come scratching around in the ruins, they will be more interested in the relics from the desert than in anything I can leave behind and rightly so."[34] The magistrate's statements are allegorical in the sense that they always have a deeper meaning

---

31 Coetzee, *Waiting*, 154.
32 Coetzee, *Waiting*, 154.
33 Coetzee, *Waiting*, 154.
34 Coetzee, *Waiting*, 155.

than the surface intentions suggest. Though the magistrate seems to be self-analytical, he tends to abandon his insights in fear of learning the truth.

There is a revengeful ironic structure of justice at work in the narrative that the magistrate does not grasp. His deepest fear, apart from dying, is that of not being knowledgeable enough. He asks the following:

> What made it impossible for us to live in time like . . . children? It is the fault of Empire! Empire has created the time of history. Empire has located its existence not in the smooth recurrent spinning time of the cycle of the seasons but in the ragged time of rise and fall of beginning and end. . . . One thought alone preoccupies the submerged mind of Empire: how not to end, how not to die, how to prolong its era.[35]

Until the end, however, the magistrate does not know that he is a body and mind of empire and that the one thought preoccupying his mind the most is how to aid and abet a lasting empire. That is why the magistrate has engaged with the men of empire, trying to understand their work in order to articulate the model of the ideal imperial man. Another vengeful scenario takes place when the magistrate's descriptions of the abused barbarian woman backfire. What he did to her is done to him at the hands of the men of empire. He is reduced to blindness, deafness, and a beggarly existence. As we cannot have empire and femininity without blood, when beaten the magistrate "swallow[s] blood."[36] A final irony is that in this narrative the women are, after all, more knowledgeable than the magistrate. The barbarian woman assumes the pain of knowing the truth of what happened to her because of empire. The magistrate's favorite knows men enough to believe in her role and perform it well. The magistrate's last lover seems to also be more knowledgeable than he realizes and makes choices of her own, as she decides how to discontinue the relationship.

The magistrate situates himself within the history of empire. He says "I was not, as I liked to think, the indulgent pleasure-loving opposite of the cold rigid Colonel. I was the lie that Empire tells itself when times are easy, the truth that Empire tells when harsh winds blow."[37] The magistrate opts for the lie in order to perpetuate the "easy" times. He denies the homoerotic bond he feels toward the colonel. He envies his virility and ability to leave marks on the girl's body and culture: '"Whom will that other girl with the

---

35   Coetzee, *Waiting*, 133.
36   Coetzee, *Waiting*, 107.
37   Coetzee, *Waiting*, 135.

blind face remember: me . . . or that other cold man with the mask over his eyes who gave the orders. . . . I must ask myself whether . . . I was not in my heart of hearts regretting that I could not engrave myself on her as deeply."[38] The magistrate's deeply felt bond with the men of empire is so strong that his last dreamlike vision is of a man, this time with well-shaped features (although of snow). The snowman has no arms, which could be a reminder to the magistrate of his impotence. Even if the snowman is meant to reflect his own image, there is still an underlying desire for Colonel Joll. After a particularly intimate contact with the barbarian woman, the magistrate reflects: "I experience no excitement . . . 'What do I have to do to move you?' . . . and with a shift of horror I behold the answer . . . in the image of a face masked by two black glassy insect eyes from which there comes no reciprocal gaze but only my doubled image cast back at me."[39] Like a schoolboy, the magistrate is infatuated with the masculine and powerful Colonel Joll. The school model is confirmed as a framework for this infatuation by the magistrate's use of the word "lesson" when he imagines the barbarian woman talking to him about Colonel Joll: "'If you want to learn how to do it, ask your friend with the black eyes.' Then she should have continued, so as not to leave me without hope: 'But if you want to love me you will have to turn your back on him and learn your lesson elsewhere.'"[40] The magistrate remains obsessed with the men of empire and their work. And *he* takes the imperial road "that may lead nowhere"[41] confirming an earlier statement: "To the last we will have learnt nothing. In all of us deep down, there seems to be something granite and unteachable."[42]

Coetzee is almost dead in this narrative. It could be that Coetzee granted the magistrate this particular viewpoint and voice because he chose to focus on unveiling for the reader the workings of an agent's consciousness to prompt critical discourse on the workings of empire. This narrative can be read in terms of what it is *not* about. It is not about penalizing empire because the institution endures, and no real barbarian uprising is staged. However, the humiliations that the magistrate is subjected to could be a sign of Coetzee's presence, as he has full control over the protagonist. The latent structure of punishment (e.g., the blood and blindness) would seem to be an expression of authorial disapproval concerning the deeds of magistrates.

---

38   Coetzee, *Waiting*, 135.
39   Coetzee, *Waiting*, 44.
40   Coetzee, *Waiting*, 135.
41   Coetzee, *Waiting*, 156.
42   Coetzee, *Waiting*, 143.

Part Four

Education, Community, and Caregiving

Chapter Eleven

Addressing Poverty and Inequality in Sub-Saharan Africa

Fostering Inclusive Education of Children with Disabilities

Serges Djoyou Kamga

Introduction

Education is essential to acquire a good job, a high income, social status, and a better life in general.[1] For persons with disabilities, education is a vehicle for improving the quality of life and addressing the "disabilization" of poverty or ensuring that disability does not lead to penury.[2] In this respect, broadening access of learners with disabilities to education would increase

---

1   Tsitsi Chataika, "Inclusion of Disabled Students in Higher Education in Zimbabwe," in *Cross-Cultural Perspectives on Policy and Practice-Decolonizing Community Contexts*, ed. Jennifer Lavia and Michele Moore (New York: Routledge, 2010).
2   Tanya Barron and Jabulani Manombe Ncube, eds., *Poverty and Disability* (London: Leonard Cheshire, 2010).

their chances of improving their standard of living. In other words, education is the equalizing factor needed to address poverty and inequality. It is one of the best weapons to combat poverty and inequality, as it empowers the beneficiaries of education to access other human rights needed to improve their well-being.

Yet, historically, children with disabilities, especially in Africa, do not have access to education. They are simply considered "uneducable."[3] To remedy the problem, international communities have adopted various international legislations such as the Standards Rules on the Equalisation of Opportunity for Person With Disabilities (adopted in 1993); the Salamanca statement and Framework for Action on Special Needs Education (adopted in 1994); the Education For All Flagship on Education and Disability (adopted in 2001); and (the only binding instrument) the CRPD, adopted in 2006 and came into force in 2008) and its Optional Protocol (adopted in 2006 and came into force in 2008). These international standards urge states to ensure that learners with disabilities are included in the education system. Article 24 of the CRPD is unequivocal in providing learners with disabilities the right to an education. And it sets the global yardstick to measure inclusive education. In this respect, it compels state parties to move toward a full right to education in inclusive settings at all levels and to ensure learners with disabilities access to education as well as the chance to develop life and social development skills. It also compels states to provide teacher training and ensure that children with disabilities have access to more than basic education.

However, the effective inclusion of children with disabilities remains elusive: these children remain at the margins and often become the face of poverty in their adult life. This chapter argues that to tackle poverty and inequality in sub-Saharan Africa, learners with disabilities must be included in the education system. This approach will show that disability is not inability, as educated learners with disabilities will not only contribute to poverty eradication but will also achieve social equality with other citizens. The chapter is divided into four parts (including this introduction). The second part deconstructs the notion of inclusive education. The third part explores avenues for advancing the inclusion of learners with disabilities in schools.

---

3   Serges Djoyou Kamga, "Inclusion of Learners with Severe Intellectual Disabilities in Basic Education Under a Transformative Constitution: A Critical Analysis," *Comparative and International Law Journal of Southern Africa* 49, no. 1 (2016): 27.

The chapter highlights the need to raise awareness of disability as an element of human diversity. It calls for the explicit constitutionalization of the right of children with disabilities to an education to ensure their visibility in the policy arena, as well as to secure better enforceability of this right. It also underlines the need to rely on local realities to further the inclusive education of learners with disabilities. The fourth part of the chapter will consist of concluding remarks.

Deconstructing the Notion of Inclusive Education

In the early days of the discourse on inclusive education, while the importance of inclusion was recognized, the challenge was to achieve satisfactory implementation. Several approaches were suggested, including the dual track system that caters to learners with special educational needs in one system and all others in another major system.[4] This approach utilized the social constructionism theory or the notion that in reality the society is a social construct, and the notion of disability is constructed to enable some to dominate others.

Besides the one-track system, there is also the multitrack system, which caters to various groups in parallel systems. This approach did not seem to be fully inclusive as it created more stigmas for learners with disabilities to deal with.[5] Moreover, the one-track system[6] posits that children have different abilities and are all gathered in the same classroom.[7] This is the position advanced by the CRPD, which calls for inclusive education. Article 24 of the CRPD provides that

> states parties recognize the right of persons with disabilities to education. With a view to realizing this right without discrimination and on the basis of equal opportunity, States Parties shall ensure *an inclusive education system at all levels and lifelong learning.*[8]

---

4   1994 Salamanca Declaration; David Mitchell, ed., "Introduction," in *Contextualizing Inclusive Education: Evaluating Old and New International Perspectives* (New York: Routledge, 2005), 5.
5   Mitchell, "Introduction," 5.
6   1994 Salamanca Declaration.
7   Mitchell, "Introduction," 5.
8   Article 24, emphasis mine.

The CRPD emphasizes the need to move toward a full right to education in inclusive settings at all levels. It urges the states parties to ensure access to education in practice and that all learners receive life-learning experience and acquire social development skills. The CPRD also emphasizes the need to train teachers to thrive in inclusive settings and compels member states to ensure that all learners are able to study beyond basic education.[9]

Based on the various elements of inclusive education, the latter is defined as a process of addressing the diversity of needs of learners through increasing participation in learning, cultures, and communities and reducing exclusion within and from education. This process involves changes in content, approaches, structures, and strategies, with a common vision that covers all children within an appropriate age range. It also embodies the conviction that it is the responsibility of the mainstream education system to educate all children.[10]

This suggests that inclusion is different from mere mainstreaming or integration. While the latter places students with disabilities in mainstream schools where they are forced to adapt to existing teaching and learning and organization of the school, the former requires adapting the system to meet the needs of the pupil/student with disabilities. In this context, the environment, teaching and learning, organization of the school, as well as the education system are systematically changed in order to remove barriers to pupils/students with disabilities so they can maximize their academic and social achievements. According to Stubbs:[11]

> Inclusive education refers to a wide range of strategies, activities and processes that seek to make a reality of the universal right to quality, relevant and appropriate education. . . . It is part of a wider strategy promoting inclusive development, with the goal of creating a world where there is peace, tolerance, sustainable use of resources, social justice, and where the basic needs and rights of all are met.

With access to inclusive education, persons with disabilities will be productive not only in their own lives as well as that of their families but will also

---

9   Paul Wehman, *Life Beyond the Classroom: Transition Strategies for Young People with Disabilities* (Baltimore: Brookes, 2006).
10 UNESCO, *Guidelines for Inclusion: Ensuring Access to Education for All* (Paris: UNESCO, 2005), 13.
11 Sue Stubbs, *Inclusive Education Where There Are Few Resources* (2002; repr. Oslo: The Atlas Alliance Schweigaardsgt, 2008), 8.

add to the development of their communities and countries. This raises the important question of how to rely on Article 24 of the CRPD to reduce poverty and inequality. Answering this question is the focus of the next section.

Fostering the Inclusion of Learners with Disabilities

This section explores what should be done to foster inclusion of learners with disabilities. Raising awareness on disability as element of human diversity, an explicit provision of the right to inclusive education in the Constitution, and the reliance on local/social context and social institutions, will be instrumental in furthering the inclusion of learners with disabilities in schools.

Promoting disability as an element of human diversity entails locating disability within other constituents of human diversities such as race, gender, sexuality, religion, language, and culture to list just a few. In this perspective, diversity can be described as the quality of being different and varied.[12] Persons with disabilities (PWDs) have the same rights as their nondisabled counterparts. However, they are generally discriminated against and are not allowed to claim their rights equally with others. Such exclusion is generally linked to societal attitudes, perceptions, misunderstandings, and lack of awareness about disabilities.[13] For instance, the false impression that PWDs cannot be productive members of the workforce may result in the refusal to consider their job application even when they are well educated or otherwise qualified for the job.[14]

Similar misconceptions are found in other groups. An indigenous child has no access to education because of language barriers—as education is conducted in English or French. Similarly, a deaf child has no access to education because of lack of sign-language interpreters in class. Both children (indigenous and deaf) face similar barriers that are environmental or societal because having interpreters will ensure their access to education. Adopting a universal learning design curriculum would actually accommodate all

---

12   *Dictionary.com*, "Diversity," *Dictionary.com*, n.d., http://www.dictionary.com/browse/diversity.
13   Janet E. Lord, ed., *Human Rights: YES! Action and Advocacy on the Rights of Persons with Disabilities* (Minneapolis: University of Minnesota Human Rights Center, 2007), 2.
14   Lord et al., *Human Rights*, 17.

learners or learners with different abilities in an inclusive classroom.[15] This suggests that just like PWDs, members of other groups face similar challenges in their daily life. For example, in many communities, women are not allowed to own property—thus discriminated against on the basis of their sex—or a person is discriminated against because of his/her sexuality, race, or religion.[16] While looking at inclusion of the marginalized and attempting to protect human dignity, PWDs shall not be forgotten. In fact, individuals with disabilities are part of the natural diversity of the human race, which includes culture, disability, language, sexuality, age, gender, religion, and spirituality.

It is important to note that all people live in a range of abilities that can change in the course of life and that no one should be ignored or marginalised because of a specific (dis)ability. Consequently, recognizing disability as an element of human diversities will go a long way in addressing the right to equality and prohibiting discrimination on all grounds for the benefit of humanity at large. This understanding of disability will certainly open doors to education for learners with disabilities who will also benefit from opportunity provided by learning.

The Explicit Constitutionalization of the Right to Inclusive Education

The explicit constitutionalization of the right to inclusive education simply calls for the express protection of this right in the constitution and, more importantly, in its binding part. The clear recognition of this right will ensure its visibility, enable disability rights to enter the policy arena, and will improve the likelihood of better enforcement.

Ensuring the Visibility of Disability Rights and the Right to Inclusive Education in the National Legal Landscape

Generally, prohibitions against discrimination on the grounds of disability are not explicitly stated in constitutions. On the contrary, there is a formal right to equality that is not practicable. This approach often prohibits

---

15   Chataika, "Inclusion."
16   Lord et al., *Human Rights*.

discrimination on the grounds of gender, race, or religion, while disability rights protection is interpreted under "other status"[17]. This approach fosters the indivisibility of disability as a sphere of discrimination. It is therefore important to remedy this visibility problem by moving from "implicit protection to explicit protection"[18] with clear and concrete protections of disability rights. From this perspective, disability rights and the right to inclusive education should be incorporated into the bill of rights or the binding part of the constitution.

The more rights to inclusive education are explicit, publicly promoted, and well-recognized, the more likely the state is to secure its financing through necessary budgetary allocation. Furthermore, such visibility is also likely to lead to the adoption of reasonable accommodation measures as well as the provision of assisting devices commensurate with types of disabilities in the classroom. In addition, securing the visibility of disability in the constitution is also expected to lead to the adoption of affirmative action policies needed to move from formal to substantive equality in the right to access education.

Disability Rights in the Policy Arena

An explicit constitutionalization of the right to inclusive education will compel the state to adopt adequate policies to give effect to this commitment under the constitution. This suggests that the disability rights discourse is likely to enter the policy arena or policy community known as a network of policy stakeholders. The latter comprises individuals, groups, government ministries (both the lead ministry and its cognate or sister ministries/departments), civic and nongovernmental organizations and other actors who dominate decision making in a given policy field.

The entry into the policy circle will propel disability issues and the right to inclusive education into the political debates with players such as political parties having to include the right to inclusive education into their program of actions, with trade unions fighting for disability rights and inclusive education in particular. In other words, the needs of learners with disabilities will be addressed. In this context, policymaking in the area of education would entail consulting those responsible for service delivery or implementation of

---

17 African Charter on Human and Peoples' Rights, Article 2.
18 Kamga, "Inclusion."

education for all, including learners with disabilities.[19] Furthermore, those who are at the receiving end or otherwise affected by the policy, such as learners with disabilities and their parents, would be also consulted.[20] In addition, this will lead to a monitoring and evaluation of the inclusive policies' impact to know whether learners with disabilities are effectively included in the education system.[21]

These policy steps for inclusion will lead to budget provisions to revise the curriculum, training of teachers, and transformation of the environment to ensure its inclusiveness. It will also provide a space for budgetary provision to establish necessary institutions and agencies needed to ensure that the right to education for learners with disabilities does become a reality.

Policies should be responsive to the inclusion of learners with disabilities. In this respect they should provide appropriate responses to the broad spectrum of learning needs in formal and other educational settings: they should put specific emphasis on those groups of learners who may be at risk of marginalization, exclusion, or underachievement; identify and remove attitudinal, environmental, and institutional barriers to participation and learning; and modify strategies and plans as well as content and approaches to learning.

Ultimately, these policy measures should ensure real inclusion and not mere integration of learners with disability. A real inclusion is

> about the child's right to participate and benefit on an equitable basis to their peers. Inclusive approaches stress the duty of schools (and educational systems as a whole) to adapt and, in principle, accept all children. A premium is placed upon full participation by all students, including (but not only) disabled children, and upon respect for their educational and wider social, civil, and cultural rights. Resources are used to encourage this participation, rather than to provide additional and separate activities. In this way, diversity in the classroom (and wider society) is embraced and viewed as an asset.[22]

---

19   Helen Bullock, Juliet Mountford, and Rebecca Stanley, *Better Policy-Making* (London: Centre for Management and Policy Studies, 2001), 42.
20   Bullock, Mountford, and Stanley, *Policy-Making*, 42.
21   Bullock, Mountford, and Stanley, *Policy-Making*, 42.
22   Sightsavers, *Making Inclusive Education a Reality* (Chippenham, UK: Sightsavers, 2011), 4, https://www.eenet.org.uk/resources/docs/16079_Sightsavers%20IE%20Policy%20Paper%202011%20-%20FINAL.pdf.

Securing a Better Enforceability of Disability Rights

The constitution is the supreme law of the land. Therefore, an express provision on disability rights in the bill of rights will elevate these rights to the same level as other fundamental rights. From this perspective, recognizing the right to inclusive education in the bill of rights would go a long way in securing its enforcement by the court of law. James Nickel[23] writes:

> there may be various degrees of supporting relations between rights, some of which are stronger than others, and that the higher the level of protection of rights in a country, the stronger the prospects of realization is rendered.

Sharing this view, Kamga[24] demonstrates that when a right is explicitly constitutionalized, it is likely to be better protected by the court. In making his case, Kamga[25] relies on the South African jurisprudence on socioeconomic rights to show that a clear constitutional protection of these rights leads to better protection by the courts.

However, even though the South African Constitution does not expressly provide for the right to inclusive education (although it guarantees the right "to education [of] everyone"), the South African courts successfully protected the right to inclusive education. In this context, the right to equality applies to the right to education, and in this legal environment, learners with disabilities are protected as demonstrated by the court in the *Western Cape Forum* case[26] where the court held that learners with intellectual disabilities are entitled to the same right to education as their nondisabled counterparts.

Nevertheless, it is important to note that in the South African context, the court is known to be independent and protective of socioeconomic rights in general, hence its ability to ensure the inclusiveness of education. This is to say that it remains essential to expressly provide for the right to inclusive education in order to guide the courts in other African jurisdictions that are not as powerful as the South African courts. Even in cases where the separation of powers is flawed and the court is unlikely to protect human rights (including disabilities rights), it could be argued that constitutionalizing

---

23   James W. Nickel, "Rethinking Indivisibility: Towards a Theory of Supporting Relations Between Human Rights," *Human Rights Quarterly* 30 (2008): 984.
24   Kamga, "Inclusion."
25   Kamga, "Inclusion."
26   *Western Cape Forum* case (2011) 5 SA 87 (WCC).

these rights will shed some light on their violation should this happen. In other words, a clear recognition of disability rights and the right to education for learners with disabilities would increase the prospect of their enforcement in Africa. Even if in some cases constitutionalizing the rights does not lead to effective protections by the court, the problem could be linked to the court's general lack of judicial independence or its incapacity to protect socioeconomic rights, as in various civil law jurisdictions.[27]

Relying on the Social Context and Social Institution

While legalism or reliance on the rule of law is important to advance disability rights and the right to inclusive education to tackle poverty and inequality, it is also imperative to address the discrimination and exclusion of learners with disabilities from school with reliance on the social construct. This means conducting an ethnographic examination in some communities and exploring how the local cultures can foster inclusive education. In this context, despite the diversity of the African continent, the communitarian way of life—the togetherness that echoes the *ubuntu* philosophy—cut across the continent.[28] The word *ubuntu* is an expression from the Nguni language whose meaning, according to Mokgoro,[29] is

> a philosophy of life, which in its most fundamental sense represents personhood, humanity, humaneness and morality; a metaphor that describes group solidarity where such group solidarity is central to the survival of communities with a scarcity of resources, where people have to rely on each other to survive.

---

27 Horace Sègnonna Adjolohoun, "Between Presidentialism and a Human Rights Approach to Constitutionalism: Twenty Years of Practice and the Dilemma of Revising the 1990 Constitution of Benin," in *Constitutionalism and Democratic Governance in Africa: Contemporary Perspectives from Sub-Saharan Africa*, ed. Thuto M. Hlalele, et al. (Pretoria: PULP, 1990), 25.

28 Ben Chigara, "The Humwe Principle: A Social-odering Grundnorm for Zimbabwe and Africa?" in *Essay in African Land Law*, ed. Robert Home (Pretoria: PULP, 2011), 117–118.

29 Mokgoro Yvone, "Ubuntu and the Law in South Africa" *Buffalo Human Rights Law Review* 4 (1998), http://www.puk.ac.za/opencms/export/PUK/html/fakulteite/regte/per/issues/98v1mokg.pdf.

Ubuntu epitomizes love and compassion for one another.[30] Hence there is the need to tap into such a culture—one characterized by love, kindness, and empathy—to advance the inclusion of persons with disabilities in general and their inclusion in the education system in particular. For this to happen, it is imperative to address the cultural belief positing that disability is a curse: this can be done not only by outlawing discrimination but also by relying on social institutions such as traditional community leaders. In this environment, it is essential to rely on what Zwart[31] calls "the receptor approach to human rights," which highlights the need to rely on local realities and social institutions to enforce international human rights standards. From this perspective, educating traditional leaders on the need to protect disability rights and inclusive education will give parents the confidence to send their disabled children to school. It is important while educating the masses on the CRPD to ensure that the discourse filters down to the grassroots level through their leaders or community organizers who have influence in communities.

The importance of traditional leaders in this endeavor cannot be neglected. According to Adewumi and Egwurube,[32]

> [T]he group referred to as traditional leaders/rulers or tribal leaders/rulers are individuals occupying communal political leadership positions sanctified by cultural mores and values, and enjoying the legitimacy of particular communities to direct their affairs. . . . Their basis of legitimacy is therefore tradition, which includes the whole range of inherited culture and way of life; a people's history; moral and social values and the traditional institutions which survive to serve those values.

Traditional leaders are the custodians of *ubuntu*, are respected in their communities and as such could be more effective than the formal legal system

---

30   Thaddeus Metz, "Towards an African Moral Theory," *Journal of Political Philosophy* 15, no 3. (2007); and Thaddeus Metz, "Ubuntu as a Moral Theory and Human Rights in South Africa," *African Human Rights Law Journal* 11, no. 2 (2011).

31   Tom Zwart, "Using Local Culture to Further the Implementation of International Human Rights: The Receptor Approach," *Human Rights Quarterly* 34 (2012): 546–569.

32   J. B. Adewumi and Egwurube Joseph, "The Roles of Traditional Rulers in Historical Perspective," in *Local Government and the Traditional Rulers in Nigeria*, ed. Oladimeji Aborisade (Ile-Ife: University of Ife Press, 1985), 20.

in addressing exclusion. Turning these traditional institutions into allies in fostering inclusion is likely to lead to a large community mobilization for inclusion: not only because it is the right thing to do but also because of the involvement of the traditional leader who is generally considered the community guide.

The involvement of the traditional institution in the inclusion of learners with disabilities will demystify disability and will normalize the acceptance of disability in the community. This will foster independent living and full inclusion of persons with disabilities not only at school but also in the communities at large. Using this method would simply be the implementation of what Zwart[33] describes as "[t]he African approach [which] focuses on collective survival, rather than pursuing individual self-interest, and therefore relies on cooperation, interdependence, and collective responsibility." In this respect, the inclusion of learners with disabilities in school becomes a collective responsibility and not the state's duty under traditional human rights discourse. This means in light of the African charter (Article 27) that provides for citizens' duty to their communities, everyone has an obligation to assist a person with a disability to ensure that he or she has access to education. In this context, inclusive education will not only be informed by the adoption of appropriate curricula, teacher training, reasonable accommodation measures, assisting devices, more disabled access to public spaces, and strong community-based mobilization.

Community mobilization produced positive results in Kenya in the 1980s when, as a result of a shortage of special schools, the community under the leadership of the Kenyan Society for the Blind developed itinerant services for visually impaired learners as well as students with other disabilities.[34] The community utilized the concept of "Open Education," which entailed convincing regular schools to register blind and visually impaired children in the local area with in-school specialist support. The sustained campaign led by the community yielded positive results, as the Ministry of Education and Teachers Service Commission got involved and sent one young and enthusiastic teacher of the blind on a three-month training course at Montfort College in Malawi.[35] Upon his return, he found full-time employment in

---

33 Zwart, "Local Culture," 555.
34 Joseph Kisanji, "Inclusive Education in Namibia: The Challenge for Teacher Education" (Rossing Foundation, Khomasdal, Windhoek, Namibia, March 24–25, 1999), 8.
35 Kisanji, "Inclusive Education," 8.

schools to foster inclusion of blind and visually impaired learners through braille reading and writing and to offer guidance in orientation and mobility. Furthermore, he assisted classroom teachers and ensured their readiness to work with disabled learners. More importantly, he also made time to "visit homes of blind children to assist with early stimulation and to prepare children and their parents for entry into regular schools."[36] Over the years, the community at large developed into a disabled-friendly environment, helping disabled learners and training more teachers to meet the needs of the schools and students.

This is indeed a localized example of fostering inclusive education. Although the state supported the initiative, the local community was responsible for implementing these disabled-friendly measures. This kind of local initiative could build on the community's obligation to provide inclusive education to its disabled learners. This was *ubuntu* at work, which is to say that an appropriate reliance on the local context should supplement formal, state-sponsored legal initiatives in fostering inclusive education.

Conclusion

The aim of this chapter was to explore ways of addressing poverty and inequality in sub-Saharan Africa. It called for the inclusion of children with disabilities in the education system as a way of combating poverty and inequality, which are the faces of "disablement." After deconstructing the concept of inclusive education, the chapter found that the best way to advance inclusive education of children with disabilities is through raising awareness of disability as element of human diversity, the explicit constitutionalization of the right to inclusive education, and the reliance on the localized social context and social institutions.

On the first point about promoting the idea of disability as an element of human diversity, it was found that linking disability with other factors of exclusion such as race, gender, immigration, or indigenous status will help shed light on educational marginalization experienced by disabled persons. This is a marginalization that stems from similar prejudicial attitudes as the exclusion of females or migrants, for instance. Such understanding can hopefully lead to tolerance and full inclusion of learners with disabilities not only at school but in the community at large.

---

36   Kisanji, "Inclusive Education."

On the second point, the need for an explicit constitutionalization of the right to inclusive education, it was found that such an approach will lead to better visibility of disability rights in general and the right to inclusive education in particular. It is also likely to propel disability rights and the right to education into the policy arena with more attention from stakeholders with the ultimate outcome being to foster the inclusion of learners with disabilities. In addition, the explicit guarantee of the right to inclusive education is expected to lead to better enforcement of that right, which will be implemented into the highest law of the land. Even though the expected outcome may not be the same—for example, in the case of weak separations of powers—the impact will remain significant in terms of standard setting.

Lastly, it was found that relying on local context will go a long way in fostering inclusion of learners with disabilities in schools. It was noted that relying on traditional institutions at the center that act as the heads of communities will be instrumental. Tapping into the local context, the chapter showed how disability rights were advanced as result of community-based mobilization in Kenya.

In sum, the chapter argued that effectively addressing poverty and inequality in sub-Saharan Africa means fostering the inclusion of learners with disabilities in the education system. Failure to do this will keep persons with disabilities at society's margins, which will only lead to increased poverty and inequality.

Chapter Twelve

Inclusive Education and Cultural Relevance in East Africa

Angi Stone-MacDonald
and Ozden H. Pinar Irmak

Inclusive Education Policies

The Convention on the Rights of Person with Disabilities,[1] the World Declaration on Education for All,[2] the Standard Rules on the Equalization of Opportunities for Persons with Disabilities,[3] and the Salamanca Statement[4]

---

1 United Nations, *Convention on the Rights of Persons with Disabilities and Optional Protocol* (Paris: UNESCO, 2006), https://www.un.org/development/desa/disabilities/convention-on-the-rights-of-persons-with-disabilities.html.
2 UNESCO, *World Declaration on Education for All* (Paris: UNESCO, 1990), https://www.humanium.org/en/world-declaration-on-education-for-all/.
3 UNESCO, *Standard Rules on the Equalization of Opportunities for Persons with Disabilities* Paris: UNESCO, 1994), https://www.un.org/disabilities/documents/gadocs/standardrules.pdf.
4 UNESCO, *The Salamanca Statement and Framework for Action on Special Needs Education* (Paris: UNESCO, 1994).

are a key series of conventions and declarations that have been enacted through the influence of the disability movement in various countries.[5]

The CRPD aims to ensure children with disabilities full participation in education and society and receive the full range of human rights.[6] Article 24 of the CRPD states that "persons with disabilities are not excluded from the general education system on the basis of disability, that children with disabilities are not excluded from free and compulsory primary education or from secondary education, on the basis of disability."[7] CRPD mandates that governments recognize disabled people's rights to an education and ensure an inclusive education system.[8]

The Salamanca World Conference, which produced the Salamanca Statement, proclaimed the need to

> recognize that every child has unique characteristics, interests, abilities and learning needs, and that education systems should be designed and educational programmes implemented to take into account the wide diversity of these characteristics and needs. . . . The statement asserts . . . regular schools with this inclusive orientation are the most effective means of combating discriminatory attitudes, creating welcoming communities, building an inclusive society and achieving education for all.[9]

A critical reading of the African union policy documents shows that disability is not clearly understood from a human rights perspective. Instead, disability issues and people with disabilities "are often seen by policy-makers as an afterthought, when compared with other minority groups, such as women and children."[10]

---

5   Oyugi, "Inclusive Education in Kenya: A Study of Special Education Teachers' Perceptions and Attitudes toward Inclusion of Children with Disabilities," University of California at Santa Barbara (2011).
6   United Nations, *Convention on the Rights of Person with Disabilities*, 7.
7   United Nations, *Convention on the Rights of Person with Disabilities*, 17.
8   T. Chataika et al., "Access to Education in Africa: Responding to the United Nations Convention on the Rights of Person with Disabilities," *Disability and Society* 27, no. 3 (2012): 385–389.
9   UNESCO, *Salamanca Statement*, viii–ix.
10 R. Lang et al., "Policy Development: An Analysis of Disability Inclusion in a Selection of African Union Policies Inclusive," *Development Policy Review* (2017).

African Union policy documents suggest that education receives a higher priority level within disability inclusion than do the other policy domains, such as health or rights protection.[11] However, upon closer review, this mention of inclusion in educational policies is generally in relation to special education services for children with disabilities in segregated settings; this is not advocating for inclusive education practices and the education of children with disabilities alongside their normally developing peers. Many special and inclusive education programs across East Africa are limited in scope within the national education systems and service provision for children with disabilities. In addition, the number of students receiving educational services in inclusive settings is low, but not many studies estimate the number of children in inclusive settings. The East African countries of Kenya, Uganda, and Tanzania have approximately 2.85 million children with disabilities.[12] There are very few statistical facts about issues concerning children with disabilities, and an exact figure denoting the number of individuals with disabilities is unavailable; student disabilities issues tend to keep a low profile in East African countries.[13] In several countries, the educational services are typically geared toward specific disabilities. A study of the situation in Ghana showed that the special and inclusive education system currently provides services for only three types of students with disabilities (deafness, blindness, and intellectual disabilities) after thirty years of work.[14] Only a fraction of 1 percent of children with disabilities were in school, and many had to wait several years for a spot in a school that could meet their needs.[15]

From a policy perspective, African governments often enact policies that assign responsibility for educating people with disabilities to government

---

11 Lang et al., "Policy Development."

12 L. Stöpler, *Hidden Shame: Violence against Children with Disabilities in East Africa* (The Hague: Terre des Hommes, 2007), https://www.ohchr.org/Documents/Issues/Women/WRGS/GirlsAndDisability/OtherEntities/TerreDesHommes.pdf.

13 Chataika et al., "Access to Education in Africa"; and G. Mukuria and J. Korir, "Education for Children with Emotional and Behavioral Disorders in Kenya: Problems and Prospects," *Preventing School Failure* 50, no. 2 (2006): 49–54.

14 L. K. Ametepee and D. Anastasiou, "Special and Inclusive Education in Ghana: Status and Progress, Challenges and Implications," *International Journal of Educational Development* 41 (2015): 143–152.

15 A. Kniel and C. Kniel, *Handbook for Starting and Running a Unit for Special Needs Children Attached to a Regular School* (Winneba: German Technical Cooperation, 2008).

educational agencies, but these agencies do not have the material or human resources to meet the demand. In fact, many struggle to meet the demand for education of typically developing students.[16] Furthermore, the complex interactions between African beliefs, cultures, and traditions on the one hand and colonial and postcolonial policy on the other influence service provisions and financial support for children with disabilities, and directives from international organizations and northern countries hamper the availability of services for individuals with disabilities. Moreover, the protection and care of children with disabilities are not prioritized.[17]

Inclusive Education Practices

Inclusive education is a global education policy[18] encouraged by UNESCO and other international policy actors, such as USAID, the Department for International Development (DFID), and the World Bank and ratified by national governments across sub-Saharan Africa.[19] In fact, some policies have gone further to say that special needs children must be educated with their typically developing peers in inclusive settings in several sub-Saharan African countries.[20] Despite political and policy commitments from various sub-Saharan African governments, the educational opportunities for

---

16 *The World Bank*, "Education for All," *The World Bank*, August 4, 2014, https://www.worldbank.org/en/topic/education/brief/education-for-all.

17 Mukuria and Korir, "Education for Children"; and Stöpler, "Hidden Shame."

18 A. Verger, M. Novelli, and H. K. Altinyelken, *Global Education Policy and International Development: New Agendas, Issues, and Policies* (New York: Bloomsbury Academic, 2012).

19 D. A. Armstrong, A. C. Armstrong, and I. Spadagou, "Inclusion: By Choice or by Chance?" *International Journal of Inclusive Education* 15 (2011): 29–39.

20 O. Abosi and T. L. Koay, "Attaining Development Goals of Children with Disabilities: Implications for Inclusive Education," *International Journal of Special Education* 23, no. 3 (2008): 1–10; L. K. Ametepee and D. Anastasiou, "Special and Inclusive Education in Ghana: Status and Progress, Challenges and Implications," *International Journal of Educational Development* 41 (2015): 143–152; and C. Howell, J. McKenzie, and T. Chataika, "Building Teachers' Capacity for Inclusive Education in South Africa and Zimbabwe Through CPD," *Continuing Professional Teacher Development in Sub-Saharan Africa: Improving Teaching and Learning* (2018): 127–150.

children with disabilities and the development of special and inclusive education are still challenging issues. In a review of inclusive practice, Pather and Nxumalo[21] found that

> developments in Africa have been aspirational in terms of models for policy and practice, although not without its challenges. Challenges which appear to inhibit inclusive education development in Africa are multifarious and point largely to systemic issues as well as attitudinal. These include poverty, limited or lack of human and material resources, large numbers of under-qualified or unqualified teachers, discriminatory attitudes, inflexible curricula, lack of clear conceptualisation of inclusion, the lack of participation of parents and community organisations in decentralised processes of decision-making, and the lack of policy integration.

The following section describes the state of special and inclusive education for five East African countries and provides a brief history of education for each to contextualize their situations. This overview is not meant to be exhaustive but rather to provide an illustration of issues and practices in East Africa commonly affecting the implementation of inclusive education.

Tanzania

In Tanzania, children with disabilities are acknowledged in policy and legislative documents as having the right to an education and to participate in their communities as active members.[22] At the same time, the Tanzania National Disability Policy openly states that the government is resource poor and cannot provide the necessary services to individuals with disabilities. Since 2008, the Tanzanian government has been working with many local organizations and outside donors to develop more inclusive practices and strategies for addressing the needs of children with disabilities in public government schools. The most recent Tanzanian data available show that between 2 percent and 40 percent of children with disabilities between ages

---

21   S. Pather and C. P. Nxumalo, "Challenging Understandings of Inclusive Education Policy Development in Southern Africa Through Comparative Reflection," *International Journal of Inclusive Education* 17, no. 4 (2013): 423.

22   Angi Stone-Macdonald and A. Fettig, "Culturally Relevant Assessment and Support of Grade 1 Students with Mild Disabilities in Tanzania: An Exploratory Study," *International Journal for Disability, Development and Education*, forthcoming.

seven and thirteen attend school, but Tanzanian policymakers believe some of these estimates are unduly high[23] As of 2013, Tanzania had twenty-one self-contained primary schools and 377 inclusive primary schools.[24]

The Tanzanian Persons with Disabilities Act of 2010 specified several basic principles for the government to enact, including full and effective participation and inclusion of persons with disabilities in all aspects of society, equality of opportunity, and accessibility. Regarding education, it stated that "persons with disabilities [of] all ages and gender[s] shall have [the] exact same rights to education, training, and inclusive settings, and the benefits of research, as other citizens."[25] Nevertheless, Tanzania is just beginning to address the needs of children with disabilities and what constitutes an equitable education and well-being for children and adults with disabilities. This question is especially complex when examining more *invisible* disabilities, such as learning disabilities and mild intellectual disabilities.[26]

In Tanzania, people often do not realize that children who do poorly in school and do not have obvious disabilities could still have developmental delays or disabilities, rather than purposefully being lazy or disobedient. Many Tanzanian teachers currently working in inclusive classrooms did not support inclusion because they believed that it would negatively impact the learning of children without disabilities; they lacked the knowledge, training, and materials to effectively teach children with disabilities and create a productive inclusive environment. [27]

Kenya

After gaining independence in 1963, the government of Kenya recognized education as a basic human right and declared free primary education for

---

23   I. J. Ruyobya and M. Schneider, *The Tanzanian Survey on Disability: Methodology and Overview of Results* (2009), http://www.statssa.gov.za/isi2009/ScientificProgramme/IPMS/1129.pdf.

24   United Republic of Tanzania, *Basic Education Statistics in Tanzania* (Dar es Salaam: MoVET, 2013).

25   United Republic of Tanzania, *The Persons with Disabilities Act, 2010* (Dar es Salaam: Government Printer, 2010), 23.

26   Stone-MacDonald and Fettig, "Culturally Relevant."

27   874 Frida D. Tungaraza, "The Arduous March toward Inclusive Education in Tanzania: Head Teachers' and Teachers' Perspectives," *Africa Today* 61, no. 2 (2014): 109–123.

all in 2003.[28] The government of Kenya has ratified various global policy frameworks in education. For example, it signed Article 26 of the Universal Declaration of Human Rights (1948), the United Nations Convention on the Rights of the Child (CRC) (1989), the African Charter on the Rights of the Child (1990), the Salamanca Statement (1994), the Framework for Action on Special Needs Education (1999), the Millennium Development goals and Education for All by 2015.[29] In addition, Kenya passed and enacted the Children's Act (2001), which was aimed at improving the well-being of all children, irrespective of whether they have disabilities.[30] However, this development has not been without major challenges, especially in relation to children with special needs and disabilities.[31]

Special needs education started in Kenya after World War II, and services were offered mainly to four categories of children with the following disabilities: hearing impairments, mental disabilities, visual impairment, and physical disabilities.[32] In Kenya in 1946, the first special needs education schools were established under missionaries and by nongovernmental organizations (NGOs).[33] Until the 1970s, when integrated programs were initiated, education for children with disabilities was offered only in special schools—mostly boarding schools and away-from-home communities.[34]

Especially in the past three decades, Kenya has exerted tremendous effort in addressing the challenges confronting students with disabilities.[35] Special and inclusive education has been expanded and now includes children with all manner of disabilities.[36] Special education is also being offered for

---

28 Republic of Kenya, Ministry of Education, *The National Special Needs Education Policy Framework* (Kiambu: Ministry of Education, 2009), http://www.unesco.org/education/edurights/media/docs/446808882707702aafc616d3a2cec918bfc186fc.pdf.
29 Ministry of Education, *Special Needs*.
30 Cited in Oyugi, "Inclusive Education."
31 Ministry of Education, *Special Needs*.
32 Ministry of Education, *Special Needs*; Oyugi, "Inclusive Education."
33 H. M. Chonge, E. N. Kiaritha, and J. O. Otieno, "Classroom Curricular Preparedness for Inclusion of Pupils with Physical Disability within Public Inclusive Schools for the Pupils with Physical Disability in Bungoma County, Kenya," *International Journal of Scientific and Technology Research* 5, no. 3 (2016): 20–24; and Oyugi, "Inclusive Education."
34 Ministry of Education, *Special Needs*; and Oyugi, "Inclusive Education."
35 Mukuria and Korir, "Education for Children."
36 Ministry of Education, *Special Needs*; and Oyugi, "Inclusive Education."

learners who are gifted, deaf-blind, orphaned, and/or living in the streets.[37] There has been a gradual increase in the number of special units and public special schools in the country, which includes vocational and technical institutions catering to learners with special needs and disabilities.[38] The availability of free primary education resulted in an increase in enrollment for all children, including children with disabilities in special schools, special units, and typical government primary schools; the government provided grants for students enrolled in special schools.[39] The government's policy on special needs education is contradictory because it offers free primary education to all citizens in principle (including children with disabilities) but fails to provide free education because there are not enough classrooms or teachers for all children to receive adequate educational services. There is no comprehensive policy on the education of individuals with disabilities, whether at the primary, secondary, or tertiary level.[40]

Kenyan schools face many of the same issues as most low and low-middle income countries in Africa: inadequate data on children with disabilities; inadequate funding, materials, and facilities; no appropriate tools and training for early identification and assessment of children with disabilities; and lack of specialized personnel and a shortage of teachers trained in inclusive or special education.[41]

Uganda

The government of Uganda recognizes the rights of persons with disabilities in its constitution, and Article 30 states, "All persons have a right to education."[42] In 1997, universal primary education offered free education for four children per family, and since 2002, free education has covered all children.[43]

---

37 Oyugi, "Inclusive Education."
38 Ministry of Education, *Special Needs*.
39 Mukuria and Korir, "Education for Children."
40 Mukuria and Korir.
41 Ministry of Education, *Special Needs*; Mukuria and Korir, "Education for Children."
42 K. Kristensen et al., "Opportunities for Inclusion? The Education of Learners with Special Educational Needs and Disabilities in Special Schools in Uganda," *British Journal of Special Education* 33 (2006): 139–147.
43 Kristensen et al., "Opportunities for Inclusion?"

In recent years, the government of Uganda has made attempts at making education accessible to all learners and adopted structure and content to promote high-quality learning for all learners' independent special learning needs.[44] To support children with disabilities in mainstream schools in Uganda, the Ministry of Education and Sport (MOES) and Special Needs Education/Educational Assessment and Resource Service programs work together.[45]

As in many other African countries, missionaries and charities played an important historical role in setting up special schools.[46] According to the current system, the commissioner is responsible for special needs education, career guidance, and counseling in MOES at the national level, and the district education officer is responsible for those with disabilities at the district level.[47]

Inclusive schools in Uganda have been grouped into clusters of fifteen to twenty, and each cluster has a special needs education coordinator who visits all schools in the cluster and provides advice on teaching learners with special educational needs. The MOES has assigned at least one teacher in each school to be responsible for inclusive and special needs education, and these teachers are expected to support other teachers who have learners with special needs in their classes in addition to their regular classroom work.[48]

As a result of universal primary education and a greater awareness regarding inclusive education, the number of learners in schools increased, requiring more resources.[49] However, the government of Uganda has not been successful in developing an inclusive education policy or providing the structural changes for inclusive education (i.e., accessible schools and

---

44 Kristensen et al., "Opportunities for Inclusion?"; and M. Suzan and P. W. Soita, "Participation Levels of Children with Special Needs in Adapted Physical Education in Selected Schools in Metropolitan Kampala, Uganda," *International Journal of Arts & Sciences* 7, no. 6 (2014): 49–60.

45 P. Lynch et al., "Inclusive Educational Practices in Uganda: Evidence Practice of Itinerant Teachers Who Work with Children with Visual Impairment in Local Mainstream Schools," *International Journal of Inclusive Education* 15, no. 10 (2011), 1119–1134.

46 Kristensen et al., "Opportunities for Inclusion?"

47 Kristensen et al., "Opportunities for Inclusion?"; and Lynch et al., "Inclusive Educational Practices."

48 Kristensen et al., "Opportunities for Inclusion?"

49 Suzan and Soita, "Participation Levels."

classrooms).[50] There is no specific budget allocated to special needs education, no special curriculum designed for children with special needs, and no critical mass of specialized trained teachers.[51] Also, most learners are not properly assessed before their admission to a special school.

In addition, according to a 2009 Foundation for Human Rights Initiative report,[52] children with physical disabilities have a high dropout rate because of inaccessibility to certain facilities and services (e.g., toilet facilities) and exclusion from play and games. Most of the special schools in Uganda are boarding schools, which hamper development toward more inclusion and more cost-effective systems of schooling.[53]

Rwanda

Christian missionaries were the first to educate children with disabilities in Rwanda,[54] where the genocide impacted services and associations of people with disabilities, so that genocide and disabilities are intertwined.[55] For all the children who witnessed the genocide, many of whom were raped, harassed, and/or separated from their parents while escaping, these experiences made all Rwandan children candidates for special needs education and inclusive education.[56] In addition, during the Rwandan genocide, many people were disabled as a result of bullets, machetes, and landmines.[57]

Rwanda ratified both the CRPD and its optional protocol in 2008 and established the National Council for People with Disabilities to act as an advocacy body, coordinate activities, and monitor progress toward this

---

50 Suzan and Soita, "Participation Levels."
51 Suzan and Soita, "Participation Levels."
52 Suzan and Soita, "Participation Levels."
53 Kristensen et al., "Opportunities for Inclusion?"
54 Education Development Trust, *A Study on Children with Disabilities and Their Right to Education: Republic of Rwanda* (Reading: Education Development Trust, 2016), https://www.educationdevelopmenttrust.com/EducationDevelopmentTrust/files/36/36a56288-d541-47d8-a14c-c3e07f713ef4.pdf.
55 Arnold Nyarambi, *A Historical Analysis of Post-Genocide Rwandan Special Education: Lessons Derived and Future Directions* (Cookeville: Tennessee Technological University, 2009).
56 Nyarambi, *Historical Analysis*.
57 Nyarambi, *Historical Analysis*.

commitment.[58] Orphans and vulnerable children are also classified in difficult circumstances in Rwanda's national policy.[59]

The government first demonstrated its interest in the education of children with disabilities and other special educational needs by setting up an office of special education in the Ministry of Education in 1997.[60] The disability program in Rwanda started in 2006 with a three-year program funded by DFID Rwanda.[61] Currently, children with disabilities are educated in both special schools and mainstream schools, but more national efforts in education are needed for all learners with disabilities.[62]

Rwanda faces the same funding challenges as other East African countries. It has limited or no funds for educating children with disabilities, schools do not have facilities to accommodate children with disabilities, sanitation is poor, and class sizes are large.[63] Moreover, policies and legislation are not well developed, and the lack of trained personnel for local implementation of inclusive education is a critical problem.[64]

Somalia

Somalia gained its independence in 1960, and civil war broke out in 1991.[65] The conflict led to the collapse of the education system, resulting in Somalia having the highest proportion of primary-school-age children not in school[66] From the late 1980s to the early 1990s, all formal education stopped, and at

---

58   Education Development Trust, *Children with Disabilities*.
59   Nyarambi, *Historical Analysis*.
60   Education Development Trust, *Children with Disabilities*.
61   S. Challoner, VSO Rwanda Disability Programme Overview (2012), http://www.ivoindia.org/Images/Rwanda-disability-overview-June-2012_tcm78-37209.pdf.
62   Education Development Trust, *Children with Disabilities*.
63   L. Talley and E. S. Brintnell, "Scoping the Barriers to Implementing Policies for Inclusive Education in Rwanda: An Occupational Therapy Opportunity," *International Journal of Inclusive Education* 20, no. 4 (2016): 364–382.
64   Talley and Brintnell, "Barriers."
65   P. Moyi, "Who Goes to School? School Enrollment Patterns in Somalia," *International Journal of Educational Development* 32 (2012): 163–171.
66   UNESCO, *Length and Starting Age of Compulsory Education for Schools Years 1998/1999 to 2004/2005* (Montreal: UNESCO Institute for Statistics, 2007), as cited in Moyi, "Who Goes to School?"

least two generations of children received little or no education or training.[67] Teachers, students, and the educated elite were forced to leave the country.[68]

After the civil upheaval in Somalia, significant steps have been taken to restore the education system.[69] The civil conflict exacerbated the country's already-dire infrastructure problems: no systematic data are available, the enrollment rate is still low, the lack of trained teachers is a serious problem, and finances are a major constraint.[70] As of this writing, the Ministry of National Education, stakeholders, and NGOs are working to provide special needs education and inclusive education; however, people's attitudes, the lack of public awareness, and limited technical and financial capacity are important barriers to the development of children with disabilities.[71]

Models of Disability and Cultural Beliefs

Models of disability shape the attitudes and beliefs of people about the care and education of individuals with disabilities. The medical model represents the view that disability is caused by a medical diagnosis, and the goal of this model is to eliminate the impairment or return impaired bodies to societal normativity.[72] For people with intellectual disabilities, "The defects that [lead] to limitations in functioning [are] treated as the basis of the disability"[73] and therefore create a negative deterministic fate. The rehabilitation model, viewing the impairment or disability as something that needs to be fixed or rehabilitated, is commonly used in low-income countries as a

---

67   Moyi, "Who Goes to School?"
68   S. A. Bekalo, M. Brophy, and A. G. Welford, "The Development of Education in Post-Conflict 'Somaliland,'" *International Journal of Educational Development* 23 (2003): 459–475.
69   Bekalo, Brophy, and Welford, "Development of Education."
70   Bekalo, Brophy, and Welford, "Development of Education."
71   Sahra Ahmed Koshin, "The Value of Educating Children with Disabilities in Somalia," *World Pulse*, February 10, 2012, https://www.worldpulse.com/community/users/sahro/posts/19524.
72   B. Simmons, T. Blackmore, and P. Bayliss, "Postmodern Synergistic Knowledge Creation: Extending the Boundaries of Disability Studies." *Disability and Society* 23 (2008): 733–745.
73   M. Parchomiuk, "Model of Intellectual Disability and the Relationship of Attitudes towards the Sexuality of Persons with an Intellectual Disability," *Sexuality and Disability* 31, no. 2 (2013): 125.

basis for services, and many NGOs operate community-based rehabilitation programs based on this framework. Doctors, social workers, and educators work to *rehabilitate* the person to function within society through training and education based on societal norms.[74] In that view, the disability occurs at the personal rather than societal level.[75] On the other end of the continuum, the social model regards disability as a normal aspect of life and not as a deviance[76] and rejects the notion that persons with disabilities are in some inherent way "defective."[77] Scholars who argue that the definition of disability is socially constructed view definitions as malleable, reflecting local beliefs about disability and the types of necessary participation in the community to be a "whole" person.[78]

In a review of literature about disability and cultural beliefs in East Africa, a variety of cultural beliefs and attitudes about people with disabilities were illustrated.[79] The review reports that individuals with disabilities are well cared for and generally integrated into the community and that services to

---

74 Deborah Kaplan, "The Definition of Disability," *The Center for an Accessible Society*, 1999, http://www.accessiblesociety.org/topics/demographics-identity/dkaplanpaper.htm; and D. Werner, *Disabled Village Children* (Berkeley: The Hesperian Foundation, 1987).

75 M. Msall et al., "Measurements of Functional Outcomes in Children with Cerebral Palsy," *Mental Retardation and Developmental Disabilities Research Reviews* 3 (1997): 197–203; and G. Mukuria, "Education for Students with Intellectual Disabilities in Kenya: Challenges and Prospects," *Advances in Research and Praxis in Special Education in Africa, Caribbean, and the Middle East* (2012): 67–85.

76 S. J. Peters, "An Ideological-Cultural Framework for the Study of Disability," in *Education and Disability in Cross-Cultural Perspective*, ed. S. J. Peters (New York: Garland, 1993), 19–35; T. Shakespeare and N. Watson, "Defending the Social Model," *Disability and Society* 12 (1997): 293–300; and S. R. Whyte and B. Ingstad, "Disability and Culture: An Overview," in *Disability and Culture*, ed. B. Ingstad and S. R. Whyte (Berkeley: University of California Press, 1995).

77 Kaplan, "Disability."

78 S. G. Harknett, "Cultural Factors in the Definition of Disability: A Community Study in Nyankunde, Zaire," *African Journal of Special Needs Education* 1 (1996): 18–24; and Whyte and Ingstad, "Disability and Culture."

79 Angi Stone-MacDonald and Gretchen Digman Butera, "Cultural Beliefs About Disability in Practice: Experiences at a Special School in Tanzania," *International Journal of Disability, Development, and Education* 59 (2012): 393–407.

help them are provided when available. In other instances, studies have found that individuals with disabilities in East Africa are ridiculed and denied services in favor of people believed to be more economically productive. The literature about disabilities in East Africa demonstrates culturally specific attitudes and beliefs that suggest a social or pluralistic model of disability is more common in East Africa than in northern countries.

First, a range of beliefs about the causes of disability is evident. Most authors document a growing awareness of the biological or genetic causes of disability, but witchcraft, the breaking of taboos, punishment by God or gods, indication of divine will, or the idea of a child as a divine gift continue to be important factors in how East Africans understand disability. Second, according to the literature, individuals with disabilities are less likely to experience stigma associated with an obvious physical deformity or a diagnostic label and more likely to face discrimination than their counterparts in northern countries if they cannot participate in the daily socioeconomic activities of the community. While the range of beliefs about the causes of disability differs from that in some northern countries, the sociocultural context in which disability as an event occurs appears as a critical feature of how disability itself is understood in East African contexts.[80]

The capabilities approach, as first discussed by Sen[81] and Nussbaum,[82] extends the social model by arguing for the just treatment of individuals with disabilities, consistent with a human-rights model focus on substantive equality and real equality of opportunity.[83] This approach considers the sociocultural context of disability within cultural and national groups. The capabilities approach, another way of looking at individuals with disabilities in society, takes into account human diversity by using education to develop "functionings" and capabilities to support individuals with disabilities to be active members of their community. Sen defines "functionings" as the actual

---

80 Stone-MacDonald and Butera, "Cultural Beliefs."
81 928 Amartya Sen. *Development as Freedom* (New York: Knopf, 1999).
82 Martha Nussbaum, *Frontiers of Justice: Disability, Nationality, Species Membership* (Cambridge, MA: Belknap, 2006).
83 Lorella Terzi, "Beyond the Dilemma of Difference: The Capability Approach to Disability and Special Educational Needs," *Journal of Philosophy of Education* 39 (2005): 443–459; and L. Terzi, "A Capability Perspective on Impairment, Disability and Special Needs: Towards Social Justice in Education," *Theory and Research in Education* 3 (2005): 197–223.

achievements of the individual through being or doing.[84] Capabilities are the opportunities or freedoms to achieve functionings that can be realized or developed.[85] Both Sen and Nussbaum use functionings in the plural to encompass all possible achievements or actions. The capabilities approach[86] views disability as one of many factors that contribute to the holistic person and promote fair and equal treatment in society.

The Capabilities Approach

The human capability approach has been defined and discussed by several scholars, beginning with Sen[87] and Nussbaum.[88] Terzi[89] further examined the capabilities approach from the perspective of disability. Her capabilities approach positions the "education of children with disabilities within the social justice debate as this diverse group has been excluded from other philosophical and political formulations of social justice."[90] Nussbaum and Terzi view education as a fundamental human right for all children regardless of their abilities and education as the key to developing their capabilities and functionings.[91] It is through education, in schools, with the family, and in the community that children gain the knowledge and skills necessary to participate fully and equally in their communities and achieve their functionings.[92] When social systems create a disadvantage, or children are unable to overcome their impairments, the capabilities approach argues for resources to support those children who need additional investment to overcome their disabilities. Nussbaum questions the idea of *normality*: "[I]t would be

---

84 Sen, *Development as Freedom*.
85 Nussbaum, *Frontiers of Justice*.
86 Nussbaum, *Frontiers of Justice*; and Sen, *Development as Freedom*.
87 Sen, *Development as Freedom*.
88 Nussbaum, *Frontiers of Justice*.
89 L. Terzi, *Justice and Equality in Education: A Capability Perspective on Disability and Special Educational Needs* (London: Bloomsbury , 2008).
90 Filiz Polat, "Inclusion in Education: A Step towards Social Justice," *International Journal of Educational Development* 31, no. 1 (2011): 52.
91 L. Terzi, "What Metric of Justice for Disabled People? Capability and Disability," *Measuring Justice: Primary Goods and capabilities* (2010): 150–173.
92 Ashley Taylor, "Addressing Ableism in Schooling and Society? The Capabilities Approach and Students with Disabilities," *Philosophy of Education Archive* (2012): 113–121.

progress if we could acknowledge that there is no such thing as 'the normal child'; instead, there are children with varying capabilities and impediments, all of whom need individualized attention as their capabilities developed."[93]

The Capabilities Approach in the African Context

In African countries, a person with a disability is usually defined as an individual who has a cognitive or physical disability that makes it difficult or impossible to complete his or her daily activities without help. Because walking long distances and manual labor are often required for survival, people with disabilities struggle with these physical activities and may be viewed as deficient because of their dependence on others; however, a disability such as dyslexia may not be viewed as a disability in an area with a high illiteracy rate, whereas someone with a minor mobility impairment may be significantly disadvantaged in a society that requires one to walk many miles during the day and carry purchased goods over long distances.[94] It is important to examine how individual societies view disability and how they conceptualize successful inclusion and participation of people with disabilities.

Furthermore, isolating disability without considering a holistic view of well-being or "wholeness" may not be functional in the local context.[95] In many African contexts, disability or ableism is not separate from one's overall well-being; it is simply a component. There is a rich literature on cultural beliefs about disability and how societies view people with disability in terms of ableism and wholeness.[96]

---

93 Nussbaum, *Frontiers of Justice*, 210.
94 Harknett, "Cultural Factors."
95 Harknett, "Cultural Factors."
96 R. Chimedza, "Disability as a Social Construct," *African Journal of Special Needs Education* 6, no. 2 (2001): 121–127; T. B. Derseh, "Meanings Attached to Disability, Attitudes towards Disabled People and Attitudes towards Integration" (PhD diss., University of Jyvaskyla, 1997); P. J. Devlieger, "Why Disabled? The Cultural Understanding of Physical Disability in African Society," in *Disability and Culture*, edited by B. Ingstad and S. R. Whyte (Berkeley: University of California Press, 1995); Brigitte Holzer, Arthur Vreede, and Gabriele Weigt, eds., *Disability in Different Cultures: Reflections on Local Concepts* (Bielefeld, Germany: Transcript Verlag, 1999); Ingstad and Whyte, *Disability and Culture*; J. Kisanji, "Attitudes and Beliefs About Disability in Tanzania," in *Innovations in Developing Countries for People with*

The capabilities approach stresses equity in education and views the functionings a person needs to develop as an individual to be successful, providing not just equality of opportunity but also equality of access. In some East African societies, disability is determined not through a medical diagnosis but by one's ability to play a role in society.[97] However, Groce and Zola state that "traditional belief systems on disability have at times proven to be quite adaptive, shifting in response to social, economic, and educational experiences gained through acculturation."[98] As cultural belief systems change, local communities are welcoming diversity and helping students with disabilities participate in public education systems. While individuals may not be aware of the capabilities approach, understanding how a person conceptualizes disability and the functionings needed in a community to be successful can help community members develop disability awareness and acceptance within their cultural local context.

The Role of Cultural Beliefs in Developing Inclusive Education Practices

Cultural beliefs and attitudes are an important part of the conceptualization of disability in any society and have a significant influence on how services are designed and developed. In sub-Saharan Africa, beliefs, particularly about the causes of disability, have historically been multifaceted. In the last twenty years, beliefs and attitudes are changing and moving toward a melded model of medical and nonmedical understandings about disability.[99] Throughout sub-Saharan Africa, the literature indicates that people with disabilities are

---

Disabilities, ed. B. O'Toole and R. McConkey (Whittle-le-Woods: Lisieux Hall , 1995), 51–70; and J. Kisanji, "The Relevance of Indigenous Customary Education Principles in the Formulation of Special Needs Education Policy" (paper, International Special Education Congress, Birmingham, United Kingdom, April 10–13, 1995).

97   Harknett, "Cultural Factors"; Kisanji, "Attitudes and Beliefs"; M. Miles, "Children with Hydrocephalus and Spina Bifida in East Africa: Can Family and Community Resources Improve the Odds?" *Disability and Society* 17 (2002): 643–658; and Talley and Brintnell, "Scoping the Barriers."

98   Nora Ellen Groce and Irving Kenneth Zola, "Multiculturalism, Chronic Illness, and Disability," *Pediatrics* 91, no. 5 (1993): 1054.

99   Angi Stone-MacDonald, *Community-Based Education for Students with Developmental Disabilities in Tanzania* (Dordrecht, The Netherlands: Springer, 2014).

cared for and receive services to help them when those services are available—which, unfortunately, is not often. Communities and families often take responsibility for their members with disabilities; however, individuals with disabilities still face discrimination regarding their ability to participate in the daily social and economic activities of the community.[100]

In Rwanda, disability is still regarded as a source of shame, and people with disabilities are commonly addressed by the type of their disability rather than their given name. Women with disabilities rarely marry, but those that are married are often mistreated and stigmatized by the widespread belief that their children must also have a disability, even when those children are developing normally; a woman who gives birth to a child with a disability is frequently abandoned by her husband.[101]

Attitudes toward people with disabilities vary according to type of disability. For example, physical disabilities are the most accepted form because of the increase of such disabilities after the genocide.[102] Children who are blind or deaf or have an intellectual impairment are at significant risk of social exclusion and suffer more discrimination than those with other types of disabilities.[103]

In Uganda, stigma is associated with disability, attitudes, and traditional beliefs about disabilities. According to Devries et al., children with disabilities and their families experience social isolation and are perceived as unworthy of dignity and respect.[104] Children with disabilities attending school are at a higher risk for violence than their nondisabled peers.

Attitudes toward individuals with disabilities in Kenya are generally negative, and these individuals have traditionally been viewed as helpless and

---

100 Harknett, "Cultural Factors"; S. O. V. P. Hartley et al., "How Do Carers of Disabled Children Cope? The Ugandan Perspective," *Child: Care, Health and Development* 31, no. 2 (2005): 167–180; Ruth Morgan, "Using Life Story Narratives to Understand Disability and Identity in South Africa," *Disability and the Life Course: Global Perspectives* (2001): 89–100; Nathan Oyori Ogechi and Sara Jerop Ruto, "Portrayal of Disability Through Personal Names and Proverbs in Kenya: Evidence from Ekegusii and Nandi," *Vienna Journal of African Studies* 3 (2002): 63–82.

101 Nyarambi, *Historical Analysis*.

102 Nyarambi, *Historical Analysis*.

103 Nyarambi, *Historical Analysis*; and Talley and Brintnell, "Scoping the Barriers."

104 K. M. Devries et al., "Violence against Primary School Children with Disabilities in Uganda: A Cross-Sectional Study," *BMC Public Health* 14, no. 1017 (2014): 1–9.

hopeless. People mostly believe that a disability is "retribution of past deeds by the ancestors."[105] Children with disabilities are hidden from the rest of society because their parents tend to be ashamed of them. According to a study by Bunning et al., causal blame is still attributed to immediate family members and often identifies women as complicit in immoral behavior because of their lower status in African society and their roles as caregivers.[106]

In addition, teachers' behaviors and attitudes are subject to outside influence and treat students with certain disabilities differently than others. For example, in a study of general education teachers' attitudes toward inclusive education in Kenya, Oyugi found that the total number of learners in a classroom encouraged the teachers to have a positive or negative attitude toward inclusion.[107]

About 98 percent of Somalis are Muslim, and religion plays an important role in people's attitudes toward and perceptions of disability. In a study carried out with Somali immigrants in the United States by Greeson, Veach, and Leroy,[108] most of the participants said that disability comes from Allah. Allah decides whether a couple will have more children and whether they will be healthy: Allah determines all outcomes. In addition, as stated by the participants, in Somalia family members care for people with disabilities, and family members and neighbors are responsible for helping people with disabilities. By contrast, according to Koshin,[109] some families see disability as a curse or punishment from Allah and keep children with disabilities indoors; some families think that girls with disabilities are more vulnerable, so parents keep them at home where it is safer.

---

105 Mukuria and Korir, "Education for Children."
106 K. Bunning et al., "The Perception of Disability by Community Groups: Stories of Local Understanding, Beliefs, and Challenges in a Rural Part of Kenya," *PLOS One* 12, no. 8 (2017): 1–20.
107 Oyugi, "Inclusive Education in Kenya."
108 C. J. Greeson, P. M. Veach, and B. S. Leroy, "A Qualitative Investigation of Somali Immigrant Perceptions of Disability: Implications for Genetic Counseling," *Journal of Genetic Counseling* 10, no. 5 (2001): 359–378.
109 Koshin, "Disabilities in Somalia."

Culturally Relevant Curriculum and the Capabilities Approach

To successfully educate students with disabilities, learners' backgrounds and the community culture, beliefs, and values must be understood. Bronfenbrenner's bioecological systems theory[110] provides a framework detailing that the interactions among aspects of the child's environment are critical to his or her development. Culture, society, and family are three of the crucial components in this model. Bronfenbrenner and Morris state, "Throughout the life course, human development takes place through processes of progressively more complex, reciprocal interaction between an active evolving bio-psychological human organism and the persons, objects, and symbols in its immediate external environment."[111] From a contextualist approach, people are embedded in the local context, and the local context is embedded in the culture.[112] Harry emphasizes that an ecocultural approach examines the specific impact of context and culture on family, school, and community interactions. Children enter school embodying the characteristics of their families, developed through familial interactions and experiences. In East Africa, the interactions that students with disabilities have with their families and their communities influence their development and ability to participate in their community. Understanding the culture and the community then informs educators and policymakers about the interactions affecting the children's development and education.

Local culture is especially important when designing curriculum for students with disabilities. This emphasis on local context encourages communities to exhibit positive attitudes and beliefs about people with disabilities and include individuals with disabilities in the schools so that they can receive an education and job training for roles in the community. Disability advocacy and culturally relevant curricula help prepare students with disabilities to be included in their families' and communities' activities. Reflecting on

---

110 U. Bronfenbrenner, "Ecological Systems Theory," in *Six Theories of Child Development: Revised Formulations and Current Issues*, ed. R. Vasta (London: Jessica Kingsley, 1992), 187–249.

111 U. Bronfenbrenner and P. Morris, "The Ecology of Developmental Processes," in *Handbook of Child Psychology*, vol. 1: *Theoretical Models of Human Development*, 5th ed. (New York: Wiley, 1998), 996.

112 B. Harry, "Trends and Issues in Serving Culturally Diverse Families of Children with Disabilities," *Journal of Special Education* 36, no. 3 (2002): 131–138, 147.

the capabilities approach, the curriculum can then be adapted using this approach in a variety of ways to draw on the strengths of children and their community while developing their capabilities and functionings that are considered valuable within their local community and context.

Funds of Knowledge

Communities and families are repositories of funds of knowledge. Using this knowledge to understand communities, local context, and how to teach students can inform our teaching practice on several levels. Gonzalez, Moll, and Amanti deploy the phrase *funds of knowledge* to denote "historically accumulated and culturally developed bodies of knowledge and skills essential for household or individual functioning and well-being."[113] While students with disabilities may be viewed as lacking basic skills and "viewed with a lens of deficiencies [and as] substandard in their socialization practices, language practices, and orientation toward scholastic achievement," the acquisition and application of these funds of knowledge may help them to be more successful members of society.[114]

The funds of knowledge were critical for the survival and community participation of children and adults in these specific families and communities. The funds of knowledge the students gain from family and the community are augmented by teachers through daily instruction on, and practice of, the most important concepts. Often, within the social context of education, there is a gap between school curriculum and daily family and community practices in the community. The funds-of-knowledge perspective attempts to narrow that gap and find points where funds of knowledge can support curriculum and families can feel supported by the school's efforts in preparing their children.[115]

---

113 Norma González, Luis C. Moll, and Cathy Amanti, eds., *Funds of Knowledge: Theorizing Practices in Households, Communities, and Classrooms* (New York and London: Routledge, 2006), 72.

114 Gonzalez, Moll, and Amanti, *Funds of Knowledge*, 34.

115 J. Messing, "Social Reconstructions of Schooling: Teacher Evaluations of What They Learned from Participation in the Funds of Knowledge Project," in *Funds of Knowledge: Theorizing Practices in Households, Communities, and Classrooms*, ed. N. González, L. C. Moll, and C. Amanti (New York and London: Routledge, 2006), 183–194.

In a study of a community in Tanzania where children with disabilities attended a special school within their community, Stone-MacDonald[116] found self-care and vocational skills were the most important skills to have for daily life. Academic skills were also important, but it is possible to survive and work with minimal academic skills—functional literacy and functional knowledge of money and counting. At the school, these skills are modeled, taught, and practiced in explicit and implicit modes of instruction. Being independent in daily life and participating in the communal work of survival is critical. With these abilities, students can participate as active members of the community regardless of their disabilities. For example, students at the school were able to care for younger siblings, independently cut grass for and feed animals, and run errands to retrieve small items at the local kiosks. Schools have an important role in preparing children to work and live as active members of their communities after they complete their schooling. To provide students with the necessary skills and knowledge, the curriculum must be culturally relevant and incorporate the funds of knowledge critical for collective participation in that culture and/or community. This is the best way to honor the local cultural and context and develop meaning capabilities in an inclusive setting.

Factors That Influence Acceptance and Community Membership

Inclusive education can help combat negative attitudes and support community membership for children with disabilities, but most countries in sub-Saharan Africa need well-trained teachers with the resources necessary to provide a quality education to all students for beliefs to change.[117] Tanzanians often attribute poor school performance from children without visible disabilities to laziness, foolishness, or poor behavior because they

---

116 Stone-MacDonald, *Community-Based Education*.
117 R. H. Hofman and J. S. Kilimo, "Teachers' Attitudes and Self-Efficacy towards Inclusion of Pupils with Disabilities in Tanzanian Schools," *Journal of Education and Training* 1, no. 2 (2014): 177–198; S. Rakap and L. Kaczmarek, "Teachers' Attitudes towards Inclusion in Turkey," *European Journal of Special Needs Education* 25 (2010): 59–75; and Tungaraza, "Arduous March."

cannot independently complete tasks of daily living or frequently need assistance and scaffolding.[118] Parents and teachers know that the school, families, and children have to work together to advocate for individuals with disabilities to demonstrate the capabilities and functionings of the students. One parent explained:

> The school is important and necessary in the community and society. When a child goes to the school his/her intelligence will be changed and his/her ability will be increased compared to if he or she never attended school. Therefore, a child going to school in the community is necessary. He or she will learn things for his or her future because when he or she is an adult, he or she will be independent, and will have an easier life compared to not going to school.[119]

This parent went on to explain that she wished her child could be in an inclusive school; however, at that time, Tanzanian schools and teachers were not equipped to handle children with disabilities or to provide sufficient resources and trained teachers. This is still the case in most of the country.[120] At the special needs school and in this community, community members were generally aware of disability, the difference between disability and disease, and current terminology, such as using *ulemavu* (disability) instead of *shida* (problem) and people-first terminology.[121] As stakeholders, parents and teachers in Tanzania all want their children to start school from a position of strength and build on those capabilities. The capability approach can support the holistic view of the child and support the growth of that child's knowledge, skills, and capabilities.

Insights from the Case Study of a School in Lushoto, Tanzania

The first case study is based on a study at a special needs school called the Irente Rainbow School. The school is located in Lushoto, a town of

---

118 Stone-MacDonald, "Cultural Beliefs."
119 Stone-MacDonald, *Community-Based Education*.
120 Tungaraza, "Arduous March."
121 Angi Stone-Macdonald, "Identification and Labels for Young Tanzanian Children: An Examination of Labels for Children with Intellectual Disabilities," *DADD Online Journal* (2015), http://daddcec.org/Portals/0/CEC/Autism_Disabilities/Research/Publications/dec2_2015%20DOJ_2.pdf.

approximately twenty-three thousand people in the Tanga region.[122] This institution is for children with developmental disabilities, where children are segregated in their education but are learning skills required for participating in the community when not in school, as it is a day school.[123] In 2009, when this research was first conducted, the Rainbow School was not inclusive but a model of how a school can prepare students for life in their community and inclusion beyond school. In 2013 the school started an inclusive preschool program that educates all children both with and without disabilities.

The school in its primary program serves around thirty children, ages six to twenty-five, with developmental disabilities such as intellectual disabilities, autism, and cerebral palsy. The preschool program serves around thirty children, most of whom do not have disabilities, although the number of children with disabilities varies each year. The education of children with disabilities helps to increase their capabilities, and the teachers and families work to educate the community about how children and adults with disabilities can participate in the community.[124]

The School Is Educating the People

The Rainbow School has been dynamic in changing the beliefs of people in the local Irente and Lushoto communities to view people with disabilities positively and to help support children with disabilities and their families. Educational services and support services through the community-based outreach rehabilitation program have occurred thanks to the work of the Lutheran church, which runs the school and the outreach program. In the local Lushoto district, students with disabilities have been slow to receive their rights to education and have fewer opportunities to participate in public primary schools even if they are able. By contrast, the local village government leaders in Irente and some areas of the outreach program have been supportive of the Rainbow School and the outreach classrooms, giving more children with disabilities the opportunity to have an education even if they cannot come to Lushoto. The outreach program is slowly changing the beliefs and access to rights for children with disabilities in the rural villages through education and medical referrals. The grassroots efforts of the

---

122 United Republic of Tanzania, *Basic Education Statistics*.
123 Stone-MacDonald, *Community-Based Education*.
124 Stone-MacDonald, "Identification."

outreach volunteers have built programs that can be sustained because of support from local leaders and community buy-in. One teacher said:

> Now many know about the school. But, sometimes when I am in town people ask about the school. They ask, "What do you do with the children who do not have intelligence?" Now, you explain that they do have intelligence, but they have a problem in their brain. So, [a student] learns certain things, but not everything. They can learn to go to the market, to help in the kitchen, to make Mother's garden, and to clean around the school and the home. So, there are things they can learn, and we explain this. [Community members] have asked me this many times.[125]

The seminars, volunteers, and personal interactions in which the school and outreach program staff engage with the community continue to raise consciousness about people with disabilities and their rights and abilities. Often interactions with people with disabilities and their families help reduce the stigma. The pastors, evangelists, and volunteers of the outreach program provide daily feedback to their communities about the importance of education and rights for children with disabilities. Their presence as community members increases the likelihood that more of the community will accept people with disabilities as full members.

Nevertheless, there are counterexamples of how Lushoto and Irente face difficulties in finding acceptance and community membership for students with disabilities. Some church leaders and diocese employees do not show respect for or value individuals with disabilities in their community. All diocese employees should be given education and disability awareness training if students are expected to successfully undertake diocesan jobs and actively participate in the diocese. People in the community make inappropriate comments, and not all parents want to send their children to school. Since the founding of the school, attitudes have been changing, but even within the church there is still much work to do. Education needs to occur in Irente and Lushoto, as well as in the entire district. At this juncture, people with disabilities must adapt to and learn the norms and expectations of the community, rather than the community learning to accept people with disabilities.

---

125 Angela K. Stone-MacDonald, "From Goats to Gardens: Preparing Children with Developmental Disabilities for Community Integration in Rural Tanzania" (PhD diss., Indiana University, 2010), 297.

Is the Community Ready?

The school stakeholders believe that students can participate in the community and within their families and are learning the necessary skills to do this. The stakeholders are the parents, teachers, community members, and local leaders whom Stone-MacDonald interviewed. They discussed these issues at training sessions, church, and in other community settings. The stakeholders also believe that the community as a whole is not ready to give the students opportunities to work and be active adults. As long as the students stay within their families and work or participate in the local areas or neighborhoods where they live, they will be accepted. The community is unsure about greater visibility for these students and needs more education and assurance about their skills and abilities. There is still a disconnect among community members between having skills and the ability to do the job. Students with disabilities from the school can demonstrate their skills to help a carpenter, clean a shop, or wash dishes. But usually when school administrators try to find jobs for these students, both in church institutions and in community institutions, people are not welcoming and worry about the risks of employing a person with a disability (e.g., poor behavior or reduced productivity). Historically, in Tanzania as in other countries, people with disabilities have been discriminated against when looking for employment, as well as when attending typical schools. As demonstrated above, these belief systems still limit people with disabilities in East African countries, particularly people with intellectual disabilities, despite national and international disability policies that guarantee equal rights for education and employment. The lack of formal employment options in Tanzania, particularly in rural areas, exacerbates this problem. The process of creating disability awareness and promoting the rights of people with disabilities has been conducted in many countries around the world, including the United States, during the past few decades. Change has occurred in Tanzania, particularly in Lushoto, during the last ten years through education and the visibility of Rainbow School students. Nevertheless, children leaving the Rainbow School are not guaranteed employment. Even ten years after this study began, very few students had formally left the school to find employment despite having vocational skills and being over the age of thirty. Even in the faith-based organization that runs the school and other institutions focused on improving the lives of individuals with disabilities, the students have trouble finding meaningful and/or paid work despite their acquired skills.

In 2009, at the time of the original study, and up to now, a typical person in Lushoto without regular contact with a disabled person would want to see such a person cared for but would not necessarily believe they could actively contribute anything to the community. The parents and teachers know that the students are capable of acquiring social and self-care skills and can help their families. Now people with disabilities are having to demonstrate that they can be useful in work outside the home.

Currently, adults with developmental disabilities are only marginally visible in the community on a regular basis. Students from the school participate in their local village or neighborhood activities and in the churches or mosques they attend. Students may go to the corner store or kiosk near their homes, but few go to the big market or participate in the community in a larger, more independent role. The school is working with a new generation of individuals with disabilities who know they have the human right to be active members of their community.[126]

Insights from the Case of an Inclusive School in Northern Tanzania

The second case is based on a study conducted at a public primary school in the Moshi area, where the NGO's and Stone-MacDonald's primary goal was to identify and support students with mild disabilities using new curriculum-based assessment. At this school, all children attend regardless of disability. When we first started working at this school, some teachers did not believe that children had disabilities, and all children were receiving the same instruction in the government classrooms. In the public primary school, there were approximately seventy students with a teacher and a teacher assistant in the morning session and another seventy students in the afternoon session.

An NGO has been working with the school principal and teachers in grades one and two to support incoming children who struggle in school. At the beginning of the school year, the NGO assesses and identifies children entering grade one who have learning disabilities, global developmental delays, intellectual disabilities, or autism and provides small-group instruction over six to eighteen months to support those students with increased intensive instruction and strategy instruction so that they can be more

---

126 Stone-MacDonald, *Community-Based Education*.

successful in their inclusive classroom. Small-group instruction occurs in a pull-out model for approximately thirty minutes three or four times a week for each student in rotating groups. Teachers working for the NGO deliver the small-group instruction with a ratio of two to four students to every teacher. The remainder of their instruction is delivered in the general education classroom by the classroom teacher. During our three-year study, with 112 students receiving small-group instruction, 90 percent of students had reached the benchmark score of 80 percent on the assessment after one year of the intervention. Thus, they were able to remain in their usual classroom and continue to complete their schoolwork at a level equal to or above their peers who did not receive additional services from the intervention or the NGO.[127] The students had demonstrated their capabilities and had gained basic literacy and mathematics skills equivalent to their peers.[128]

One could argue that it is incorrect to call this an inclusive school: the students do not receive any special education services for a disability, and the school did not recognize the disabilities or delays of students until the NGO intervened. It is inclusive either because the children have not yet been identified or labeled and/or they have not yet been excluded from the classroom based on a disability or developmental delay; but it is not inclusive in the sense that children with disabilities receive services in a classroom with their typically developing peers. In this community, parents and teachers are still just beginning to learn about disability and the differences between disability and disease and what it means for children to have a disability. At the same time, they are negotiating the cultural beliefs and norms around capabilities and functionings and what it means in their community for an individual to be "capable." Parents of children with mild intellectual disabilities in this study saw their children as unrelated to children with other developmental disabilities (e.g., cerebral palsy and autism). According to US definitions, this school is really "mainstreaming" (not inclusive) because all children are being served together regardless of disability or needs but without any additional support for children with special needs.[129]

In this study, Tanzanian primary classroom teachers explained that they did not have knowledge about students with special needs and therefore could not specifically identify or support these students without outside help. Teachers thought of students with special needs or disabilities as

---

127 Stone-MacDonald and Fettig, "Culturally Relevant."
128 Nussbaum, *Frontiers of Justice*; Terzi, *A Capability Perspective*.
129 Stone-MacDonald, "Identification and Labels."

students with physical or multiple disabilities, or outward markers of cognitive disabilities. One teacher stated that there were no children with disabilities (*ulemavu*) in the school because there were no children with noticeable physical disabilities or other obvious signs, such as unique facial features found in some genetic disorders. When specifically asked, she stated that she did not view mild intellectual disabilities or learning disabilities as actual disabilities but as a character deficit that the student was willfully exhibiting. In analyzing the interviews, we found a lack of understanding among adults about disability and repeated use of words like *lazy* to describe children with suspected disabilities. Teachers were not knowledgeable about students with disabilities. Their conceptions of disability were associated with physical or multiple impairments—or other outward markers of intellectual disabilities. These results are supported by existing research in Tanzania that demonstrates the need for continued disability awareness efforts.[130]

In this study, we examined not only how the assessment could help us to identify students who needed support but also how to provide for their needs holistically. Using the principles of the capabilities approach framework, these students are viewed as more able to participate as successful adults after school: this is because with the intervention, they can more successfully complete their schoolwork and demonstrate reading, writing, and mathematical skills.[131] In Tanzanian society, capability and disability are intricately intertwined, where individuals need to demonstrate both academic abilities and daily functional life skills to be seen as *whole*.[132]

Conclusions

Societal views are shifting in sub-Saharan Africa regarding children with disabilities. In particular, Hui, Vickery, Njelesani, and Cameron found that participants in their meta-analysis examining studies from across Africa expressed the need to include children with disabilities in local education,

---

[130] Kisanji, "Indigenous Customary Education"; Tungaraza, "Arduous March"; and Stone-MacDonald, *Community-Based Education*.

[131] Terzi, "Beyond."

[132] Harknett, "Cultural Factors"; and Stone-MacDonald, *Community-Based Education*.

and some also agreed that both girls and boys with disabilities should be viewed and treated equally in inclusive education policies and practice.[133]

As stakeholders, parents and teachers in Tanzania want young children to start school from a position of strength and build on those capabilities. The capabilities approach can support the holistic view of the child as well as the growth of that child's knowledge, skills, and abilities. Inclusive education cannot just be another policy or directive from northern countries or international organizations offering money in exchange for implementation of this practice. Stakeholders must be listened to, and inclusive education must be integrated into East African education practice with a culturally relevant curriculum, cultural beliefs, and community funds of knowledge. Mitchell argued that the centralized educational systems in East African countries are not yet responsive to the individual needs of students with disabilities and not sensitive to the cultural context in each country or community:

> The highly centralised systems which persist in postcolonial states are characterised by a lack of teacher and school-level autonomy, which act as barriers to local, needs-based adaptation. For example, a "one size fits all" curriculum is commonplace, often encapsulated in a single textbook per subject/grade. . . . Students' progression through the grades is generally dependent on the memorisation of a stable body of state-authorised knowledge, assessed through multiple-choice questions; this is not compatible with a skills-based, contextually adaptable programme of study for a diverse student body.[134]

At the local and community level, advocates of inclusive education are necessary to change long-standing beliefs and practices.[135] This is supported by evidence that attitudinal change is more important than specific skills and competencies for inclusive education. Training that boosts teachers' confidence to work with children with disabilities is more important than

---

133 N. Hui et al., "Gendered Experiences of Inclusive Education for Children with Disabilities in West and East Africa," *International Journal of Inclusive Education* 20, no. 5 (2017): 1–18.

134 R. Mitchell, "Inclusive Education in Sub-Saharan Africa," in *Inclusive Education in Uganda: Examples of Best Practice*, ed. E. Sarton et al. (2017), 4, https://www.researchgate.net/publication/315740656_Inclusive_education_in_sub-Saharan_Africa.

135 Mitchell, "Inclusive Education."

developing specific skills.[136] Positive teacher attitudes toward inclusive education are associated with enacted inclusive education practices and their positive experiences with inclusive education.[137]

Education is of central importance to the capabilities approach as it provides "social opportunities . . . not only for the conduct of better lives" but "for more effective participation in economic and political activities."[138] Inclusive education aims to provide equitable educational opportunities that support social opportunities, better lives, and full participation in economic and social life within communities. A culture or community can support or deny the rights of individuals with disabilities but shifts in approaches and access to rights are possible through individual and collective action. That shift is visible in individual communities throughout East Africa, where individuals with disabilities and their families have agency to develop their capabilities and participate as active, full members of their community. Through inclusive education and changes in mindsets, more communities can experience these shifts, which have been seen in both words and actions in places like Lushoto, Tanzania.

---

136 P. Mittler, *Working towards Inclusive Education: Social Contexts* (London: David Fulton, 2000).

137 E. Avramidis and B. Norwich, "Teachers' Attitudes towards Integration/Inclusion: A Review of the Literature," *European Journal of Special Needs Education* 17, no. 2 (2002): 129–147; K. Urton, J. Wilbert, and T. Hennemann, "Attitudes towards Inclusion and Self-Efficacy of Principals and Teachers," *Learning Disabilities: A Contemporary Journal* 12, no. 2 (2010): 151–168.

138 Sen, *Development as Freedom*, 39.

Chapter Thirteen

Youth, Women, and Disability in Africa

Economic Empowerment and Community Strategies to Leave No One Behind

Ntombekhaya Tshabalala,
Elizabeth Ladjer Bibi Agbettor,
and Theresa Lorenzo

Introduction

Africa has a youthful population, many of whom are unemployed. The United Nations Convention on the Rights of Persons with Disabilities[1] recognizes the right of disabled persons to have the same rights as nondisabled people in the workplace. However, the inequality gap in employment between disabled persons and those without disabilities is still wide, especially for women and

---

1   United Nations, *Convention on Rights of Persons with Disabilities* (New York: United Nations, 2006), Article 27.

youth, both male and female, in Africa.[2] The United Nations[3] recognizes that without access to financial services, many are unable to increase their incomes. Access to economic services is thus seen as key to achieving this goal. Work is the means by which an individual can secure the necessities of life.[4] The right to decent work, employment, and financial inclusion is a fundamental human right recognized by the Sustainable Development Goals (SDGs) for the attainment of a holistic global development for all.[5]

Despite achieving some of the Millennium Development Goals (MDGs) noted in 2015, an estimated 825 million people were reported as living in extreme poverty, and eight hundred million people suffer from hunger.[6] The assessment of progress toward the MDGs highlighted that the poorest along with those disadvantaged because of gender, age, disability, or ethnicity are often bypassed.[7]

Building on the MDG achievements, the 2030 Agenda for Sustainable Development Goals (SDGs) aims to completely eliminate extreme poverty by 2030. While the SDG 1 stresses the eradication of extreme poverty by ensuring social protection for the poor and vulnerable through increased access to basic services and support, the SDG 8 promotes the right to full, inclusive, sustainable, and decent work for all through the eradication of inequalities of unemployment. These policies echo the fact that an environment that enables the generation of income, including opportunities for employment and decent work, should be made available for all on an equal basis.[8]

---

2 Arne H. Eide, "Education, Employment and Barriers for Young People with Disabilities in Southern Africa," *Education for All Global Monitoring Report* (UNESCO, 2012).

3 United Nations, *United Nations Millennium Declaration* (New York: United Nations, 2000), https://www.ohchr.org/EN/ProfessionalInterest/Pages/Millennium.aspx.

4 World Health Organization, *Community Rehabilitation Guidelines* (Geneva: WHO, 2010).

5 United Nations, "The 17 Goals," *United Nations*, 2015, https://sdgs.un.org/goals.

6 United Nations, "17."

7 United Nations, "17."

8 T. Lorenzo and V. Janse van Rensburg, eds., *Disability Catalyst Africa*, series 5, *Monitoring Disability Inclusion and Social Change* (Cape Town: Disability Innovations Africa, 2016).

From a cultural perspective, Tshabalala[9] notes that personal experience indicates a gap between the Western and African schools of thought around managing and dealing with money. She suggests that financial systems need to address cultural dynamics to be inclusive of and accessible to the African population. This approach will positively impact people's ability to manage finances. Furthermore, the issue of language presents a challenge to most rural Africans whether they are literate, illiterate, or with disabilities. Financial inclusion encompasses "convenience." This inclusion requires that the operations of financial institutions become convenient for South Africans irrespective of ability, culture, or religion.[10] Financial inclusion that takes into account vulnerability in terms of social, cultural, gender, and disability perspectives is the draw-in to the provision of equal access to economic services, to fulfill the principle of leaving no one behind in the Agenda 2030.

This chapter explores the right of all people to decent work[11] and the right to access services and participate in economic, social, and political development. This chapter also uses the Community-Based Rehabilitation (CBR) guidelines as they recommend economic services and empowerment for persons with disabilities using a multisectoral approach. We present and analyze how people with disabilities operate their economic empowerment strategies as well as assess life changes as a result of engaging such strategies. Impact is measured by assessing the accessibility of the five elements of the livelihood component that enable participation of youth and women in development opportunities, together with some of the social and empowerment components. These indicators capture the situation of people with disabilities in areas where disability-inclusive development is carried out in order to contribute to the efforts of promoting inclusion, as requested in

---

9   Ntombekhaya Tshabalala, "Savings, Investments and Credit Groups: A Holistic Approach to Community Upliftment," in *The Walk Without Limbs: Searching for Indigenous Health Knowledge in a Rural Context in South Africa* [*Internet*] (Cape Town: AOSIS, 2019).

10 Pindie Nyandoro, "Taking Financial Services to Africa's Poorest Consumers," *Guardian*, July 15, 2013, https://www.theguardian.com/global-development-professionals-net-work/2013/jul/15/financial-inclusion-africa-banking.

11 United Nations, *Convention*, Article 27.

the Global Disability Action Plan through generating evidence concerning the effectiveness of CBR.[12]

Community-Based Rehabilitation Guidelines as the Operational Strategy of the CRPD

CBR is a multisectoral development approach that aims to equalize opportunities and include people with disability in all aspects of community life. Its implementation and success rely on joint efforts of people with disability themselves, their families and communities, and the relevant service sectors.[13] For ease of implementation and monitoring progress, the CBR Matrix highlights five key elements: health, education, livelihood, social life, and overall empowerment. Each of these elements has five components linked to them, as indicated in the figure 13.1 below. The guidelines provide a framework for an inclusive approach to social, economic, and political empowerment.

CBR identifies three strategies for achieving equal opportunities for persons with disabilities—namely, rehabilitation, poverty reduction, and social inclusion. Max Neef's[14] Human Scale Development framework maintains that development is people driven. He has identified nine fundamental human needs that are the same in all cultures and across history. Subsistence is the preeminent human need, while the other eight needs are interrelated and not hierarchical.

An unmet need can become a resource and motivation that mobilizes people to take action to change their circumstances. The ways that people meet their needs, which differ across age, cultures, gender, and contexts, are defined as "satisfiers." Satisfiers can be singular or synergistic. Deprivations occur when human needs are not satisfied, which leads to human poverty. A potentiality exists when the unmet human needs become a resource. The dynamic interconnectedness between the deprivation and potentiality of our fundamental human needs is the stimulus that could break the vicious cycle of poverty and disability. The case stories shared in this chapter connect the

---

12 World Health Organization, *WHO Global Disability Action Plan 2014–2021: Better Health for All People with Disability* (Geneva: World Health Organization, 2014).
13 World Health Organization, *Community Rehabilitation*.
14 Max Neef, *Human Scale Development* (New York: Apex, 1991).

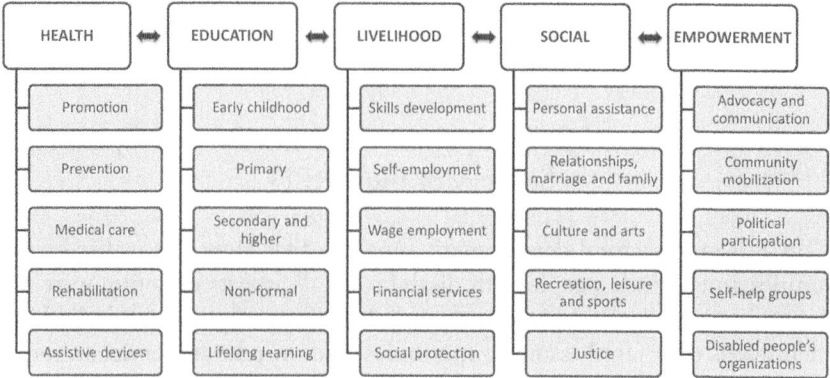

Figure 13.1. Matrix of CBR Guidelines. *Source:* World Health Organization, *Community-Based Rehabilitation: CBR Guidelines* (Geneva: WHO 2010), https://www.who.int/publications/i/item/9789241548052.

elements of self-employment through foundational, business, or core skills development, together with financial and family support.[15]

Livelihoods Programs of Ghana Blind Union

The case studies of the Ghana Blind Union employment programs share the experiences of youth and women with visual impairments in the attainment of SDG 8[16] and the practicality of leaving no one behind.

The Ghana Policy Context

In Ghana, access to decent work and employment continues to be a challenge, and progress in this area reflects the performance of successive governments in power. The promotion of equal opportunity for employment of persons with disabilities is affirmed in Article 8 of the National Disability Act 715. This act commits the government to the provision of rehabilitation centers in all ten regions of Ghana to offer career counseling and skills

---

15   World Health Organization, *Community Rehabilitation*.
16   [1001] The right to full, inclusive, sustainable, and decent work for all through the eradication of employment inequality.

training for persons with disabilities. Also, Article 8 grants tax exemption to private companies that employ persons with disabilities.

In addition to Act 715, the District Assembly Act (Act 455) has provisions for persons with disabilities. This act provides 7.5 percent of the total revenue of Ghana to the District Assemblies for local development. Section 2 of Act 455 mandates the allocation of 2 percent of the 7.5 percent to the support and development of persons with disabilities and their livelihood activities in the districts. In committing to the implementation of this act, the government developed a guideline for the disbursement of the fund as well as the establishment of fund management committees in all the districts nationwide. Persons with disabilities should have direct representation on all committees.

This initiative is confronted with problems such as untimely release of funds, diversion of funds into different programs by the District Assemblies, low capacity of persons with disabilities in the districts to hold the District Assemblies, and fund management committees for accessing the fund. These issues undermine the effectiveness of the fund.[17]

The government of Ghana, in its quest to address rampant youth unemployment, has created and implemented various employment models for youth under the National Youth Employment Authority. In order to create equal opportunities for all, special models were designed for persons with disability in 2015.[18] The government's flagship program, Nation Builders Corps (NABCO), was launched in May 2018 to create employment for young graduates in the formal sector. Of this, a 10 percent quota is reserved for persons with disabilities, and women with disabilities are given special preference. These initiatives are intended to create equal work opportunities for persons with disabilities.

Aside from the government's initiatives to be more inclusive, organizations of persons with disabilities such as the Ghana Blind Union (GBU) have recently implemented various programs geared to improving the economic status of blind and partially sighted persons in Ghana. This multisectoral development approach to inclusion in economic services is recommended by

---

17 "Shortfalls in Disability Act Working," *Ghana Web*, May 7, 2014, https://www.ghanaweb.com/GhanaHomePage/NewsArchive/Shortfalls-in-Disability-Act-worrying-357191.

18 "Name and Shame Vote Buying Parliamentary Aspirants-GACC Tells NPP, Ghana News," *Ghana News*, June 16, 2015, http://www.ghananews24.com/news/name-and-shame-votebuying-parliamentary-aspirantsgacc-tells-npp.

the CBR Guideline that encompasses the development of core skills, savings groups, family support, and financial services.

Skills Development for Informal Employment and Entrepreneurship

GBU has involved blind persons in training programs, and their interaction with sighted or other beneficiaries in similar training has reduced prejudice against visually impaired persons and promoted visually impaired persons' access to the labor market. Since 2012, this program has created livelihoods for 289 women and 426 youth in Ghana.

The Story of Francis

Francis is thirty-one years old and a native of Bekwai. He has no formal education, totally blind, and unmarried. Francis had been retailing mobile phone recharge cards for a living before becoming a beneficiary of the GBU inclusion project. The project disbursed an amount of GHC 370 to Francis to help expand his business.

At the initial stages, he started with a wooden booth where he placed his recharge cards for sale. With the financial support from the project, he remodeled this into a glass booth to make it attractive for his customers. In the course of running the business, Francis faced a number of challenges. He had engaged his nephew to take care of the business, but the nephew was mugged by unknown assailants, perhaps because he was young and could not defend himself. Additionally, people took advantage of Francis's blindness by using fake currency to make purchases. In all these circumstances, Francis lost some money but did not give up. He had some savings that helped him bounce back when he decided to take sole charge of his business. Initially, he had engaged the nephew because he was busy with church activities as a youth leader. Although he has not abandoned his church activities, he closes his shop any time he goes for a church activity and reopens when he returns.

Home Workers Schemes

Home workers schemes promote livelihood development through the acquisition of foundational skills and family support. Under this scheme, blind persons are encouraged to undertake ventures chosen from a list of options provided by trainers within their home environs. This strategy means that training is provided within the home setting. To make this effective and supportive, a family member or relative is included in the training. This support ensures that if the blind person encounters challenges in the process of production or sales, there is immediate help available.[19] Notwithstanding this backup support, care is taken to emphasize the blind person's control of the entire production process. Apart from ensuring manual dexterity, this approach also helps to boost the self-confidence of the blind individual. Some of the ventures include soap making, snail farming, mushroom production, and weaving. While accurate statistics of the total number of visually impaired persons using this approach are not available, it was found that more women with visual impairment in the project districts benefited from the intervention.[20]

In cases where the blind individual did not have a strong character or personality, family members invariably took over the ventures, due to over-protectiveness or exploitation. In the delivery of this approach, there was little or no collaboration with other connected organizations or individuals in similar ventures. Consequently, there were limited avenues for sharing experiences and learning. This approach concentrated on reaching the individuals in their homes and overlooked the importance of involving community leaders. It meant that issues of awareness and including attitudes of pity hampered marketing of the products.[21]

Community Farms

Another strategy to the provision of livelihoods development is community farms. These farms provide livelihoods for visually impaired persons, especially youth, through foundational and core skills development and community support. A large plot of land is acquired, usually from the traditional authorities. This plot is subdivided between blind persons who are given training in small-scale or dry-season farming. Blind persons have their own individual plots. They receive training with a family member whose role is to assist when required. Beneficiaries choose which vegetables to grow. A volunteer from the community is chosen by the blind persons

---

19 P. Obeng-Asamoa, *Economic Empowerment Strategies for Sustainable Employment of the Blind* (Accra: Salt and Light, 2018).
20 Obeng-Asamoa, *Economic Empowerment*.
21 Obeng-Asamoa, *Economic Empowerment*.

themselves to supervise. Training is also extended to harvesting and marketing of products. The driving principle is that the more you work, the more you harvest.

Though this approach has provided livelihoods for visually impaired persons—especially the youth because of their energy levels—they were not fully empowered. The drawback of the community farms approach is that it was limited to rural farming communities. Blind persons were not provided with options of what kind of livelihood activity to undertake. They were all compelled to engage in agriculture that was rainfall dependent. They could do much work during rainy seasons and have no work in lean seasons.[22]

The Story of Emmanuel

Emmanuel Osei Asibey's life is a testament to how financial services can help redefine the lives of many blind people. His first attempt at accessing credit from Odotobiri Rural Bank to start a poultry farm was refused. Eventually, when he was able to convince the bank officials by leveraging on GBU's initial capital to begin the poultry farm on a small scale, the bank was more than willing to grant Emmanuel credit in excess of his requested sum. He paid back his initial loan in record time, has taken additional credit, and has a good repayment record. Today, Emmanuel is doing wonderfully well with his farm, raising birds to feed the community and contributing to safeguarding the food security of this country.

Strategies for Creating Inclusive Financial Services

Financial services can greatly improve livelihood because they teach others how to make investments and manage money.[23] These case studies share the practical experiences of women and youth with disabilities in accessing financial services for livelihood activities.

---

22   Obeng-Asamoa, *Economic Empowerment.*
23   World Health Organization, *Community Rehabilitation.*

Revolving Loan Schemes

The GBU runs a revolving loan scheme to provide financial support for visually impaired youth and women starting their own businesses. Beneficiaries were required to apply for loans to undertake their chosen ventures. Applications were vetted by a committee, and loans were disbursed. Beneficiaries were expected to pay back the loans over an agreed period with profits accrued from the enterprises. Funds received were to be recycled and given to new applicants.

Individual Financial Support and Social Protection

Another approach entailed directly targeting blind persons, especially women, through the provision of individual financial support. With this approach, individuals apply for funding to undertake income-generating ventures. Training does not form part of the process. It is assumed that individuals have already had experience in their field of preference or have received past training. Funding may be required for commencement of new ventures or expansion of existing ones.

This funding targets youth and women/girls who have received training from rehabilitation or vocational centers. Their ventures are mostly petty trading and production. Funding support is provided once, and the recipient is required to manage the venture. Where the beneficiary has natural business acumen, the economic venture flourishes. But where this is not the case, bookkeeping challenges arise. There are also instances where beneficiaries are unable to build their capital reserves and thus require additional financial support. Where such support is not available, the venture collapses. Consequently, individuals are not easily weaned off family and organizational support.

Partnerships with Rural Mainstream Banks

This approach explores the inclusion of women and teenage boys and girls with disabilities into mainstream financial services. Since 2012, the GBU has partnered with rural banks to extend financial services to visually impaired women and youth. Services such as credit and short-term loans are granted to visually impaired women and youth in flexible terms. As a result, these individuals entered into ventures such as petty trading, poultry farming, and palm oil production. One notable success of the partnerships was that all beneficiaries were able to open bank accounts and for the first-time access general and tailormade facilities of banks.

The Story of Dorcas

Dorcas is twenty-one years old and currently living in Ashaiman in Greater Accra. Dorcas did not have any livelihood activity prior to joining the GBU project, although she was a casual worker at Justices Printing Press. While working with Justice Akwesi, Dorcas was informed about the GBU project through other blind members. Dorcas benefited from training on how to establish and manage her own business. In addition to this training, she was also given a grant of GHC 400 (approximately $68) as start-up capital and advised to open a bank account with Ada Rural Bank. Dorcas failed to open a bank account and instead used the grant to procure utensils for her bakery. As a result of this, Dorcas could not access a loan from the Ada Rural Bank. This limitation contributed to Dorcas's liquidity challenges. Thankfully, during a review meeting, Dorcas was advised again to open a bank account, and she did. Although she did not have additional funds to fully set up her business, she was able to use the knowledge she had gained through entrepreneurial skills training to get modest orders from friends for cookies. With access to a loan from Ada Rural Bank, Dorcas has diversified her trade activities to also selling cooked noodles.

Challenges of Inclusive Financial Services

If financial help is provided without training for beneficiaries, several pitfalls could occur. For example, it is presumed that all applicants possess business acumen and management techniques. As a result, businesses had auspicious beginnings, but the enterprises could not be sustained. Experience showed that most beneficiaries were unable to repay their loans, and their ventures tended to collapse due to limited knowledge of sound business principles.

Inclusive Financial Services in South Africa

South Africa is widely known as a rainbow nation, an indication of the diverse population, currently estimated at fifty-two million people of various cultures, languages, and religions. According to the latest statistics, Africans form about 80 percent of the population, the majority residing in rural areas.[24] Cultural dynamics and language barriers play a prominent role in how Africans manage money and relate to financial institutions.[25] This situation is particularly pertinent for disabled people and those who have not had a full education. Financial institutions need to become accessible to South Africans, irrespective of language or other barriers.[26] The Employment Equity Report revealed that disabled people are only represented in 1.4% of top management positions.[27] As a result, disabled people often end up depending on others, including government disability grants. Existing research confirms that it is still difficult for disabled people to get financial support to start off their businesses as they often rely solely on the disability grant as their main source of income.[28]

The Savings and Credit Group concept explored in the following case studies provides an ideal alternative model to supporting and empowering community-based economic development strategies.

Savings and Credit Groups (SCGs) in Rural Communities

In SCGs, members regularly contribute an agreed-upon amount to a group account, and each member either receives a lump-sum payment or payments

---

24 Statistics South Africa, *Census 2011* (Pretoria: Statistics South Africa, 2012), http://www.statssa.gov.za/publications/P03014/P030142011.pdf.
25 Tshabalala, "Savings."
26 Nyandoro, "Financial Services."
27 Statistics South Africa, *Census*.
28 Lorenzo and Janse van Rensburg, *Disability Catalyst*; J. M. Cramm et al., "Disabled Youth in South Africa: Barriers to Education," *International Journal on Disability and Human Development* 12, no. 1 (2012): 31–35; and T. Lorenzo et al., *Disability Innovations Africa*, 3: *Youth, Disability and Rural Area: Facing the Challenges of Change Disability Catalyst Africa* (Cape Town: Disability Innovations Africa, 2013).

from profits generated over time from group savings. Through group cohesion, members manage to do things they could not afford to do on their own. Studies conducted in 2010 and 2017 revealed that the poor who want to get out of debt use group savings and income generation in the form of small businesses to build their wealth.[29]

What is unique about the Savings and Credit Group model is its method of pulling people out of poverty. Savings groups and microcredits in the form of small loans with affordable interest rates have the potential to enable the poor to actively participate in their communities and change their socioeconomic situations for the better. In most cases, women are facilitators of socioeconomic support in their families. Disabled people, on the other hand, tend to depend on family and social grant support for most of their lives. For these reasons, it is important to ensure that economic empowerment initiatives are inclusive of women and disabled youth if we are to create sustainable local economies.

Participants in savings groups are able to supplement their social grant through savings generated by participating in SCGs, informal jobs, and small businesses. Members joined savings groups with expectations of what their savings would help them achieve. They wanted to achieve financial security to build or improve their homes, supplement family income, start or boost businesses, or secure money to pay for their children's education.

Participation in savings groups does not always solve all problems. Some members may meet the costs of building their homes but still struggle to furnish them. Members get distracted from building their savings as they find themselves having to buy necessary household equipment or struggling to pay for emergency needs such as unexpected medical costs.

Most important to members across the groups that participated in phase one and two of this study is that most of them managed to settle loans owed to loan "sharks," which brought a sense of freedom. Savings groups offer a supportive space where members find it easy to share frustrations and reflect on their actions, which they find difficult to do when going through difficult times in their households.

---

29 Save Act, *Annual Report 2010*, http://saveact.org.za/wp-content/uploads/2010/04/SaveAct_annual_report_2.pdf; and Tshabalala, "Savings."

Identified Challenges for Inclusive Economic Empowerment

Findings from a previous study[30] confirm that participation in savings groups has positive effects on health, relationships, and confidence. These positive effects are due to increased financial capacity to deal with risks. Additionally, the banking sector and government have a vital role to play in supporting savings and credit groups. Savings groups are essential to local economic development, and therefore their participation in assisting local integrated development plans (IDP) is important. In partnership with savings groups, local economic development (the conduit for implementation of policies at the local level) can cover more ground in creating a financially inclusive society. But there are reasons why savings groups resist working with banks. These reasons include lack of understanding of financial benefits for SCGs and not being aware of how the financial sector operates.

Low Self-Esteem and Fear of the Unknown

In savings groups, resistance to acceptance of more members was attributed to fear of the unknown and uncertainty about whether members would be able to address challenges that could come with change and a larger group. In addition, low self-esteem and self-belief deterred members from trying alternative ways of doing things. They expressed fear that they might lose the little they have. Understanding the context in which the savings groups operate enables the unfolding of a holistic, people-centered, appreciative, multisectoral, and sustainable development process. Such a process values local people's knowledge and acknowledges that they are the experts in their own development. They need to be supported with the necessary skills to unleash their abilities. Findings on experiences of savings group members indicate that such groups are valuable assets both financially and socially. Participants joined savings groups in order to supplement family income, which was mainly derived from government social support grants. This extra income enables achievements that were previously impossible.

With the support from local government—the Social Development and Local Economic Development Unit in particular—relevant strategies can support efforts of group members and protect them from being victimized by loan sharks.[31]

---

30   Save Act, *Annual Report*.
31   Tshabalala, "Savings."

Discussion of Community-Based Economic Empowerment Strategies for Disability-Inclusive Development

Experiences from both Ghana and South Africa indicate that there is a need for an appreciative approach when it comes to working with communities to build on what people already have. This process allows for inclusive, reciprocal relationships between practitioners and the communities they work with. Most importantly, this reciprocity will ensure sustainable projects.

While it is important to focus on "financial inclusion," it is equally vital to promote the concept of "financial mobility." *Financial inclusion* is the process of providing needed support and access to financial services for everyone—irrespective of color, income, context, language—or a bridge between economic opportunity and outcome.[32] *Financial mobility*, on the other hand, is the ability to move from one form of income to another while also being able to recover in times of financial difficulty.

In need of support are communities' efforts to find relevant paths to financial freedom in ways that do not create dependency on others. The ideal is to foster an ability to move between employment and ownership status, thus ensuring sustainable solutions to local economic development.

As demonstrated in the GBU case studies, although financial inclusion and financial mobility may enhance individual self-employment, these must be accompanied by training in foundational and entrepreneurial skills. Without these, self-employment start-ups and efforts to be financially mobile may fail. The onus is on development practitioners and state actors to adequately address the needs of women and youth with disabilities before designing livelihood interventions and poverty alleviation strategies.

Disability-inclusive economic empowerment requires shifting perceptions, harnessing personal financial management, and maximizing limited work choices.[33] Being vulnerable is an everyday experience for many

---

32 Mitsuhiro Furusawa, "Financial Inclusion: Bridging Economic Opportunities and Outcomes" (presentation, Conference on Financial Inclusion in West Africa, September 20, 2016), https://www.imf.org/en/News/Articles/2016/09/20/sp092016-Financial-Inclusion-Bridging-Economic-Opportunities-and-Outcomes.

33 T. Lorenzo et al., "Mapping Participation of Disabled Youth in Sport and Free-Time Activities to Facilitate Their Livelihoods Development," *British Journal of Occupational Therapy* 82, no. 2 (2019), https://doi.org/10.1177/0308022618817281.

people as stigma still exists related not only to impairments but also to cultural differences. Lorenzo and colleagues[34] also found a strong sense of the importance of family support for youth to succeed, which is demonstrated in these case studies. Some participants saw themselves as equal to nondisabled people and maintained a sense of interdependence. Self-respect started among the disabled youth themselves and spread to their families and community.

Extensive and active community support networks provide spaces for making friends and developing life skills that may foster success in job seeking and employment. NGOs focus on self-development to promote participation in livelihood development. NGOs also provide a strong sense of familial belonging and create spaces where social networks facilitate friendships.

In order to support entrepreneurship, newspaper classifieds are used to find jobs. Mothers of disabled children are encouraged to organize themselves into self-help groups and explore possibilities of job sharing that would provide alternative support for childcare.

Savings, Investments, and Credit Groups (SICGs) are mainly run by mothers to address family health needs, invest for their children, cope with crisis situations such as funeral costs, and start small businesses to generate income. Current research by Imijelo Yophuhliso[35] indicates that with constant awareness of disability inclusion, SICGs are beginning to consciously involve disabled people in their communities. This participation by people with disabilities in savings groups not only boosts confidence among disabled people but also raises awareness in families and communities; they see that if given an opportunity, people with disabilities can manage their incomes as well as make informed decisions about ways to contribute to their family incomes.

Community-Based Work as Social Enterprise

The search for employment among youth resulted in community-based workers considering ways in which they can generate income using skills and knowledge accrued from community experiences. These workers have extensive knowledge and skills to provide community-based care services. Savings group options are considered relevant forms of financing income-generating initiatives and of self-help start-up finance opportunities.

---

34   Lorenzo et al., "Mapping."
35   Tshabalala, "Savings."

Partnerships between Disabled People's Organizations and Financial Institutions

The Ghana Blind Union is a merger between the Ghana Society for the Blind (GSB) (established in 1957) and the Ghana Association of the Blind (GAB) (established in 1963). These organizations rendered services to blind and partially sighted persons and merged in 2010 to pool their resources, widen their service delivery, and avoid duplication. Before the merger, for many decades GSB and GAB promoted livelihood development of persons with visual impairments, especially women and youth, in the informal sector.

The GBU collaborated with other state institutions to provide training in financial literacy. This collaboration sought to provide livelihoods for visually impaired women and youth, promoting similar conditions for self-employment as those enjoyed by sighted colleagues. To make this approach successful, partnerships were forged with governmental organizations like the National Board for Small Scale Industries, as well as some rural banks. The approach provided beneficiaries with a resource base for the expansion of their business ventures. It also provided training in management of their enterprises.

Participatory Tools for Monitoring Economic Empowerment

Making environments and services available and accessible is a complex undertaking and needs coordinated effort between governments, NGOs, and higher education sectors. The environmental factors influencing participation need to be monitored. One of the categories of the environmental factors influencing participation in the ICF classification is Services, Systems, and Policies.[36] The case studies reflect the essential need for accessible and available information. Communication of financial services, transport, education, and employment are also discussed. Inclusive systems are synergistic satisfiers of people's fundamental human needs, which reduces poverty and develops self- and collective reliance.

---

36 World Health Organization, *International Classification of Functioning, Disability, and Health: Children & Youth Version: ICF-CY* (Geneva: World Health Organization, 2007).

The Wheel of Opportunities for Participation[37] is a participatory tool for monitoring barriers and facilitators of participation and the implementation of disability inclusive policies. Narrative action reflection workshops[38] involve a process of continuous storytelling and action learning cycles with participants of programs and service providers in urban and rural communities; these workshops can be held on a quarterly basis to monitor implementation and impact.

A study on SICGs[39] utilized a reciprocal, participatory Indigenous Knowledge Systems (IKS) approach, which enabled us to cautiously share knowledge while being aware of the fact that the communities we engage with are experts in local knowledge. This relevant approach for community engagement programs is based on equally reciprocal partnerships. The Sustainable Livelihoods Framework allowed for identification of the support necessary for savings groups to achieve their goals, thus improving efficiency and contributing to the upliftment of the communities at large.

Environmental Factors Influencing Participation in Economic Empowerment Opportunities

The case studies shared in this chapter have highlighted how the categories of Support and Relationships, Attitudes and Services, and Systems and Policies[40] are critical factors to monitor. Accessibility presents a challenge to the majority of rural Africans who are at least able to read; the situation is even more challenging for those who cannot read.

Accessible information and communication of financial and social protection systems: blind and deaf youth use mobile technology to access major banks and South African Social Security Agency (SASSA) for grants; youths

---

37 T. Lorenzo, "Collaborative Reasoning: Teaching and Learning to Facilitate Disability Inclusion in Policy and Practice," in *Global Perspective on Professional Reasoning*, ed. M. Cole and J. Creek (New York: SLACK, 2016); and T. Lorenzo et al., *Disability Catalyst*.

38 T. Lorenzo, "Listening Spaces: Connecting Diverse Voices for Social Action and Change," in *New Approaches for Qualitative Research: Wisdom and Uncertainty*, ed. M. Savin-Baden and C. Howell Major (New York and London: Routledge, 2010), 131–144.

39 Tshabalala, "Savings."

40 World Health Organization, *International Classification*.

with intellectual disabilities are more marginalized.[41] Financial systems need to address cultural dynamics that impact people's understanding and ways of dealing with finances. Personal financial management skills are a valuable starting point for people with disabilities and their families. Savings group members are supported in creating household financial diaries and learning about how investments work. They also develop skills to manage finances and pursue short- and long-term investments. Information about skills development opportunities and financial support needs to be made accessible for those with learning disabilities as well as hearing and visual impairments.

Transportation systems: Inaccessible transportation systems, especially in rural communities, reduce the chances of economic empowerment for youth and women, especially those with disabilities. Lorenzo and colleagues[42] found that family and friendship networks operated more effectively in urban areas where there was more public transportation or where parents and family members were able to provide transportation.

Education systems: Further education and training for skills development, as well as opportunities for skills transfer and ongoing learning, need to be captured systematically. Accreditation and articulation in training for career development need to be addressed. Members of savings groups and families can benefit from basic financial management skills that higher education institutions can offer. Community engagement programs and courses aimed at empowering community-based organizations would in turn train savings group members and families. In addition, caregivers and managers running the Early Childhood Development (ECD) centers can benefit from programs that aim at developing their understanding of inclusive education. This will promote inclusion, stimulation, and retention of children with disabilities in ECD centers and local schools. Ultimately, such programs will help form communities that are inclusive of people with disabilities as well as create opportunities for unemployed disabled youth.

Employment systems: mixed provision of informal, formal, or supported employment in urban areas, as well as informal or self-employment on rural farms and towns, must all be considered, taking into account the unique needs of the beneficiaries and the diversity in cultural systems. For example, many mothers give up work to look after their disabled children. In this regard, their business preferences, needs, and focus may be affected. Training in business skills and mentoring for income-generating initiatives or for

---

41   Lorenzo et al., "Mapping."
42   Lorenzo et al., "Mapping."

starting social enterprises will enhance the economic status of mothers with disabled children as suggested by savings groups in South Africa.

From the GBU experience, self-employment for persons with disabilities both in rural and urban areas requires a multisectoral approach. This approach includes building stronger networks and partnerships with both state actors and the private sector, involvement of family and community, provision of social support, and training in entrepreneurial and foundational skills.

Conclusion

We have shared experiences of livelihood development for visually impaired persons and, by extension, all persons with disabilities. The case studies have unveiled the potential of a multisectoral approach to leveraging employment opportunities for persons with disabilities. Social opportunities can also promote economic ones. In addition, when a community becomes aware of their attitudes to the disabled, more inclusion can result. The collaborative efforts of savings groups and income-generating shared projects raise awareness and help people reach greater heights than they could have done individually. These strategies continue to address root causes of inequalities that hinder inclusive, honest work.

The CBR guidelines provide a framework for monitoring implementation strategies that help achieve decent and sustainable work for persons with impairments. It is imperative that state agencies, development partners, and DPOs implement collaborative approaches to inclusive livelihood development for all.

Acknowledgments

Research team of *Sports4Work Project of DIA* at Inclusive Practices Africa, a collaborative research unit at University of Cape Town (UCT), which included the alumni of the Higher Certificate in Disability Practice (UCT).

Funding received from the National Research Foundation (NRF) enabled research on *Sports4Work*.

The University Research Committee at Southern Africa Labour and Development Research Unit at University of Cape Town (SALDRU, UCT) and NRF contributed financially toward the work conducted with SCIGs in the Eastern Cape Province, South Africa.

Chapter Fourteen

Caregiving and Support in African Context

A Personal Perspective

Frances Emily Owusu-Ansah

Introduction

Careful reflection has convinced me to write this chapter as a hermeneutic discourse on caregiving and support for the elderly disabled in the Ghanaian African context. I believe it is important to write not solely from an academic or empirical stance, but also drawing from over a decade of personal experience as a caregiver for an aged, visually impaired mother. My experiences as a clinical psychologist also inform the perspectives shared in this chapter.

I believe my journey with my mother will add to knowledge on caregiving for the elderly disabled, as well as inform the formulation of policies and support services for caregiving in the African context. I share reflections from the experience not only to emphasize the personal growth it has afforded me but also because I believe that my experience may resonate with and benefit caregivers in Ghana and beyond who are in similar situations. Therefore, in this chapter, I discuss issues related to caregiving in Ghanaian society—and by extension the African context—from a personal perspective and, where appropriate, supported with empirical evidence.

Aging can be complex and accompanied by deterioration of functioning. Many elderly persons experience various forms of disabilities—mental (e.g., dementia) and physical (e.g., mobility and visual impairment). Throughout the chapter I will use the term "elderly disabled" to refer to elderly persons whose functioning is compromised by age-related complications such as loss of vision, mobility, and/or mental capacity.

This chapter will examine the challenges and opportunities in caregiving and caregiver services. Challenges include social obstacles and family dynamics that affect caregiving. Opportunities will include caregiver support in the caregiving experience, with suggestions for ways forward.

Background

I am the youngest of seven children, yet for many years I played a leadership role among my siblings, particularly in caring for our now ninety-four-year-old mother. My journey with Mother, as her primary caregiver, began soon after my father died suddenly in 1999 at the age of eighty-five. Before that, my parents lived together in our family home. After my father died, Mother lived alone with two domestic helpers while we (her children) lived outside Ghana. This was a lonely and emotionally difficult time for her. The unexpected passing of my father shocked her, and she aged quickly after his death. Within a year, her health deteriorated, and she developed high blood pressure and diabetes. The combination of the two, particularly the diabetes, gradually impaired her vision with glaucoma and cataract complications that eventually rendered her visually impaired. She has been afflicted with this impairment for almost fifteen years now. When these changes began, we realized that Mother needed support and care.

My older siblings decided to take Mother to the United States so they could care for her there. All of them except one lived there. Managing Mother's care was not as easy as they thought. They juggled the demands of their personal lives—family and job—by sharing the responsibilities of Mother's care through what I call a "home rotation system." Mother was frequently moved from one home to the other depending on which of my siblings had time off work to take her in for a few days. In 2001 when I visited Mother in Texas, she was miserable and wanted to go back to Ghana, but my siblings could not honor her wishes because none of us would be at home to care for her. Mother had to stay another year in the United States even though she was desperate to come back home and fearful she would die in a "foreign land." It broke my heart to see Mother that unhappy, and that was when I made the personal decision and commitment to take care of her.

I returned to Ghana in 2003 and, being her only daughter in the country at the time, Mother's total care rested squarely on my shoulders—mostly by choice and partly by default. At that time, I had only a vague idea where this "journey" was going to take me and how drastically the decision to be Mother's caregiver was going to change my life. It has been a journey of faith and transformation that has come with great personal costs and sacrifices to my academic career, health, and relationships. The cost of my caregiving choices has significantly affected my career. There have been many opportunities for advancement that I had to reject as I prioritized Mother's care. The constant fatigue, stress, and emotional drain have taken their toll and affected my health, too. Relationships with siblings have been strained, repaired, and transformed.

I have learned that every crisis brings opportunity. The caregiving experience, difficult as it is, has changed my outlook on life. As I struggle with daily choices between my career, personal life, and my mother's care, I have had to reappraise my life's purpose and redefine "success" as an academic. I now appreciate the positive impact I have had on my mother's life. I consider my caregiving for her as my most prized accomplishment because through it I have received many gifts that were initially "wrapped" in tattered covers. My interest in disability work and research, for example, came through my experience of caregiving. The crucible of providing care for my mother has changed my life in ways I could not have imagined. I bring these experiences to bear on this chapter not because they are unique but because I believe they illustrate some of the challenges and opportunities related to caregiving and the importance of care for the caregiver.

Informal Caregiving: Societal and Familial Challenges

Ghana, like many African countries, has seen much social change in the last few decades. Ghanaian society is slowly but surely becoming Westernized, socially fragmented, and individualistic. Some of the changes are readily visible while others are more insidious. The less perceptible ones include changes in Ghanaian social values and the concept of family. More and more collectivist values are gradually being eroded and replaced with individualistic tendencies. Hitherto, the concept of family was extended—both in theory and practice. It included first, second, and third cousins; nephews;

aunts; and uncles. In some cases, it even included persons from the same village community and clan. Presently, this broader familial concept seems to exist only during family gatherings such as funerals. The outward behavior of many Ghanaians suggests that the concept of family is now basically nuclear. More and more people seem to be "closing in" when it comes to the provision of support (financial and otherwise) and active interest or participation in "family matters."

This social change and the gradual fragmentation of families are seen even in recent architectural designs of homes. These days, the homes are built smaller and with just enough space for the immediate family. The strong family bonds and social support networks that characterized Ghanaian society—and on which many relied for informal caregiving for the elderly—are extinct. Communal values of sharing and collective interdependence are becoming a thing of the past.

Another consequence of the deterioration in extended family cohesion is empty homesteads and resultant lack of care for the aged. In the past, entire families lived together—a practice that made support and companionship for the aged readily available. Nowadays, care and companionship for the disabled elderly in Ghanaian society have been adversely affected by the rapid migration of young people to seek better life opportunities. Consequently, many elderly disabled people live by themselves or with hired house help. Though Ghanaian society is rife with newly built homes by "children abroad," these homes are occupied by aged parents who are desperately in need of companionship and care. Most are cared for by nonfamily hired domestic help. A few have children who provide care; many others are lonely and neglected. The quality of care provided by these mercenary nonfamily caregivers is fraught with problems. Sometimes the children who live in Ghana are unable to provide quality care for aged disabled parents because of their busy life demands and work responsibilities. Adult children who are able to provide care do so under great constraints and immense sacrifices because of lack of governmental and family support.

In the Ghanaian cultural context, not unlike other African contexts, informal caregiving is common. Care for the elderly is undertaken by family members, particularly by one's own children. Among the Akan of Ghana, for example, care for aged parents is the filial responsibility of the eldest daughter. When she is unable to fulfill this duty, then younger siblings may take up that role. This practice is reflected even in the language of the people thus: "*obi hwe wo ma wose fefe a, wo nso wo hwe no ma nese tutu*"—literally meaning: "*If another takes care of you to grow teeth, you must also take care of him/*

her till their teeth fall out." Therefore, care for the aged parents (who may also be disabled) rests with family members and is primarily informal, unlike in societies with greater availability of caregiver support services.[1]

Institutional structures or government-funded support services for the elderly disabled are practically nonexistent in Ghana. As far as I know, there are no government-funded support services specifically designed for the care of the elderly disabled. Likewise, I am unaware of any well-established and functional care institution, such as a nursing home for the elderly or a hospice facility for the elderly disabled in the country.

The few private agencies in existence assist families who need to engage the services of a caregiver. However, these few support services are mostly found in the big cities and are privately owned and quite expensive. The average Ghanaian can neither access nor afford these services. In the absence of any well-established professional care facilities, informal caregiving, done mostly by family members, is the common practice. Yet this is fraught with many challenges because the sociocultural support systems that hitherto sustained informal caregiving are vanishing. In present-day Ghana, informal caregiving is hampered by urban migration, infiltration of and acculturation to Western lifestyles and values, and families separated by job demands.

In this situation, sometimes family caregivers face the challenge of making caregiving decisions at great personal sacrifice. In my experience, to reduce the stress of the daily commute to Mother's home and the associated inconveniences, given my full-time job at the university plus other personal life responsibilities, I arranged for her relocation to my home on the university campus. For eight years we lived together, as I managed her care with all my other life responsibilities. It was far from easy. I was often physically exhausted, frustrated, and emotionally drained.

When Mother's vision got worse and she could no longer move around on her own, this living arrangement was no longer possible. Consequently, I had to hire some help and relocate her to the family home, which could be renovated to suit her needs. I had to train the domestic helpers to assist

---

[1] M. R. Janevic and C. M. Connell, "Racial, Ethic, and Cultural Differences in the Dementia Caregiving Experience: Recent Findings," *Gerontologists* 41, no. 3 (2001): 334–347; J. C. Chow et al., "Types and Sources of Support Received by Family Caregivers of Older Adults from Diverse Racial and Ethnic Groups," *Journal of Ethnic and Cultural Diversity in Social Work* 19, no. 3 (2010): 175–194; S. Whitter, A. Scharlach, and T. S. Dal Santo, "Availability of Caregivers Support Services," *Journal of Aging and Social Policy* 17, no. 1 (2005): 45–62.

her. I frequently commute to visit her, supervise her medication and daily care, and provide for her other needs (e.g., I take holy communion to her and pray with her). So, in many ways, even though my mother does not live with me, I still play the role of caregiver. The psychological "burden" of care sometimes extends beyond physical boundaries, and the caregiver can be psychologically tethered to the care recipient even from a distance.

Relationships with siblings can sometimes be severely strained by caregiving. We sometimes had disagreements and had different perceptions of the seriousness of Mother's situation and what caregiving response was appropriate. Some felt that as long as they supported Mother financially or sent some material goods, they were providing "good" care for her. For many years, I felt this was not what was needed. As Mother was adjusting to losing her sight, there were many emotionally difficult and lonely days, and we both needed the gift of presence that my siblings could not afford. During that time, sometimes all I needed was someone to take my place for a short while so I could travel or take a short break. When this was not possible, I felt frustrated, stressed, and emotionally alone. My siblings eventually began responding better—taking turns to be with Mother even for a short time. The challenges somewhat changed our relationships, and I pray that after Mother's death we emerge intact and stronger. These family challenges are part of the cost families must bear during caregiving: a systemic family cost.[2]

Caregiver-Care Recipient Dynamics

Caregiving, however motivated, impacts both caregiver and care recipient. It is a complex phenomenon that produces both psychological rewards and mental distress.[3] It changes the quality of life of both caregiver and care recipient.[4] Some caregivers who undertake it voluntarily discover

---

[2] E. Kearns, "The Caregiving Crucible: Crisis and Opportunity," in *Family Caregiving in the New Normal*, ed. Joseph E. Gaugler and Robert Kane (London: Elsevier, 2015), 43–53.

[3] A. Turner and L. Findlay, "Informal Caregiving for Seniors," *Statistics Canada Catalogue* 23, no. 3 (2012): 1–5.

[4] S. Savage and S. Bailey, "The Impact of Caring on Caregivers' Mental Health: A Review of the Literature," *Australian Health Review* 27, no. 1 (2004): 103–109.

strengths, fulfillment amidst challenges,[5] and resilience. Others are negatively affected to the point of burnout.[6] Moderating factors related to the extent and nature of impact include age, attachment,[7] cultural background,[8] intrapersonal resources, financial status, health or disability, and level of dependence of care recipient.[9]

In the process of caregiving, both caregiver and care recipient experience emotional transitions and adjustments. The caregiver wrestles with life changes brought on by the caregiving role. Combining care for Mother with academic responsibilities required giving up some leisure activities and a change of sleep patterns to accommodate her needs.

The psychological state and mood of the care recipient affects the caregiver. Mother became completely visually impaired over a period of years. She underwent several eye surgeries, hopeful for a restoration. During this phase, she struggled with getting used to the "new" her—deteriorating sight and needing assistance to do many of her activities of daily living (e.g., bathing, feeding, and moving around). Being this dependent was often emotionally difficult for her. The gradual loss of her sight frightened her, and she sometimes expressed her fears in sadness and irritability or both. There were "good" days and "not so good" days. On her good days, her mood was cheerful, and she seemed to accept her blindness. The difficult days were filled with long silences, anhedonia, and changes in her eating and sleeping patterns. None of us were quite sure what triggered the emotionally difficult days. We simply lived it together until it passed. Seeing Mother sad and irrevocably changed by her illness—along with my inability to alleviate it—evoked a deep sense of helplessness. I would go to my room and cry.

---

5 O. Akintola, "Perceptions of Rewards Among Volunteer Caregivers of People Living with AIDS Working in Faith-Based Organizations in South Africa: A Qualitative Study," *Journal of the International AIDS Society* 13, no. 1 (2010).

6 Savage and Bailey, "Impact."

7 M. D. S. Ainsworth, "Attachments Beyond Infancy," *American Psychologist*, 44, no. 4 (1989): 709–716.

8 S. Sorensen and Y. Conwell, "Issues in Dementia Caregiving: Effects on Mental and Physical Health, Intervention Strategies and Research Needs," *American Journal of Geriatric Psychiatry* 19, no. 6 (2011): 491–496; M. I. Wallhagen and N. Y. Mitani, "The Meaning of Family Caregiving in Japan and the United States: A Qualitative Comparative Study," *Journal of Transcultural Nursing* 17, no. 1 (2006): 65–73.

9 Savage and Bailey, "Impact."

Caregiver Care

Care for the caregiver is critical to the subjective well-being of the caregiver as well as the quality of care for the care recipient. Support in the various forms—financial, emotional, and physical presence, particularly from significant others—can be a formidable source of strength and solace for both care recipient and caregiver. This way the task of providing care, however difficult, is less burdensome.[10]

Aside from empirical evidence in previous works, as a caregiver and psychotherapist having worked with informal caregivers as clients I have learned firsthand how caregiving comes at great personal cost and does not leave the caregiver unscathed.[11] My clinical observations show that many caregivers struggle with depression; conflicting emotions of guilt, anger, and helplessness; a perceived lack of appreciation by family members; physical and psychological fatigue; and a search for meaning in the caregiving experience. Some have to change jobs or give up work completely. Others give up relationships and relocate to be near the loved one who needs care. These challenges, observed in the Ghanaian context, are not uncommon among other informal caregivers elsewhere.[12] Yet, in a context in which government-

---

10 S. K. Lutgendorf and M. L. Laudenslager, "Care of the Caregiver: Stress and Dysregulation of Inflammatory Control in Cancer Caregivers," *Journal of Clinical Oncology* 27, no. 18 (2009): 2894–2895.

11 Kearns, "Caregiving."

12 Kearns, "Caregiving"; S. H. Zarit and J. M. Zarit, "Family Caregiving," in *Psychology and Geriatrics: Integrated Care for an Aging Population*, ed. Benjamin A. Bensadon (London: Elsevier, 2015), 21–43; F. E. Owusu-Ansah, "Sharing in the Life of Person with Disability: A Ghanaian Perspective," *African Journal of Disability* 4, no. 1 (2015); S. Rizk, K. Pizur-Barnekow, and A. R. Darragh "Quality of Life in Caregivers of Children with ASD," in *Comprehensive Guide to Autism*, ed. Vinood B. Patel, Victor R. Preedy, and Colin R. Martin (New York: Springer, 2014), 223–246; F. McClelland, "How Caregiving Impacts the Caregiver: Influences in the Caregiving of Elderly Family Members," *Research Link* 5, no. 1 (2013); R. Aziz, A. Salama, and F. A. Abou-El-Soud, "Caregiver Burden from Caring for Impaired Elderly: A Cross-Sectional Study in Rural Lower Egypt," *Italian Journal of Public Health* 9, no. 4 (2012): 1–10; U. O. Okoye and S. S. Asa, "Caregiving and Stress: Experience of People Taking Care of Elderly Relations in South-Eastern Nigeria," *Arts and Social Sciences Journal* (2011); P. R. Juster and M. F. Marin, "The Stress of Caregivers," *Mammoth Magazine* 10, no. 3 (2011): 1–12;

funded structures and support services are lacking, the essential task of caregiver care is often neglected. The outcome is caregiver burnout and lower quality of care given to the elderly disabled.

Literature on caregiving and supportive communities in African contexts is relatively scant. Evidence from other studies consistently affirms the buffering effects of support on caregiving[13] and emphasizes that "one size" does not fit all in the provision of caregiver support. Ethnic and cultural groups differ in what forms of support they access, utilize, and find meaningful.[14]

This is why caregiving experiences and challenges must be examined in context for a better understanding and conceptualization of suitable context-specific interventions. This way, meaningful and culturally appropriate interventions of caregiver support can be initiated. What does the Ghanaian context (and by extension similar African contexts) reveal about caregiving and support for the caregiver? What challenges and opportunities are present in the African context, and how many of these can be addressed and/or harnessed?

Akintola, "Perceptions"; S. L. Lavela and N. Ather, "Psychological Health in Older Adult Spousal Caregivers of Older Adults," *Chronic Illness* 6 (2010): 67–80; S. C. Reinhard et al., "Supporting Family Caregivers in Providing Care," in *Patient Safety and Quality: An Evidence-Based Handbook for Nurses*, ed. Ronda Hughes (Rockville: Agency for Healthcare Research and Quality, 2008); Mary Jo Gibson and Ari Houser, "Valuing the Invaluable: A New Look at the Economic Value of Family Caregiving," *Issue Brief (Public Policy Institute (American Association of Retired Persons)* IB82 (2007); M. Pinquart and S. Sorensen, "Correlates of Physical Health of Informal Caregivers: A Meta-Analysis," *Journal of Gerontology* 62, no. 2 (2007): 126–137; R. E. Rambough, E. L. Howse, and W. J. Bartfay, "Caregiver Strain and Caregiver Burden of Primary Caregivers of Stroke Survivors with and without Aphasia," *Rehabilitation Nursing* 31, no. 5 (2006); Wallhagen and Mitani, "Meaning"; P. P. Mwinituo and J. E. Mill, "Stigma Associated with Ghanaian Caregivers of AIDS Patients," *West Journal of Nursing Rese* 92, no. 3 (2006): 409–413; Savage and Bailey, "Impact"; M. Navaie-Waliser, "When the Caregiver Needs Care: The Plight of Vulnerable Caregivers," *American Journal of Public Health* 92, no. 3 (2006): 409–413.

13 R. F. Young and E. Kahana, "The Context of Caregiving and Well-Being Outcomes among African and Caucasian Americans," *Gerontologist* 35, no. 2 (1995): 225–232; and P. Dilworth-Anderson, S. W. Williams, and T. Cooper, "The Contexts of Experiencing Emotional Distress among Family Caregivers to Elderly African Americans," *Family Relations* 48, no. 4 (1999): 391–396.

14 Chow et al., "Types."

In my years of caregiving, I have seen how totally oblivious and unprepared Ghanaian institutions—hospitals, health professionals, and even faith communities—are in responding to the new reality of growing numbers of aging disabled persons in need of support services beyond what their families can offer. This situation needs to evoke responsible social and governmental responses because the need for elderly care will continue.

Some of the suggestions outlined in Kearns[15] are applicable to the African context. The government needs to provide funds to make caregiving support sustainable and community based. For example, government-funded counseling support programs in workplaces could be initiated for caregivers. Part of the caregiver support could be to help caregivers understand that inherent in the costs of caregiving are opportunities for profound growth. Likewise, critical attention needs to be paid to education and training of medical practitioners and other health professionals to equip them with the necessary skills.

African societies must harness inherent resources—human, physical, spiritual—in their contexts to enhance caregiving. African culture is highly religious, and Ghanaians are no exception. Being religious and having membership or affiliation with a faith community is valued. Given the plethora of churches and faith communities in many African societies, consistent and well-organized responses from these communities would go a long way to relieve the distress of caregiving. Faith communities need to renew commitment to support caregivers and care recipients by frequent home or hospital visits.

Although many African communities are being Westernized and values are changing, there is still a modicum of respect for the elderly in many contexts. Age and filial piety are still valued. For example, in the absence of well-functioning social security support structures, children are the primary "social security" for parents, and many do well to provide financially for their parents. Building on these values, some initiatives can be undertaken. For example, families and social groups need to develop intergenerational programs that enforce extended family values and systems through which the youth engage older persons and develop an appreciation for the complexities of aging. Such programs may help bridge the gap between age groups and between families and sustain motivation for better caregiving and support. This is important because informal caregiving is undertaken by family members and often motivated and sustained by sociocultural values and

---

15   Kearns, "Caregiving."

expectations. In the wake of modernization in society with resultant job stresses, migration, and fragmentation of families, this is constrained. Yet informal caregiving is the only option available. Therefore, support for and a renewal of the extended family practice and collectivist values of interdependence would be a great support for both caregiver and care recipient.

Conclusion

The number of elderly persons will continue to increase as science and medicine advance. More aged persons will need care. How prepared are African societies for this upward trend? The experience of caregiving in the African context may not be that different from caregiving elsewhere. Yet it holds context specific challenges and opportunities, given the lack of formal government-funded support systems. The empirical evidence, as well as my own personal and clinical experiences, provide opportunities to contemplate the direction of social change. African societies have a wealth of resources and indigenous knowledge for the initiation and implementation of these initiatives.

Note: The author's mother passed in November 2019, after the completion of this chapter.

Part Five

Activism and Barriers to Inclusion

Chapter Fifteen

So That the Stew Reaches Everybody

Women's Negotiations of Leadership and Power in Ghana's DPOs

Denise M. Nepveux

> *The transformative potential of a movement is only as present as the strength or voice of the most marginalized.*
>
> —Emi Kane

This chapter reports on a qualitative study of disabled women's challenges and strategies in carrying out leadership roles in Ghanaian DPOs. A growing literature documents and theorizes experiences of disability oppression in Global South countries. Likewise, a growing body of literature explores policy needs and measures outcomes concerning disabled people[1] in African countries. A smaller but growing literature documents the experiences, needs, and aspirations of disabled African women[2] and economic

---

1 Maxwell Peprah Opoku et al., "Extending Social Protection to Persons with Disabilities: Exploring the Accessibility and the Impact of the Disability Fund on the Lives of Persons with Disabilities in Ghana," *Global Social Policy* 19, no. 3 (2018).

2 Denise Nepveux, "'In the Same Soup': Marginality, Vulnerability and Belonging in Life Stories of Disabled Women in Accra, Ghana," (PhD diss.,

disparities between disabled women and their male counterparts.[3] Only a few studies, however, document the impact of DPOs in accomplishing social and policy change or influencing the lives and identities of their members.[4] There is a dearth of literature on the internal power dynamics of DPOs and the challenges less-empowered members, particularly women, experience when they attempt to take leadership roles in these typically patriarchal organizations.

Women with Disabilities in Development and Human Rights Agendas

As other writers in this volume have illustrated, poverty, exclusion, and invisibility are pervasive for people with disabilities across the African continent. In Ghana, as elsewhere in Africa, people with disabilities live insecure and often shortened lives due to educational and economic exclusion, barriers to health care and transportation, underinvestment, low expectations of their families, and vulnerability to violence, harassment, and stigmatization.[5]

In the late twentieth century, despite growing attention to disability as a form of inequality, girls and women with disabilities were rarely addressed at the policy level. Although specified as an underrepresented and "vulnerable group" by the UN Committee on Discrimination against Women General Recommendation 18 in 1991, disabled girls and women were not mentioned in the Convention on Discrimination against Women (CEDAW) and continued to be overlooked in national data collection and international development initiatives.[6] This began to change with the Fourth World Conference on Women in Beijing in 1995, which saw vocal representation

---

University of Illinois at Chicago, 2009); B. Dhungana, "The Role of Self-Help Groups in Empowering Disabled Women: A Case Study in Kathmandu Valley, Nepal," *Development in Practice* 20, no. 7 (2010): 855–865.

3   A. Naami, "Disability, Gender and Employment Relationships in Africa: The Case of Ghana," *African Journal of Disability* 4, no. 1 (2015).

4   Nepveux, "Soup."

5   A. Naami and Reiko Hayashi, "Empowering Women with Disabilities in Northern Ghana," *Review of Disability Studies* 7, no. 2 (2007); Naami, "Disability"; and Nepveux, "'Soup.'"

6   Tina L. Singleton et al., "Gender and Disability: A Survey of InterAction Member Agencies," (Eugene, OR: Mobility International USA, 2013), http://wwda.org.au/wp-content/uploads/2013/12/gendismiusa1.pdf.

by women with disabilities from both Global North and Global South countries. The resulting document explicitly mentioned concerns of women with disabilities in a number of areas.

Since that time, researchers, policymakers, and funding bodies began attending to the intersection of gender and disability. Mobility International USA led this charge by convening several international meetings of women with disabilities and issuing reports that challenged international development funders to begin targeting and tracking disability and gender among all of their efforts. Ghana's ratification of the Convention on the Rights of Persons with Disability in 2012, as well as the continual efforts of the International Disability Alliance and other national and international disability advocacy groups before and since that time, have brought disability, including a strong gender focus, onto the radar screen of national and international development efforts.

The Women's Manifesto for Ghana, written by a wide coalition of women's groups in Ghana that included disability representation, recognizes disabled women as being "among the most vulnerable groups in Ghanaian society" and acknowledges that these women "continue to experience oppression and violation of their basic human rights in all aspects of life."[7] It acknowledges that disabled men and women in Ghana encounter disabling barriers to entering and using buildings, facilities, and public spaces. This manifesto also recognizes discrimination and inequality of access to health care, employment, education, and social security. With regard to women and girls, the manifesto identifies social exclusion and discrimination in "all manner of social and sexual relationships, including marriage" and vulnerability to "violence and abuse."[8]

In the gender policy of Ghana, which was not yet published at the time of data collection for this study, "limited attention to issues and aspirations of women with disability" is identified as one of the key challenges to gender equality and women's empowerment: "There is insufficient . . . understanding of the situation of WWD and this affects the planning, implementation, and monitoring of women's initiatives with the WWD lens."[9]

---

7   Women Manifesto Coalition, *The Women's Manifesto for Ghana* (Accra: Coalition on the Women's Manifesto for Ghana, 2004), 59, https://library.fes.de/pdf-files/bueros/ghana/02983.pdf.
8   Women Manifesto Coalition, *Manifesto*, 59.
9   Ghana Federation of the Disabled, *Gender Policy: Integrating Gender Perspectives in the Work of Member Organizations* (Accra: Ghana Federation of

DPOs and the Disabled People's Movement in Ghana

For decades now, DPOs have played crucial roles in promoting the social, political, and economic rights of persons with disabilities in Ghana, as in many other African countries.[10] DPOs provide unique spaces of camaraderie and mutual support among disabled youth and adults. They enable collective self-representation[11] where previously there was only a charitable or paternalistic voice. The efforts of the GFD and its member groups have brought disability to the attention of news media, politicians, policymakers, and the public; this has helped reframe disability as an issue of inclusion, social justice, and human rights.

In Ghana, people with disabilities were subjects of (limited) rehabilitation schemes by the British Colonial Government and under Nkrumah.[12] Two member organizations that currently participate in the Ghana Disability Federation (GFD) are direct descendants of British royal societies. Others self-organized for mutual survival during the famine of the 1980s, and still others have organized and incorporated more recently.[13] Current membership of the GFD includes DPOs by and for persons with visual disabilities, hearing disabilities, physical disabilities, albinism, mental health concerns, and neurological conditions. It also includes the Ghana branch of Inclusion International, which primarily represents parents of children with developmental disabilities like autism. These organizations employ national and regional staff, as well as voluntary boards of directors. The membership of each organization and the GFD elects district, regional, and national officers every four years. Organizations also have "wings" or caucuses that represent particular subgroups. Most organizations have women's wings, and several also have youth, workers, and sports wings. The wings also elect national, regional, and district level officers. Funding for the federation and its constituent groups is largely grant-based, including support from Ghanaian banks and other businesses, Ghanaian foundations such as Star Ghana, and

---

the Disabled, 2010).

10   Nepveux, "Soup."

11   R. Young, M. Reeve, and N. Grills, "The Functions of Disabled People's Organisations (DPOs) in Low and Middle-Income Countries: A Literature Review," *Disability, CBR and Inclusive Development* 27, no. 3 (2016): 45–71.

12   Jeff D. Grischow, "Kwame Nkrumah, Disability, and Rehabilitation in Ghana, 1957–66," *Journal of African History* 52, no. 2 (2011): 179–199.

13   Nepveux, "Soup."

significant transnational funding from DANIDA, USAID, and the Boston-based Disability Rights Fund.

In 2010, the GFD issued a gender policy that applied to all of its member organizations. It acknowledged significant disparities in membership representation and set out mechanisms for this. In the CRPD, which Ghana ratified in 2012, DPOs are considered "representative organizations" with whom governments must confer when making legislation. This obligation to involve DPOs in policymaking raises the stakes on the participation of women in DPOs and their opportunities to voice their concerns via these organizations.

Diversity and Inequality within Ghanaian DPOs

Ghanaian DPOs have great internal diversity on a number of axes of identity and inequality.[14] Members tend to come from lower income backgrounds and have extensive material, human development, and psychosocial needs.[15] But they cover a wide spectrum in terms of rural versus urban living, gender, age, ethnicity, religion, language, literacy, education levels, family and marital status, employment and income, and relative security of housing.[16]

Educational differences play a large part in the challenges of group cohesion and effective leadership. A few members have university degrees; many have middle school or secondary school education; and many others—particularly women members—have only primary school or no formal education. Written information is generally in English, and group leaders tend to lead meetings in what they perceive to be the majority language of the group. In Ghana's multiethnic and multilingual environment, this tends to

---

14   The content of this section is based upon intermittent participant observation with Ghanaian DPOs and multiple conversations with their members over several years.

15   Opoku et al., "Extending."

16   I have yet to encounter a DPO member who openly identified as gay, lesbian, bisexual, or transgender. Although GLBT communities exist, for example Sassoi communities, identities that stray from cisgender and heterosexual remain largely shunned and thus difficult and dangerous to openly express. Same-sex intimacy remains illegal in Ghana. Vigilante violence toward gay and transgender people is documented in the news media.

mean that many members—particularly women—are excluded from information and dialogue.

International and transnational funders have impressed upon DPOs the need to equalize opportunities for women, resulting in a GFD gender policy. Their presence seems to have had complex and contradictory effects. It has reinforced hierarchies based on formal education and has meant that the agenda is set (or perceived by members to be set) based on funder priorities, which have involved human rights advocacy, specifically advocacy for legislation to bring Ghana's national laws into line with the CRPD. On the positive side, it has enabled leaders to access information, pursue educational opportunities abroad, and participate in international developments. European volunteers have also contributed significantly via Voluntary Service Overseas (VSO). Transnational funders have discouraged the prior DPO emphasis on "employable skills training" in favor of particular understandings of "empowerment," "capacity building," and "advocacy."

Gender inequalities in DPOs are significant. Because of educational inequalities at the household level, particularly among older generations (and because of ongoing educational barriers for girls such as poor provision for menstrual periods), women in DPOs tend to have fewer years of formal education than their male counterparts. Many have low levels of ability in English, which is the language of education, government, and commerce. Many of the older women have received extensive training in trades such as seamstress work or weaving that are no longer (or have never been) viable livelihoods. Some women earn a living through "trading" (i.e., selling) in markets, along roadsides, or at a table in front of their houses.[17] Some survive through piecing together a living that may include transactional sex. Many find themselves raising children without the support or involvement of the children's fathers. As women who are marked as less valued, they are particularly at risk of rape, domestic violence, and abandonment by partners.[18]

Inequalities among women in DPOs are also significant. Educational differences are sometimes correlated with socioeconomic differences. Educational inequalities among disabled women are common, even among

---

17   Naami, "Disability."
18   Mobility International USA, *Loud, Proud and Prosperous! Report on the Mobility International USA International Symposium on Microcredit for Women with Disabilities* (Eugene, OR: MIUSA, 1998), https://digitalcommons.ilr.cornell.edu/gladnetcollect/296/; and Singleton et al., "Gender and Disability."

a single impairment group, given that many girls with disabilities have not been able to gain access to even primary school, yet others have gone as far as university. Impairment type matters. For example, girls who are partially sighted may struggle in mainstream education with few or no accommodations and eventually drop out of school, whereas girls who are labeled "blind" may have access to residential schools for blind students, followed by senior secondary school and even teacher training using braille. Away from the major cities, however, even a JSS (Junior Secondary School) education is a significant advantage for women with disabilities.

The significant educational and socioeconomic class differences among women in the DPOs, particularly in major cities, are reflected in the elected offices women are able to attain as well as the respect they are (or are not) afforded once elected. Leaders are more likely to have salaried jobs or a small business and are more likely to be married. They also enjoy the social status among their peers that made them more electable, particularly to regional or national office. This often (although not always) means that top officers have completed secondary school education or beyond, whereas many members—particularly women—have little or no formal education. Educational inequality significantly affects women members' access to information because organizational business, workshops, and training are sometimes conducted in English.

As discussed in later sections, however, higher education can also distance women leaders from members and other leaders—present and past—who have less formal education. Specifically, tensions seemed to be rising at the time of the study between older, more experienced (but less formally educated) women leaders and their younger, university-educated peers. At times these tensions played out in a younger woman losing a reelection bid in favor of a senior peer. When such intergenerational struggles occurred within a women's wing of a DPO, younger women had (and often took) the option of leaving and channeling their energy in a youth wing where they believed they would be more valued.

About This Study

The purpose of this study was to learn about the experiences and perspectives of women who have occupied leadership roles within Ghana's DPOs at local, regional, or national levels. Specifically, I wanted to know what challenges women experienced within their leadership roles and how they responded.

Kathryn Geurts and I, two US-based researchers who had several years of experience with Ghanaian DPOs on other research projects, convened a group of eight women DPO leaders in June 2010 to seek guidance on study questions and approaches. This gathering affirmed and helped to clarify our focuses on challenges and strategies employed by women in leadership. Over the following five weeks we conducted individual semistructured interviews with fifteen women leaders through a snowball sampling method. Geurts and I collaborated on most of the interviews, but a few were conducted by only one of us. Interviews were conducted in the Greater Accra and Eastern regions, in homes of participants and other locations as per their preferences. Ghana Blind Union, Ghana Society of the Physically Disabled, Ghana National Association of the Deaf, and Ghana Association of Persons with Albinism were represented among interviewees as well as in the initial meeting. Fortunately, we were able to interview several leaders from more distant regions during visits to the Greater Accra region that happened to coincide with our fieldwork. Most of the interviews were conducted in English, as per the preference of participants. Interviews with several deaf participants were conducted with Ghanaian Sign Language interpretation. Our interviews followed an interview guide derived from review of the literature and our knowledge of Ghanaian DPOs. We employed the interview guide flexibly in order to follow individual participants' interests and emphases. Interviews were digitally recorded with the consent of participants and were later transcribed verbatim. Transcripts were uploaded into Atlas.ti software and analyzed for a priori and emergent themes.

This study was approved by the Research Ethics Board of York University in Toronto, Canada. All participants gave informed consent. We assured participants that their names would not be used without their permission. A few participants did want their names to be used, but none are identified here because most preferred confidentiality. Also, because these are small organizations, because disability type may identify the organization participants belong to, and because matters discussed here are politically sensitive within the DPOs, specifics of disability are rarely mentioned in this chapter.

Participants and their Paths to Leadership

Participants either self-identified or were identified by others as a leader at the local, regional, or national level of a DPO in Ghana. During the time the research was carried out, most held elected positions in their district or region, or they served at the national level. Participants were serving members in the Greater Accra, Volta, Eastern, and Upper East regions. Most had held various positions for over ten years. Several had been members for at least five years but were holding office for the first time. Two were elders in the disability movement who had salaried jobs and no longer occupied formal roles in DPOs; they were often called upon to consult on DPO issues or to chair events. One was currently a staff member in a DPO national office but had held a number of elected offices.

Participants were generally longtime DPO members before they ran for an elected position. Most had joined the organization as youths in order to connect with others' experiences and resources. It was through the DPOs that one could register as a disabled person, which would qualify them to receive government benefits. For women we interviewed, secretary, financial secretary, or treasurer positions were common entry points to leadership. A number of women who began as secretary or treasurer went on to hold "first vice" or president positions. Several women also developed leadership skills through participation in elected roles in women's wings of their district DPO. They then moved up to regional- and national-level office or ran for positions in their district or regional DPO group.

In accordance with the GFD gender policy—parts of which had been adopted years earlier through advocacy by women in some DPOs—some organizations had set aside specific elected positions to ensure women's presence in leadership at all levels. This had recently opened up opportunities for more women, not only for elected positions but also for representing their local group at workshops or gatherings.

Women's Leadership Priorities and Contributions

Participants in our study were consistently enthusiastic about the value of women's leadership to the movement as a whole and specifically for the benefit of women members. Contrary to our initial expectations, however, our conversations did not tend to revolve around political advocacy efforts. Instead, women emphasized their efforts to improve the internal functioning of their organizations. For example, women said they tried to increase the flow of information within their organization, improve accounting for funds, and increase participation opportunities. These were the concerns that apparently motivated women to pursue and continue leadership roles.

Participants frequently emphasized fairness and accountability as contributions women leaders made to both women's wings and the DPO. One said that women are realistic and attend to the needs of the whole group. Another described women as "dynamic," "firm," "honest," and as people who "will get the work done, irrespective of whatever." Another commented that women are more trustworthy, less corrupt, more sharing of information, and more inclusive and fairer than men in their dealings with members.

Our participants were acutely aware of barriers and resistance to women's success in leadership roles, both within and outside the disability movement. Some of this resistance came from men in the DPOs. One leader recounted that ten or fifteen years earlier, men in the disability movement had greatly resisted women's bids for leadership. Her organization had conducted a national referendum on a proposal to reserve all "first vice" positions for women, and it had generated much debate. When asked about their opposition, she recalled, "They think inferior of a woman." From her perspective, such an attitude "all boils to ignorance [and] lack of education." This leader said that men in Ghana see women as "not at par" with men and "not strong enough" or deserving of the right to make decisions. Power was seen as men's natural endowment while women were associated with weakness.

A number of our participants observed that despite increased gender discourse since the 1995 Beijing summit, men continued to dominate DPO leadership for the most part, and both male and female members were ambivalent at best about women's prospects for leadership. Yet despite this larger context, the leader we interviewed felt that there was currently adequate support for women's leadership within the disability movement, if only because more women could run for positions. She felt that internalized oppression stemming from both gender and disability played a role in deterring women: "I don't know whether they are afraid of or they feel shy . . . But nobody is telling them to take positions." Although direct and open resistance to women's leadership may have diminished in recent years, it became clear from our conversations with women leaders that there were many subtle ways in which their leadership was consistently undermined. We sought to identify these ongoing hindrances to women's leadership and ways in which leaders thought about, anticipated, and worked against or around them.

Criticisms of Women's Leadership

When we asked participants, "What are some things people say about women leaders?" they tended to point to a few common criticisms they had heard but did not agree with: bossiness, arrogance, and pride. They said that these were gendered stereotypes, not unique to women in DPOs but commonly applied to women who moved up in any power hierarchy in business or government. They faced these stereotypes within their DPOs as well, both from grassroots members and men in leadership.

Women leaders were criticized by both men and women members for behaving in a way that was "too knowing." Leaders were expected to be knowledgeable and capable. They also had to bring knowledge from higher echelons of the organization. But there was a danger of alienating members by showing contempt for less educated or less informed viewpoints.

One leader reflected that she had learned—at times through making painful mistakes—how to offer help or suggestions to group members in a way that would not insult them. She reflected: "They don't want you to make them feel low. . . . If you do that, they will make you miserable in their midst. . . . With a genuine heart I'm trying to help. But they think [I am trying to put] them down."

Women who were assertive or directive also risked being labeled "bossy." One leader commented to us that "bossiness" was not the sole province of women but a characteristic of leaders generally—and for good reason. Both men and women leaders must be firm, confident, and assertive. To her, "Everybody is kind of bossy" when in a leadership role. However, she observed, "We live in a patriarchal society which views men as people that should occupy the top role. . . . And if you are a woman and you want to insist on the right things being done . . . people would often say that 'oh she's trying to be bossy.'"

Another participant shared an anecdote about a workshop for women's wing members of her organization. After lunch, a number of women would drift off to their rooms for naps rather than return promptly for the afternoon session. A leader began walking throughout the building, shouting that everyone should wake up from their naps. "And then there's conflict!" she concluded. From her perspective, the leader was simply trying to ensure that the goals of the workshop were met. But members resisted her authority.

As another leader pointed out, members experienced exclusion and discrimination at home and felt relief to be among others who shared their perspectives. They also labored continually at home to survive with few resources and little support. Thus, in the small spaces of relative equality and freedom afforded by DPO gatherings, they resisted being told what to do.

"Too Big in Your Shoes": Backlash to Women's Power

Another of the most common criticisms of female leadership was "pride," which held several meanings. One was social climbing (i.e., rejecting one's former [grassroots] peers). One participant mimicked the allegations her members would raise about recently elected women leaders: "If they see you, it's as if they don't know you. They won't visit you, they won't mind you. Even if I'm calling that I'm coming, [they] leave."

She commented that when women members were first elected to a leadership role, their peers were particularly vigilant, looking for any sign of arrogance or social disregard. They would observe that in her newfound leadership role, "She is too proud." This seemed to be particularly a concern among women rather than a critique from a male perspective.

A second use of "pride" referred to women's stepping beyond their rightful places *as women*. In contrast to using the concept to indicate snobbery, other participants spoke of "pride" as a violation of expected roles and power relations, particularly with respect to gender and age. "Pride" signaled something particularly threatening to men's power and the social power structure. Indeed, among the labels/criticism women leaders confronted, this meaning of "pride" seemed to be the most serious allegation and the one that would prompt the strongest backlash. The fear of being so perceived hindered women's ability to confidently navigate their relationships with members, other leaders, and organizational staff.

A young woman leader described a moment when she was seeking information from the organization's head office about her youth wing's finances in relation to a grant. She was rebuked for being assertive:

> I think I have to ask so that I will know and get right information for my people. And they were denying me from getting such information. . . . But they think they can just snub me because I just came [into office, and they were saying,] "You are . . . just a youth . . . so who are you to talk?" But I didn't permit them so it was like some kind of small hatred for me.

Reflecting on earlier days of women's leadership in her organization, an older leader recalled the misgivings members and leaders expressed about designated positions for women leaders: "They say that women leaders . . . are too proud. There is pride in them. The pride means the bluff. So when they give leaders [positions] to them, they'll be bluffing the men. And they will not respect them." "Bluffing" was a name for acting arrogantly or aggressively in excess of one's given status or authority. So to say that women in leadership would be "bluffing" the men would be to say that women would be claiming authority beyond their due *as women*, and doing so in a way that did not spare men's pride (i.e., their need to have their sense of superiority publicly validated). Perhaps the public nature of the perceived power grab was the most threatening aspect because of the resulting humiliation.

Such power-grabbing behavior by women was not only condemned but accompanied by existential threats. One participant said that the stereotype of women who are "given such an opportunity" to lead both women and men is being "too big in your shoes." Such behavior will doom you to be forever unwed because "no man will even make an attempt to approach you." I asked this participant if such sayings held truth, and she mentioned it was true of some women but not all.

"Pride" could be used as a weapon to silence women when they questioned men's actions or insisted on being part of the decision-making process. One female leader told us about a consequential instance in which men in her organization planned a budget for a workshop that would include a number of women. When she and others questioned the adequacy of some budgetary line items that would affect women participants, the men became angry, and there was a backlash. "Now it seems that they have seen that the women are proud, so they've washed their hands of the women," she commented. She said that the support and training that the fledgling women's wing had previously received from men in the executive council ceased, and men in leadership began to exclude women officers from planning and decision making.

Thus, although there was significant support for women in leadership roles, women leaders were asked to walk an impossible line: once elected, they needed to fulfill their roles as leaders while also remaining unchanged and taking a fully egalitarian stance in terms of peer relationships, assertions of power, and assertions of knowledge. They also had to guard against backlash, particularly from their male counterparts, who could block their ability to function. In the following section we consider how women leaders managed these seemingly contradictory expectations.

Women's Ways of Leading: Humility, Transparency, Accountability, Engagement

Women leaders in our study said they prioritized relational aspects of leadership in order to make their work possible. Especially in light of the misgivings they experienced or anticipated among their members, they felt they could not afford to simply assume authority to promote an action agenda or they felt they would face backlash if they simply assumed authority to promote an action agenda. Instead, they needed to build rapport and trust with their members.

Humility

One leader spoke of being "free" (i.e., friendly and informal) with her members. Several others spoke of "lowering" themselves. One district-level leader commented that she and other women leaders in her region all used a similar approach: "We are just one [with the members]. . . . When you come and we are sitting down, we're just chatting like the same. . . .Because the leaders, they bring themselves down, they lower themself." Making oneself humble and accessible to members was important especially because of the educational inequalities between them. Another observed, "I am very down to the earth. Like I discuss things easily with them and they come [to my office] any time they want, they get closer to me, I get closer to them, we are like family, and to be frank any time I come for a meeting I have some joy within, I just get satisfied, and I'm happy when we have a meeting." This leader was university educated, had a salaried job, and was living in a town. She was leading a group of disabled subsistence farmers that she had organized through outreach. But the fact that she had organized them did not compel their ongoing consent to be governed.

> When I asked another university-educated leader about what helped her to be effective, she had much to say on the matter. She said, "I drop myself." She practiced an ethic of respect and openness to learning from members. She also resisted feelings of shame or embarrassment at moments when she recognized that her education, which she valued, had not prepared her for things she needed to do as a leader. She talked about allowing herself to be vulnerable and to not know—and to be open about not knowing so as to learn: I think my education has been helping me a lot. Because I am educated, I seem to learn fast. And also my ability to drop myself and go along with others. . . . For instance, I finished

university. And they said, "Oh, she finished university, she knows how to write reports." I felt it was shameful that I . . . didn't know how to write a report. But I dropped myself. I dropped all the things about university and I opened myself.

Transparency

Crucial to the process of gaining members' trust was a cluster of behaviors and commitments that some of our participants called "transparency." For our participants, transparency included some combination of consistent truthfulness and information sharing, seeking input and consent before taking action, and reporting back to members after attending a meeting or event. Many had been to internationally sponsored training sessions where this concept would have been discussed. This influence was felt in participants' discussion of the concept and in the frequency with which it was raised. For one leader, the word "transparency" encompassed every important leadership trait and practice. She defined transparency as truthfulness, consistency, and information sharing.

Reporting to local members on events outside the district was important to one local leader. She said that prior to the formation of a district women's wing, all local leaders in her area had been men. The women's wing became a vehicle for women's leadership development, such that women later also began to run for office in their district groups. With men at the helm, hardly any information had been reaching members about what their elected leaders had learned in training sessions or what was going on in the organization at the national level. She portrayed women leaders in her area as a unified voice for transparency. She emphasized that leaders "should make [information] accessible."

One experienced leader who had also worked as a staff member also took a strong stance on information sharing: "Well in this type of organization I don't think there is anything that is secret or that should be considered classified. . . . Information should be put in the domain of the people. Let them get the information irrespective of it, whatever happens."

Accountability

Another leader emphasized that information-sharing promoted trust: "Once they trust you, it makes you a good leader of course." One leader whose DPO had developed more recently and had undergone crises in leadership also said that information sharing was a major topic of her group's meetings as they influenced their leadership's behavior: "If you say, 'I'm in power,' then you can go just directly to the office and do whatever you like. We don't like that. . . . So when you are going to do something you have to let . . . all of us know that this is going on before you go and do it."

Engagement

It was not adequate for a leader to act and then report. Instead, a leader needed to consult other leaders and members before taking action. A district president also stressed that transparency was a key leadership quality. For her, however, this meant consulting other elected officers (who together formed an executive council or "the executive") and welcoming their suggestions rather than planning and making decisions alone. She said, "A leader must be transparent. When you do something, you ask the executive and you sit down with them, 'How should we do these things?' You should all bring your mind and . . . share your ideas. And that is what we have been doing." She offered an example of seeking consent before applying for money for a project: "Even before I would take a step to do something, I tell them, 'This is what I want to do. Is it good?' . . . If they say 'not a good idea,' we boycott it, but most of the time they've seen that my suggestions are always good." Thus, from this leader's perspective, a good leader will share her ideas and plans with members—even those ideas that she knows will be supported. As discussed previously, she believed that this approach built trust.

Another leader emphasized collective decision making. She said that a leader needs to be aware of members' "needs, what they want, what they like" and "their perception of the whole thing you want to do." Her definition of transparency was also about sharing information and ideas with members and soliciting their consent. These practices would ensure that all shared either the credit for success or "blame" if outcomes were poor. She said that she had picked up these leadership approaches from her formal education and from programs she had attended but also from assessing her own expectations as a group member. "I think sometimes too you have to use yourself as [an] example. . . . So if I expect my leader to do [something] then I have to also be like that."

Some leaders we interviewed did identify what they saw as understandable limits on, or acceptable exceptions to, transparency and collective decision making. Some were logistical (e.g., occasions when a quick decision was needed between meetings). "Sometimes there will be some cases—instant cases—that you need to take a decision before you tell your people. But where there is room, you have to give information for them to give their consent."

Other exceptions to transparent practices were about avoiding unrest within the group when privileges were not equally distributed. For example, when grant funding for a workshop did not cover interpreters, only those members considered competent in English would be invited. Leaders might quietly select and invite participants in order to avoid conflict with those not invited. This latter example, however, was linked to concerns some participants expressed about fairness. They spoke of tendencies of those in power to concentrate resources and opportunities among "the elite" (i.e., over-resourced members who needed them the least).

One participant, who grew up in poverty and could only afford to complete a middle school education, was unhappy about what she perceived as elitism and favoritism in her organization. She had held regional leadership positions, such as treasurer and secretary, but—in relation to the national officers—considered herself a "floor member" nonetheless. She said that the "leaders are not free and fair with their floor members, and they are not transparent." She did not feel that women in leadership had fulfilled their promise (whether stated or unstated) to disrupt this tendency. She gave an example of how members were chosen to represent the organization at national or international meetings:

> When there is a chance, for example to go somewhere, they will only . . . give the chances to them[selves]. But [for] me, a floor member, [it] is always difficult. And at times too, even when they come to the floor [members], they will look for the one they love much.

Favoritism and cronyism by the elite were problems not only because attending a national or international meeting would have been an invaluable opportunity to learn and contribute but also because those who attended failed to report back to the floor members. Accountability was lacking. This participant lamented, "All the time, it is the national people who go there. And whenever they [return], for me I don't feel they impart all that they have from there to us."

Failing to share what was learned at a national or international meeting signaled petty corruption: use of this privilege only for personal enjoyment or gain rather than for the good of the organization, its members, and its purpose. These were not "wonky" or theoretical matters for this leader and others but highly significant emotional issues that made them question their investment in the organization and the legitimacy of the entire endeavor. Yet few, if any, alternative organizations existed. Many times, over years of fieldwork, I have had informal conversations with members of various organizations in which they expressed their disgust with leadership and staff behavior, as well as a sense that those in elite levels of DPOs had little contact with or concern for their struggling and impoverished membership.

Empowerment

> Leaders have power. If you [exercise] that power [over members], it's as if you are controlling them. You have to feel like them, throw the question on them. If you want to dictate, they won't come to meetings. We share powers.

Before data collection for this study began, I had visited a meeting that one of our eventual participants led. She called for volunteers for a number of ceremonial and practical roles within the meeting (e.g., opening prayer) and seemed intent on maximizing participation throughout. This was qualitatively different from other meetings I had witnessed that were led by men: these followed a formal structure in which people with titles made their reports, and the meeting facilitator used the majority of the time. When I interviewed her a few weeks later, this older woman leader did not name "empowerment" as a goal but spoke extensively about how she engaged her members in the work of the group. She emphasized sharing power and engaging participation as much as possible.

One leader, who was a petty trader with a middle school education, used both "empowerment" and "capacity building" when she spoke of her goals as a women's wing leader in a district distant from the capital. For this leader, "capacity building" described her efforts to educate the public, for example through local radio programs about blind women's abilities to fulfill the roles of wives and mothers. Concerning empowerment, she said that she tried to serve as an example of how women could speak out and lead others. She emphasized a process of "encouragement"; she said that women should instill courage in one another to "come out" and "put things into action." She tried to do this through role modeling and encouraging interactions with members. She also saw empowerment workshops as helpful in supporting women to learn public speaking.

To a younger and university-educated leader, empowerment meant an internal process of self-recognition: "Accepting the disability and wanting to come out of their shells. People who have believed in themselves, that, 'irrespective of my disability I still have a part to contribute.'" Although she herself was university educated, she said that she did not prize formal education in leaders over self-acceptance and recognition of one's own potential. She averred that this was the most important preparation women leaders could have.

One participant, new to leadership but a DPO and women's wing member for decades, disparaged the shift she had witnessed from employable skills training workshops to empowerment workshops. She was one of the few women in her local group who earned reliable income from a small sewing business, which she ran out of her family of origin's house. Her business made her a visible and relied-upon member of her family and neighborhood. She had attended one "empowerment" workshop and concluded it was a waste of time and money. She said she could not understand the content of a workshop she had attended, which was conducted in English. And from her perspective, real empowerment of women DPO members would be training in skills that would earn them money. By earning money through work, she reasoned, they would also earn respect from family and neighbors.

There was no agreement about the extent to which mentoring occurred among leaders, but some of our participants felt that some senior or formally educated women held their positions too long—not because they were pursuing a clear agenda but because they had become accustomed to the perks of the position—and that they were reluctant to mentor others or even share what they learned when sent to a meeting:

> Because of the qualification, every day they will be there. Instead of giving the chance to somebody else, no! . . . And such people too, they don't share things with other people. . . . For example, this meeting that we went [to] today, what we learned from the National Commission on Women and Development, instead of imparting the other people when we come to our meeting, we will keep it for ourselves. So do you think we are doing in the favor of the group or our own benefit? You see?

There was also a sense that the social divisions between age cohorts and (especially) women with different educational levels influenced whether mentoring would occur or not. Some pointed out that when university graduates were among the membership, they would unfailingly be elected over others with more experience in the group. One participant emphasized that other factors were more important: "There shouldn't be anything like 'you are university graduate, and I am not,' so when there is any post, you have to be taking and leave me out. While maybe you may not get the time to do it, or you may not be able to do it. And I can be able to do it and do it well." Some of the younger, university or polytechnic-educated women expressed frustration with the slow turnover of leadership in the women's wings. Observing little action, they hypothesized that those women who repeatedly ran for and held positions were motivated by the occasional perks of the position rather than the potential to organize for change. They gravitated toward youth wings, seeing them as a more dynamic alternative. And they emphasized their own commitment to practices of empowerment. As one young leader commented:

> Yes, to me [empowering the members] is part of our job as a leader. We have to. Because if tomorrow we are not there, . . . Who is to take the seat? Who is to advocate? . . . Anything can happen at any time, so whilst we are there, we shouldn't keep all the knowledge . . . in us! We should give it out! Because even when we become old like our fathers have become old now, it's the youth who will have to be taking decisions, worrying, troubling the government to put things in place. But if you don't tell them their rights and the right thing to do, meaning . . . we die with whatever we know, there will be nobody to be there to fight for those who are coming.

Discussion

Women leaders grappled with many significant challenges, including members' contradictory and unrealistic expectations of leaders; patronage politics; entrenched leadership and resistance to new approaches within DPOs; abject poverty and need among members; frustration and anger over government unresponsiveness and lack of tangible change; barriers to accessing elected officials and ministers; and unrealistic government expectations that local groups would somehow meet the welfare, human development, and entrepreneurial needs of their members.

As was pointed out previously in this chapter, the Ghanaian government's legal obligation to involve DPOs in policymaking raises the stakes on the participation of women in DPOs. In order to influence the agenda, women need opportunities to play active and influential roles in district, regional, and national levels of their DPOs. Our conversations with women leaders suggested that they were not, at the time of this study, primarily concerned with shaping or engaging in an advocacy agenda. Instead, women leaders focused on improving functioning within groups, emphasizing that their male predecessors had often failed to engage "floor" members actively and had operated in unaccountable ways. Issues of fairness and accountability within the organizations were very much on members' minds. These issues centered on distribution of three key resources: knowledge, money, and power.

Women leaders—all of whom were likely to have participated in empowerment, advocacy, and capacity-building training that were regular features of DPO activities at the time of this study—seemed to find concepts such as "transparency" and "empowerment" helpful to their thinking about how to engage most effectively with their members as leaders. Their interpretations of these concepts seemed flexible and varied, yet consistent in terms of emphasizing a greater and more egalitarian engagement with membership.

When women with disabilities took on leadership roles, they entered a liminal position in relation to other women with disabilities and were called upon to demonstrate where their loyalties were: whether they would be using their position to further the well-being of the group or seeking their own advantage. "Pride" as well as "bossy" and "knowing" worked as threats to stifle women's agency as leaders. The real or imagined possibility that members would dislike elected women leaders or even reject, undermine, or recall them required extensive efforts toward social-relational aspects of leadership. While this was perhaps good for group spirit and cohesion, it was also over and above the advocacy, educational, and economic development agendas that their groups intended to pursue.

In some cases, intergenerational and class conflict among women also preoccupied women leaders. Members were sensitive to hierarchy and inequality within their disabled people's organizations, particularly at the local or district levels, and particularly among women. Women leaders thus faced a nearly impossible challenge in terms of impressing and reassuring members—some of whom may have seniority in terms of age or tenure in the group—that they are competent and powerful enough to lead the group, yet not asserting superiority or aloofness. Women identified several strategies that they used to navigate members' misgivings and foster their trust.

The sociable and egalitarian approaches described by these leaders also took into account the sensitivities of members who had been neglected by their families, communities, and the larger society. The neglect and harm had led them to impoverishment, ill health, and few life chances. For many, there were ongoing experiences that undermined members' senses of safety, self-respect, and well-being. Women leaders thus understood that they needed to lead by example, particularly in terms of respectful and egalitarian interactions and nonviolent conflict resolution. At the same time, some women leaders acknowledged that because they came from relatively privileged backgrounds or encountered disability later in life, they did not have direct experiential knowledge of the social suffering of many of their members.

Women leaders faced significant surveillance, doubt, and even harassment and undermining from DPO members, and specifically from male leadership, on the basis of gender bias.[19] In some cases, male leadership withdrew their support entirely from women leaders once women gained enough confidence to question the status quo. Power was understood by some male leaders to be a zero-sum game; if disabled women gained power, disabled men would surely lose, rather than enjoy shared empowerment with respect to the larger struggle. Women's experiences of resistance from male leaders in Ghanaian DPOs are consistent with research on masculinities in Ghana, which are deeply entrenched in feelings of pride, shame, and honor.[20]

Women who sought power within the disability movement were confronted with harsh and gendered stereotypes meant to force choices between being powerful and being recognized as a woman, or indeed as a Ghanaian. Labeling women as "culturally deviant" (thus culturally dangerous) was a way of shutting down their political aspirations. These dynamics reflect women's experiences in other political arenas in the ways in which "African culture" and "the family" are portrayed as under threat when women acquire power.[21] Indeed a few years prior to fieldwork for this study, presidential candidates from major parties had engaged in lively public discussion about marital rape and concurred on the potential danger to Ghanaian families and

---

19 Naami and Hayashi, "Empowering Women."
20 M. Adinkrah, "Better Dead Than Dishonored: Masculinity and Male Suicidal Behavior in Contemporary Ghana," *Social Science & Medicine* 74, no. 4 (2012).
21 Saida Hodžić, "Unsettling Power: Domestic Violence, Gender Politics, and Struggles Over Sovereignty in Ghana," *Ethnos* 74, no. 3 (2009): 331–360; and S. Razavi and M. Molyneux, "United Nations Research Institute for Social Development," in *Gender Justice, Development, and Rights*, ed. Maxine Molyneux (New York: Oxford University Press, 2002).

culture if it were to be recognized as a criminal act.[22] Echoes of this discussion were present in our conversations with disabled women leaders about their experiences within the disability movement—ostensibly a movement for the liberation of all disabled people.

Conclusion

The women leaders we interviewed showed great tenacity and imagination in how they approached their roles in a conflictual, fraught, and under-resourced context. The work of leadership is not simply a matter of strategic effort but a learning process that also can be highly emotionally demanding.

Women reckoned with significant barriers in meeting the expectations of their members and even in being allowed to lead. The need to gain the trust and respect of their members and to set up more transparent and accountable systems within their organizations meant that women leaders focused more on internal matters than on advocacy for structural or social change. This behind-the-scenes work at the time of this study seemed to gain them little support, recognition, or visibility even within their own organizations, as men continued to occupy more visible positions and tended to be the ones engaging in public advocacy.

At the same time, the women's wings, where women ostensibly could be free of patriarchal barriers, were entrenched in intergenerational and class-based battles to hold power and set agendas. These centered partly on whether women's wings would focus more on direct economic empowerment of their poorest and least educated members or embrace a broader and more advocacy-focused agenda.

Women DPO leaders need to work across yawning cultural divides within their organizations. These are divides that originate partly from socioeconomic differences and differing gendered and generational perspectives but also reflect the cultural tensions and shifts underway in Ghana more generally.

As Abena Busia points out, "African women's ways of negotiating the world are . . . frequently invisible and assumed to lack significance." Women's experiences of leadership within Ghanaian DPOs shed much light not only on their own contributions but also on the complexities of gender and disability in contemporary Africa.

---

22 Hodžić, "Unsettling."

Acknowledgments

This study was completed under a postdoctoral training grant from the US Department of Education through the Center on Human Policy in Syracuse, New York. Extensive thanks to Ghanaian women DPO leaders who gave their time, efforts, and insight to this study. Much appreciation to Kathryn Geurts for arranging initial meetings and extensive participation and collaboration in interviews for this study; to Christine Malec, Chris-Mike Agbelie, and Anne-Marie Bourgeois for transcription assistance; and to Sarah Anderson for linguistic interpretation and interpretive help. All errors and shortcomings in the work are my own.

Chapter Sixteen

Disability Policy, Movement Activism, and the Nonenforcement of a Disability Act

The Case of Ghana

Emmanuel Sackey

Methodology

The purpose of this chapter is to examine how disability is to analyze the factors accounting for the nonenforcement of the Ghana Disability Act since its adoption in 2006. Data was generated through personal interviews with thirteen Ghanaian activists of the disability movement between 2016 and 2017, a content analysis of official policy documents of the state, and a review of secondary literature. The policy documents reviewed include the National Disability Act 715, the 1992 Constitution, the National Disability Policy adopted in 2000, official documents of the Ghana Federation of Disability Organizations (GFDO), the Ghana Blind Union, the Ghana National Association of the Deaf (GNAD), the Ghana Society of the Physically Disabled (GSPD), and media reports. In addition, I relied on my field experience (acquired between 2008 and 2012) in the disability sector during my role as former director of GNAD and a research and information officer of the GFDO.

Background of Disability Policy in Ghana

In postindependence Ghana, the genesis of disability policy can be traced to the early 1960s, when Kwame Nkrumah's Convention's People's Party (CPP) adapted the British social orthopedics model of rehabilitation.[1] As a disability policy, the central objective of the social orthopedics model is to make the disabled population employable. The initiative of the government was informed by the outcome of national surveys in the 1950s that showed that the majority of street beggars were persons with disabilities (PWDs). Thus, between 1961 and 1966, the integration of PWDs into the workforce became the central focus of National Disability Policy. This was coupled with emphasis on special education. The Education Act of 1961, for instance, made provision for the special needs of PWDs.[2] Besides, the rehabilitation policy of the CPP government encompassed the generation of a database of PWD, the establishment of Rural Community Rehabilitation Centers with Urban Industrial Rehabilitation Units (IRUs), and the employment of graduates of the community rehabilitation centers by the IRUs.[3]

For equating disability with unemployment, the disability policy of the Nkrumah regime could be criticized for its capitalist bias, which contradicted the regime's prosocialist claim. In view of the severity of certain physical and

---

[1] According to Grischow, the original British model of *social orthopaedics* was initiated in response to labor shortages in wartime and geared toward the integration of disabled British soldiers into the labor force. See Jeff D. Grischow, "Kwame Nkrumah, Disability and Rehabilitation in Ghana, 1957–1966," *Journal of African History* (2011): 179–199.

[2] Victor C. Anson-Yevu, *A Caste Study on Special Education in Ghana* (Paris: UNESCO, 2008), https://unesdoc.unesco.org/ark:/48223/pf0000094448. The University of Education at Winneba trains professional teachers in special education. More recently, the Center for Disability Studies (CEDRES) at the Kwame Nkrumah University of Science and Technology (KNUST) was established (in 2009) to provide higher education in rehabilitation.

[3] "On the Worlding of Accra's Rehabilitation Training Centre," *Somatosphere*, April 27, 2015, http://somatosphere.net/2015/on-the-worlding-of-accras-rehabilitation-training-centre.html/.

sensory impairments, not all categories of PWDs may be employable. This creates tension between the principle of citizenship and the rights of PWDs to state welfare. Besides, compared to the current era, the co-optation of the DPOs did not create an enabling environment for movement activism. The shortcomings of the disability policy of the CPP government also included a lack of gender balance in the rehabilitation programs and persistent unemployment among a significant proportion of the graduates of the IRUs. Grischow attributes the latter to a lack of capital and marketing opportunities for the products produced at the special industrial centers. Nonetheless, the policy initiatives of the CPP government regarding disability were considered unique and progressive compared to those of other independent African states.

Subsequent governments pursued various disability laws and policies. These include the adoption of a National Mental Health Policy in 1972,[4] the Beggars and Destitute Act (392 of 1969), and the NLCD Legislative Instrument (LI) 632, which sought to criminalize begging and compel disabled people to explore skills training and job opportunities offered by the Regional and Community Based Rehabilitation Centers.[5] The insights from the previous state interventions informed the adoption of a new National Disability Policy in 2000. In order to grant the impetus for enforcement of the policy, the disability movement advocated for its transformation into a law. This culminated in the passage of Act 715 in 2006.

The literature review shows a correlation between changes in international disability rights protocols of the United Nations and disability policy reforms in Ghana. For instance, the UN Policy Guidelines on Inclusive Education influenced the onset of inclusive education in the country.[6] Similarly, the UN's *Standard Rules on the Equalization of Opportunities for Persons with Disabilities*[7] influenced the content of the National Disability Policy adopted

---

4   A. D. Awenva et al., "From Mental Health Policy Development in Ghana to Implementation: What Are the Barriers," *African Journal of Psychiatry* 13 (2010): 184–191.

5   Alexander Kwesi Kassah, "Begging as Work: A Study of People with Mobility Difficulties in Accra, Ghana," *Disability and Society* 23, no. 2 (2008): 163–170.

6   Maxwell Preprah Opoku et al., "Decade of Inclusive Education in Ghana: Perspectives of Educators," *Journal of Social Inclusion* 8, no. 1 (2017).

7   United Nations, *Standard Rules on the Equalization of Opportunities for Persons with Disabilities* (New York: United Nations, 1993), https://www.independentliving.org/standardrules/StandardRules.pdf.

in 2000.[8] As with other sectors, disability laws and policies have not been static but have undergone periodic amendments. In the current democratic dispensation, the disability movement has played a major role in legal and policy reform.

Impact of the Disability Movement

As part of the socialist inclinations of the first postindependence government, the voluntary organizations in the disability sector were incorporated into the institutional apparatus of the Social Welfare Department.[9] The foremost DPOs that were co-opted by the state include the erstwhile Ghana Society of the Blind (GSB) and the Ghana Society for the Deaf (GSD). Following the end of the socialist experiment, the DPOs became independent from the state. Grischow observed that the CPP government's nurturing and funding of the DPOs laid the foundation for the subsequent emergence of a vibrant disability rights movement in Ghana. Social movement scholars postulate that a movement emerges when three core conditions are prevalent: namely, an agenda for change concerning aspects of the socioeconomic and political structures; the prevalence of clearly defined opponents; and a network of groups, individuals, and organizations that share a collective identity under which they mobilize for collective action.[10] These theoretical assumptions hold for the Ghanaian context.

The establishment of the Ghana Federation of Disability Organizations (GFDO) in 1987 solidified the country's disability movement. Since then, the member organizations of the umbrella body have increased from three founding organizations to eight DPOs. These include the Ghana Blind Union (GBU), the Ghana National Association of the Deaf (GNAD), the Ghana Society of the Physically Disabled (GSPD), the Mental Health Society of Ghana (MEHSOG), and the Ghana Association of Persons with Albinism (GAPA). The rest are Inclusion Ghana (IG), a pro–children's rights

---

8   Ministry of Employment and Social Welfare, *National Disability Policy* (Accra: DELARAM, 2000); and B. I. Koray, "The Strengths and Weaknesses of the Constitution in Relation to Persons with Disabilities," in *National Mini-Consultation for Persons with Disabilities* (Accra: DELARAM, 2010), 1–8.
9   Grischow, "Nkrumah."
10 Donatella Della Porta and Diani Mario, *Social Movements: An Introduction* (Oxford: Blackwell, 2006).

organization with a focus on intellectual disability; Share-Care, an organization of persons with autoimmune health conditions; and the Ghana Burns Survivors Foundation (GBSF).

I attribute the recent vibrancy of the disability movement to three factors. Firstly, after several years of military rule, the return to democratic governance in 1992 opened political spaces for the participation of civil society organizations (CSOs) in the process of national development. The DPOs took advantage of the new political environment to mobilize for policy reforms. Secondly, the resurgence of the disability movement has been facilitated by financial and technical support of donors and development agencies. As a result of the new policy agenda that emphasizes the participation of CSOs in the development process, the DPOs attracted significant support from foreign donors and international development agencies. The initial organizational development of the GFDO was, for instance, enhanced through the funding from NORAD, the Norwegian Agency for Development Cooperation.[11]

Thirdly, I posit that when compared with the current era, the previous incorporation of DPOs by the state and the dependence on government for sponsorship made the disability movement less radical in its advocacy engagements. Thus, the autonomy from the state granted the movement an impetus to engage in a more radical advocacy. Even though the GFDO is recognized by the state as the representative body of DPOs in the country, the membership of the movement transcends the federation. The members of the GFDO forge alliances for policy advocacy with other CSOs through the National Disability Network. While the movement is dominated by associations of PWDs, there are nondisabled persons who associate with the movement because of their commitment to social justice, their personal connection to PWDs through family or other relationships, or their status as professionals whose career involves working in the disability sector.

As a constituent of Ghanaian civil society, the disability movement has been very influential in legal and policy reform. Besides the National Disability Act 715, the movement influenced Parliament's ratification of the United Nations Conventions on the Rights of Persons with Disabilities and the passage of the National Mental Health Act 846 in 2012. The success of the movement also includes contributions to the formulation of Ghana's

---

11   Geurts, "Worlding."

second (2006–2009) Poverty Reduction Strategy[12] and improvement in the political participation of PWDs in national elections (as voters). The persistent advocacy through lobbying of Parliament and engaging with state ministries, stakeholder forums, media engagements, and occasional street protests contributed to the movement's success. Among the successes of Ghana's disability rights movement, the passage of Act 715 remains the most remarkable, for it serves as the cornerstone of current disability policy in Ghana.

Act 715 and the Institutional Framework for Its Implementation

Ghana's 1992 constitution emphasizes nondiscrimination and the rights of citizens to access social services and to participate in all spheres of national life on an equal basis.[13] Article 29 of the constitution specifically emphasizes that subsidiary legislation be promulgated to ensure a comprehensive mainstreaming of disability aspects into national development. In the early 2000s, the disability movement invoked the constitution to advocate for the enactment of the National Disability Act 715, which was passed by Parliament in 2006. To a significant extent, the act remains the most comprehensive legal document pertaining to the rights of PWDs in Ghana. Building on the previous National Disability Policy,[14] Act 715 guarantees the rights of PWDs to participate equally in education, health care, employment, political participation, and acessibility to public transportation. It also provides for equal access to information and communication as well as, among other things, an accessible environment and recreation.

The Major Actors

The process leading to the promulgation of Act 715 involved a number of institutional actors. These include the Ministry of Social Protection, Ministry of Justice, the National Parliament, and the DPOs comprising the disability movement. While it took the advocacy initiative of the movement

---

12   International Monetary Fund, *Ghana: Poverty Reduction Strategy Paper* (Washington, DC: International Monetary Fund, 2012), https://www.inf.org/external.pubs/ft/scr/2012/cr12203.pdf.

13   Government of Ghana, *Constitution of the Republic of Ghana* (Accra: Assembly, 1992).

14   Ministry of Employment and Social Welfare, *National Disability Policy*.

to place the legislation on the agenda of Parliament, the mandate to submit disability-related bills to Parliament falls under the jurisdiction of the Ministry of Social Protection. On the other hand, the drafting of national laws is the responsibility of the Ministry of Justice. Following a series of legislative forums, which encompassed various stages of drafting and parliamentary deliberations, the act got presidential assent in 2006. Among the prerequisites for enforcement was the establishment of a National Council for Persons with Disabilities (NCPD), which occurred three years later. The formulation of comprehensive legislative instruments (LI), which would spell out the details of the enforcement modalities, became the remaining condition for enforcement.

In accordance with Act 715, in formulating the LI, the NCPD is expected to collaborate with the attorney general's department; other state ministries, departments, and agencies (MDAs); and representatives of the disability movement. The inputs of the MDAs are deemed necessary because disability mainstreaming is a multisectorial process. Thus, for the LI to be comprehensive, it must include provisions generated in consultation with MDAs such as the Ministry of Education, Ministry of Employment and Labor Relations, the Ghana Standard Authority, Ministry of Health, and the Judicial service, etc. Even though the formulation of the LI began, the process was halted in 2012 when the advocacy of the movement led to a shift in agenda from the formulation of the LI to an amendment of Act 715 in order to align it with the CRPD. The amendment process began in 2010.

Accounting for the Stagnation

In the following sections, I examine the extent to which the degree of government commitment to disability mainstreaming, the institutional and technical constraints on the effectiveness of the NCPD, and the role of the disability movement contributed to the stagnation of the enforcement of Act 715.

Government Commitment to Disability Mainstreaming

Among the representatives of the disability movement, there is a wide perception that the nonimplementation of Act 715 is due to lack of state commitment to disability mainstreaming. This perception is based on the fact that since the NCPD was established to monitor the implementation of Act 715, it has not been adequately resourced to fulfill its mandate. However, it would be an overimplication to attribute the problem to lack of commitment on the part of the state. As shown in the introductory sections, succeeding governments have made various attempts through state policy to make development inclusive for the disabled population. Presently, the most outstanding evidence of state commitment to disability mainstreaming is the innovation of a disability component of the District Assembly Common Fund (DACF). The DACF is a local development fund created under Article 252 of the 1992 constitution stipulating that not less than 5 (currently 7.5) percent of the national income be allocated to all District Assemblies to enhance local development. In 1993 the District Assembly Common Fund Act (455) was enacted to set out the detail modalities for the disbursement of the fund. Between 2005 and 2006, a revision of the DACF included a clause that mandates the district assemblies to allocate 2 percent (currently 2.5) of their quarterly allocation to PWDs.

Other state interventions include a 2017 initiative by the Ministry of Road and Transport to reserve a 50 percent quota of road toll collecting jobs along the country highways to PWDs. Besides, coupled with the use of sign language interpretation services at state-organized events,[15] GBC-TV, the state broadcaster, has mainstreamed sign language interpretation services into its news programs to bridge the communication barrier for the deaf. Besides, the Ministry of Education adopted an inclusive education policy in 2015, whereas the Ghana Accessibility Standard was adopted in 2016 to make the environment accessible to people with mobility impairments.

Lack of resources is to blame for the non-implementation. Inadequate funding is a wider challenge across the MDAs and not only confined to the disability sector. For instance, even though the provision of social services is an obligation of the state, the piloting of inclusive education in the country was funded by UNESCO and UNICEF.[16] The funding challenges of public agencies are largely due to the underdeveloped economy and the fact that

---

15   The initiative is facilitated by the Ministry of Information.
16   Opoku et al., "Inclusive Education"; Wisdom Mprah, Michael Amponteng Kwadwo, and Isaac Owusu, "Barriers to Inclusion of Children with Disabilities in Inclusive Schools in Ghana," *Journal of Disability Studies* 1, no. 1 (2017): 15–22.

national expenditure tends to exceed the national income.[17] A significant proportion of Act 715, such as the component that requires making all built environments accessible for PWDs, requires enormous financial resources on the part of both the state and the private sector.

Arguments for the state's noncommitment, on the other hand, could be tenable in the case of the elements of the legislation that do not require financial resources for implementation. For instance, the enforcement of section 10 of Act 715, which makes provisions for tax rebates for corporate entities that employ PWDs, requires political willingness on the part of government leaders. Similarly, the implementation of sections 32, 33 and 40 of Act 715 are not contingent on the availability of resources. Revising the curriculum of existing educational institutions mainly requires political commitment more than resources. From this perspective, the various governments can be criticized for not demonstrating adequate commitment to the implementation of the legislation. Nonetheless, states' resource constraints represent a global phenomenon. Even in the United States, resource constraints remain a challenge to disability mainstreaming.[18] It is primarily due to resource constraints that section 60 of Act 715 grants a ten-year moratorium on the reconstructing of all social infrastructure. Therefore, the state's lack of interest is not the primary concern.

Institutional Constraints on the Effectiveness of the NCPD

An effective implementation of Act 715 requires that the various MDAs factor a disability mainstreaming component into their budget. For instance, since 2012, the National Electoral Commission (NEC) has established a disability unit and formulated an action plan that makes it possible for PWDs to vote in national elections. This has been possible because the NEC makes budgetary allocations to support the implementation of accessible voting centers and inclusive election mechanisms, such as the provision of tactile ballots for the blind and sign language interpreters for the deaf. Unlike

---

17   Ministry of Finance, *Annual Debt Management Report for the Year 2016* (Accra: Ministry of Finance, 2016).
18   Jeb Barnes and F. Thomas Burke, "Making Way: Legal Mobilization, Organizational Response, and Wheelchair Access," *Law and Society Review* 46, no. 1 (2012): 167–198; and Eilionoir Flynn, *From Rhetoric to Action: Implementing the UN Convention on the Rights of Persons with Disabilities* (Cambridge: Cambridge University Press, 2011).

the Mental Health Act (846), which prescribes the imposition of a special national levy for psychiatric care, the implementation of Act 715 is not tied to any specific financial allocation. As for other state agencies, the NCPD board is supposed to receive its budgetary allocation from the Ministry of Finance. But the leadership of the NCPD often complains about delayed and inadequate subventions from the national treasury.

In accounting for the anomaly, an ex-member of the NCPD attributes the scenario to the Ministry of Social Protection's lack of mandate to authorize other state agencies with jurisdiction over disability matters:

> What needs to be done is for the Council to be placed directly under the office of the President as . . . in other countries. . . . In that case the various ministries can be authorized from the office of the President, for the enforcement of disability provisions, then the Council coordinate and report to the office of the president. In my opinion this would facilitate disability mainstreaming better than what we currently have.[19]

In accordance with the 1992 constitution, all MDAs must report directly to the office of the president. Placing the NCPD under the office of the president would therefore be more pragmatic because it would enhance the mandate of the NCPD to ensure compliance from the MDAs. Such a bureaucratic arrangement is not unprecedented. Agencies such as the National Development Planning Commission (NDPC) and the Department for Public Private Sector Partnerships (PPPs) operate under the aegis of the president. As emphasized by the ex-board member of the NCPD, similar institutional arrangement is a contributing factor to the relative success of South Africa's national Disability Council. I therefore posit that the legal and institutional framework under which the NCPD operates remains a major contributory factor to the nonenforcement of the National Disability Act.

Technical Constraints of the NCPD

The NCPD was established in 2009 in accordance with the stipulations of Act 715. As a subsidiary agency of the Ministry of Gender and Social Protection, the core function of the NCPD is to coordinate, monitor, and evaluate all disability policies of the state. The NCPD also advises the government on

---

19   1083 Personal Communication, Ex-Board Member, National Council NCPD, 15 September 2017.

disability issues. However, human resource constraints, particularly lack of technical expertise, also accounts for the inability of the NCPD to ensure the implementation of Act 715:

> As we speak now, the Council does not have a Board, so the Council does not exist. It's only a secretariat. How many permanent staff are there? The Executive Secretary was seconded from the Social Welfare Department. The secretariat does not have technical staff that can ensure the implementation of the Act 715.[20]

Salient in the above quotation is the assertion that the NCPD does not have the number of staff with the technical expertise required to fulfill its mandate. Section 43 of Act 715 demands that the board of the NCPD be composed of representatives of the Ministry of Health, the Department of Social Welfare, the Ministry of Local Government and Rural Development, Ghana Employers' Association, the Ministry of Education, the Ministry of Youth and Employment, the Ministry of Social Protection, and three representatives of DPOs. The board members of the NCPD are expected to have varied professional experience relevant for disability mainstreaming.

While not constitutionally stipulated, it would be ideal that the staff members of the NCPD possess expertise in fields such as disability law, accessibility standards, inclusive and special education, and rehabilitation. This would allow the NCPD to fulfill its mandate. Yet currently only the executive secretary is familiar with the *nitty gritty* of the disability sector. Prior to the secondment of the current executive secretary from the Department of Social Welfare about three years ago, only one technical director had a professional background related to disability.[21] Thus, the lack of adequate staff with the requisite technical expertise impacted negatively on the effectiveness of the NCPD and contributed to the stagnation of the enforcement of the Disability Act.

---

20 Personal communication, Chairman Ghana Disability Forum, September 16, 2017.

21 The technical director is professional audiologist. This medical background is limited in relation to the mandate of the National NCPD's scope and needed to be complemented with other experts ranging from rehabilitation, inclusive and special education, inclusive employment and labor experts, disability law, etc.

Culpability of the Disability Movement

The disability movement has played a key role in promoting the rights of PWDs in Ghana. As noted in the preceding sections, it was the advocacy initiatives of the movement that set the pace for the promulgation of Act 715. However, there are two grounds on which the movement can be faulted for the delayed enforcement of Act 715. The first is the lack of willingness to use legal means to seek redress, despite having the opportunity to do so. The second is the premature call for amendment, which led to further delays in the implementation of the legislation.

The only known legal suit pursued as part of the advocacy strategy of the movement is the case of *Franklin Jantuah v. the Ghana Disability Forum*. Following the 2016 presidential CPP nomination of Ivor Greenstreet, a disabled lawyer and businessman, Mr. Jantuah, the last surviving member of Ghana's first cabinet in the postindependence era and member of the party, remarked that a disabled person should not have been elected as the flagbearer of the CPP.[22] The statement was condemned by the various DPOs aligned with the disability movement. The Ghana Disability Forum filed a legal suit against the veteran politician, which is currently pending at the Human Rights Court in Accra. Two relevant issues emerge from the use of legal suit as an advocacy strategy, namely the cost of legal services as an obstacle to litigation and the lack of willingness to engage in court litigation.

In the pursuit of the aforementioned case, members of the forum had to mobilize voluntary financial contributions for the services of a lawyer because financial constraints account for the hesitancy to use legal means. Besides, a section of the movement opines that there should be more education on and awareness of the disability laws before the use of legal action. They argue for a gradual approach to the use of legal action because most Ghanaian individuals and organizations are not aware of the stipulations of the disability act. The gradualists also maintain that in certain instances what some PWDs perceive as violations of their rights may actually be misconceptions due to ignorance of the law. For instance, it was unclear to the Ghana Disability Forum whether a local airline that refused to board PWDs with crutches and wheelchairs was actually in violation of the law. PWDs may sometimes be culpable for the perceived discrimination, perhaps in situations where they do not follow administrative procedures such as indicating the need for

---

22   "Disability Forum Sues Jantuah Over 'Scandalous Statements,'" *Rainbow Radio*, June 9, 2016.

special assistance when booking flights. Thus, for a section of the gradualists in the disability movement, the decision to opt for legal action should be contingent on the availability of resources, as well as rigorous technical knowledge of the disability laws.

On the other hand, a segment of the movement contends that legal action remains the most pragmatic approach to advocacy in a resistant society.[23] The latter for instance maintains that even though Act 715 gave a ten-year moratorium for compliance with accessibility components of the law, the grace period has elapsed. Thus, for such members, legal action against entities that violate the rights of PWDs would be a more ideal option.

It is arguable that while court litigation could help ensure compliance with disability laws, it cannot guarantee anything without an optimum level of public awareness about the legislation.[24] Even so, in a resistant society, legal action offers a pragmatic approach to advocacy. Yet the cost of legal services remains a major challenge for this option. To overcome the obstacle, it would be realistic for PWDs to have access to legal aid through a collaboration between the NCPD and the Commission for Human Rights and Administrative Justice, as well as the Ghana Legal Aid Department for pro bono services. But so far, the movement has done very little in this regard.

Secondly, following Parliament's ratification of the CRPD in 2012, the movement petitioned Parliament through the NCPD for amendment of Act 715. The objective of the proposed amendment is to harmonize the provisions of the act to the protocols to the CRPD. This occurred at a time when the work on the legislative instrument to guide the enforcement was ongoing. While the revision of Act 715 is necessary, there should have been sequencing within a timeline that could grant the impetus for its implementation to begin. Even though the CRPD makes it obligatory for a state that ratifies it to conform to its provisions, compliance with the CRPD requires enormous resources on the part of the state and the private sector. Considering the underdeveloped nature of the economy,[25] it is not certain that Ghana can comply with the protocols of the CRPD.[26]

---

23 This implies society that continues to discriminate against PWDs despite public awareness of disability rights.
24 Barnes and Burke, "Making Way."
25 Ministry of Finance, *Debt*.
26 Even the United States, which is economically developed, has not ratified CRPD due to a commitment to the ADA promulgated in 1990. See Mike Pickup Davis, "The US Should Not Sign UN Disability Convention,"

Furthermore, whereas the participation of PWDs is necessary for the formulation of disability law and policies, the initial legislative forums were predominantly composed of PWDs, out of which only one had expertise in disability law. At various times the legal expert acted both as member of the movement and representative of the attorney general's department. This afforded limited opportunities for an alternative legal perspective. Subsequent recruitment of the services of another legal consultant led to the discernment of enormous gaps between Act 715 and the CRPD. Thus, if the GFDO, which led the movement, had established an inclusive legal and policy committee with membership criteria that transcended disability identity, the undue delay could have been avoided. Moreover, since all laws and policies are subject to periodic amendments, it would have been more pragmatic to begin the implementation of Act 715, with the revision process to follow. By halting the previous implementation process and setting a new agenda, the movement also contributed to the delay of the law's implementation.

Political Actors and Strategic Response to Institutional Pressures

The passage of laws and policies without implementation is not an unusual phenomenon in Ghana. This form of institutional decoupling transcends the disability sector. For instance, a recent study on local government and development policy indicates the prevalence of institutional building traps, whereby a cycle of policy reforms is enacted without compliance with their prescriptions.[27] Neo-institutional sociology offers a framework through which these dynamics could be properly understood. Among the core propositions of the model is that institutionalized practices tend to diffuse in a given environment, as a result of a logic of appropriateness rooted in the need for legitimacy.[28] Thus, for neo-institutionalists, the conformity to insti-

---

The Hill, September 21, 2014, http://thehill.com/blogs/congress-blog/healthcare/218254-us-should-not-sign-un-disability-convention.

27 Matthew Sabbi, *Local State Institutional Reforms in Ghana: Actors, Legitimacy and the Unfulfilled Promise of Participatory Development* (Baden-Baden: Nomos, 2017).

28 John W. Meyer, "World Society, Institutional Theory, and the Actor," *Annual Review of Sociology* 36 (2010): 1–20; Georg Krucken and S. Gili Drori, "World Society: A Theory and Research Program in Context," in *World Society: The Writings of John Meyer*, ed. Drori Georg Krücken and Gili S. Drori (Oxford: Oxford University Press, 2009), 3–35; Richard Scott, *Institutions*

tutional standards is not just induced by the instrumental reasons for rewards or the motivation to avoid sanctions. The implication is that certain institutional practices are adopted not only because they are considered efficient by the actors that adopt them but also because they are considered socially acceptable.

In accordance with this perspective, institutional actors may engage in decoupling or maintaining an appearance of conformity (without actual compliance) when the socially acceptable standards are found to be technically inefficient. Decoupling therefore becomes a strategy of balancing the tension between the need for technical efficiency and legitimacy from the institutional environment. Meyer observed that the dynamics of globalization have put nation-states and organizations under obligations to conform to legal and policy standards of their counterparts in other regions around the world.[29] As a result, some developing states adopt policies promulgated in the economically developed regions, despite the lack of capacity for implementation.

In a revised model that synthesizes assumptions of both the old institutional and neo-institutional perspectives, Oliver[30] postulated five core passive and active responses that organizations adopt to deal with pressures from their institutional environment. These comprise acquiescence, compromise, avoidance, defiance, and manipulation. In accordance with Oliver's analytic framework, acquiescence implies conformity without any objection. Acquiescence is assumed to be the preferred strategy of organizations in the context of uncertainty about the consequences of not adopting the dominant trends. For Oliver, compromise remains a preferable strategy to institutional pressures when actors are confronted with incompatible demands from multiple stakeholders. As a strategic response to institutional pressures, *defiance* implies the rejection of demands of stakeholders when organized entities perceive that they can succeed without significant negative consequences

---

and Organizations: Ideas and Interests (Los Angeles: SAGE, 2008); Walter Powell and Paul DiMaggio, "Introduction," in *The Neo-Institutionalism in Organizational Analysis*, ed. Walter Powell and Paul DiMaggio (Chicago: Chicago University Press, 1991), 1–38; and Paul DiMaggio and Walter Powell, "The Iron Cage Revisited: Institutional Isomorphism and Collective Rationality in Organizational Fields," *American Sociological Association* 48, no. 2 (1983): 147–160.

29 Meyer, "World Society."
30 Christine Oliver, "Strategic Responses to Institutional Processes," *Academy of Management Review* 16, no. 1 (1991): 145–179.

for noncompliance. In accordance with Oliver's model, manipulation comes when organizations seek to transform or neutralize the influence of the institutional demands confronting them.

When these theoretical propositions are applied to the empirical case in focus, the dynamics of disability policy formulation and nonimplementation in Ghana depict policy adoption as a strategic response of the state in order to maintain an appearance of being socially responsible. This enhances the legitimacy of the state in the eyes of its disabled population and the international community. Thus, the promulgation of Act 715, the ratification of the CRPD, and the current ongoing process to align the act to the protocols of CRPD are manifestations of institutional isomorphism. On the other hand, the failure to enforce the legislation eleven years after its passage suggests institutional decoupling. Being part of the global disability movement, advocacy of the Ghanaian DPOs forms part of a wider transnational phenomenon. Similarly, the state, being a member of the United Nations, came under a normative influence to sign the CRPD. Having ratified the convention in 2012, the state then came under pressure from the disability movement to conform to the CRPD and amend the Disability Act.

However, there is a logic of instrumentality underlying this form of institutional decoupling. The extent to which institutional actors respond to the pressures to conform to certain standards is contingent upon the degree to which their survival depends on the source that the pressure is emanating from. In Ghana, the emergence of a competitive multiparty system has generated an environment for politicization of social issues, which the disability movement also appropriates to push its agenda.[31] I argue that the Disability Act was not adopted only because of a logic of appropriateness on the part of Parliament but also because the failure to meet the demands of the disabled population comes with political cost to the various parties. PWDs comprise a significant percentage of the national population.[32] Even though

---

31 Andrew Downing, "Power and Disability in the Global South: A Case Study of Ghana's Disability Rights Movement" (master's thesis, University of Lund, 2011).

32 The estimates are based on the current (updated) estimates of the Ghana Statistical Service. The 2010 National Housing and Population Census indicated that PWDs comprise 3 percent of the national population. According to the last census report, this represents 737,743 out of a projected twenty-five million people—a figure the disability movement has contested as being too low. See Ghana Statistical Service, *2010 Population and Housing Census: A Summary Report of Final Results* (Accra: Ghana Statistical Service, 2012).

the official estimate shows that PWDs form 3 percent (over 800,000 people) of an estimated 29.6 million population, it is mathematically possible for PWDs to influence the outcome of national elections[33] should they decide to vote on the basis of the extent to which the governing parties respond to their interest.[34]

As a case of institutional decoupling, the passage and nonenforcement of the twelve-year-old legislation defy a monocausal explanation. If the implementation is currently on hold because of the proposed amendment to align it with the CRPD, then the institutional perspective holds. Even then, it is the regulative and normative pillars of institutions at work because Ghana has ratified the CRPD and therefore comes under obligations to enforce its protocols. Yet the initial passage of Act 715 was preceded by street protests organized by the disability movement. Following the promulgation of the act, there has been evidence of budgetary constraints. By passing the law, the state strikes a compromise, for it maintains an appearance of being socially responsible to its disabled population. This pacifies the populace and reinforces the legitimacy of the state. Thus, in the context of limited resources, the adoption and nonenforcement of Act 715 may be a strategic response aimed at balancing the tension between the demands of the disabled population and the political survival of the governing parties.

Conclusion

The preceding sections show the multidimensional nature of institutional decoupling pertaining to the stagnation of the enforcement of Ghana's Disability Act 715. I give primary consideration to the institutional factors because, even if all MDAs were adequately resourced and the technical gaps were remedied, the current legal-institutional framework under which the NCPD operates would still not be enough for the council to compel the MDAs to factor disability aspects into their action plans and budgets. The alternative option is for the NCPD to take legal action against entities that violate the provisions of Act 715. Yet the legal option is not possible until

---

33 Emmanuel Sackey, Dynamic Tensions Civil Society and Development of the Disability Rights Movement (Munster, Germany: Lit, 2018).
34 There have been two election roundoffs since 2000. In the case of the 2008 presidential elections, only forty thousand votes separated the winning party and the runner up.

the detailed legislative instruments to guide the implementation are completed. Furthermore, without the legal authority to compel the MDAs to allocate specific proportions of their budget to disability mainstreaming, Act 715 would only remain a legal document. To overcome this challenge, an alternative approach is to place the NCPD under the office of the president.

I have also emphasized that while the disability movement helped facilitate passage of Act 715, the movement also contributed to the delay of its implementation. Even though the state has ratified the CRPD and comes under obligation to revise Act 715, in order to harmonize it with the international protocols, there must also be an admission that the state lacks the resources for the implementation of the CRPD protocols. The advocacy strategy of the movement could therefore have been sequenced in such a way as to reflect this reality. In the absence of the requisite resources, the state strategically responds to the movement agitations by adopting policies and laws that are not enforced. By maintaining an appearance of being socially responsible to its populace, the governing parties garner political support.

Subsequently, the disability movement ought to be more pragmatic in terms of which advocacy issues to confront. In a context where the DPOs could also use portions of their resources to provide some of the basic services required by their members, using enormous resources to advocate for issues the state cannot address is imprudent. This does not imply that certain advocacy initiatives such as the call for amendment of Act 715 were not necessary. It implies that the movement could strategically sequence their agitations within a relatively convenient time frame such as when government is not obliged to conform to austerity measures. Ultimately, the institutional and technical limitations that obstruct the goals of the NCPD would also have to be rectified in order to overcome the nonenforcement of the National Disability Act.

Chapter Seventeen

Students with Disabilities' Lack of Opportunity for Sport and Recreational Activities

The Case of South African Universities

Desire Chiwandire

Introduction

The South African government has enacted various policies that oblige universities to provide conducive environments for the equal participation of students with disabilities (SWDs) in sport and recreational activities (SARAs). Despite this, research indicates that SWDs have low participation opportunities in comparison to their nondisabled peers in SARAs on campuses, with universities focusing more on the academic needs of SWDs than on their social needs. In order to describe and assess the measures being taken by South African universities to promote the participation of SWDs in SARAs, twenty-eight qualitative interviews with disability unit staff members (DUSMs) were conducted. Data were analyzed using a theoretically derived qualitative content analysis in which othering was employed as a theoretical lens. The study found three broad responses: those who objected strongly to the participation of SWDs in SARAs; those who wanted to see SWDs participating in SARAs but expressed concerns over barriers; and those who fully supported the participation of SWDs in SARAs and who argued that it promotes positive academic outcomes, is a basic right, and is part of a healthy lifestyle. It is the contention of this researcher that universities should prioritize the equal participation of SWDs in SARAs as a holistic way of creating an enabling environment for SWDs.

Disability Sport: An International Context

According to Patricia Miller, every person has a right to participate in sport that is governed by rules based on equality and has sufficient access to any necessary resources.[1] The rights for PWDs to participate in sport and recreation are enshrined in such international human rights instruments as the CRPD.[2] Article 30 of the CRPD provides for the participation of PWDs in cultural life, recreation, leisure, and sport. Section 5(b) of this article specifically obliges signatories to take appropriate measures to ensure that PWDs have the same opportunity and provision of resources, including coaching, as their nondisabled peers in order to participate in disability-specific sport and recreational activities.[3] Disability-specific sport refers to any organized competitive or recreational physical activity that PWDs participate in, "whether it is in an integrated or disability-specific setting."[4] Sports that are commonly available for PWDs include "track and field, table tennis, wheelchair tennis, wheelchair dance, chess, judo, 5-a-side soccer (for the athlete with visual

---

1 Patricia Miller, *Fitness Programming and Physical Disability: A Publication for Disabled Sports* (Champaign. IL: Human Kinetics, 1995).
2 United Nations, *Convention on the Rights of Persons with Disabilities and Optional Protocol* (New York: United Nations, 2006), http://www.un.org/disabilities/documents/convention/convoptprot-e.pdf.
3 United Nations, *Convention*.
4 Marit Sørensen, "Integration in Sport and Empowerment of Athletes with a Disability," *European Bulletin of Adapted Physical Activity* 2, no. 2 (2003): 1; Oluseyi Dada and Christiana Ukpata, "Sport Participation and Facilities as Predictors of Marketable Skill in Sport for Persons with Disability in Nigerian Universities," *European Journal of Special Education Research* 2, no. 5 (2017): 136.

impairment), 7-a-side football for athletes with cerebral palsy, swimming, wheelchair basketball, wheelchair rugby, and cycling."[5]

Globally, PWDs continue to be generally excluded from mainstream sports.[6] Barriers include negative psychosocial factors, such as nondisabled persons' negative attitudes, prejudices, stereotypes, and stigmas toward PWDs.[7] Other barriers include limited information on issues of disability sport,[8] lack of funding because of the belief that disability sport is costly,[9] and architectural barriers, such as inaccessibility of sport facilities[10]. These barriers are more prevalent in developing countries[11] as PWDs face major barriers that limit their access to and participation in sport.[12] Barriers such as shortage of available accessible sport for all programs, a lack of financing for accessible sport, a paucity of accessible sport facilities, lack of accessible sport-specific equipment, and limited or no capacity to host major disability

---

5   Christa Rohwer, "Benefits of Sport for People with Disabilities," Health24, May 13, 2013, http://www.health24.com/Fitness/Exercise/Benefits-of-sport-for-people-with-disabilities-20130531.

6   Karen DePauw and Susan Gavron, *Disability Sport* (Champaign, IL: Sports and Recreation, 2005); Claudine Sherrill and Trevor Williams, "Disability and Sport: Psychosocial Perspectives on Inclusion, Integration and Participation," *Sport and Science Review* 5, no. 1 (1996): 46–64; Giseal Kobberling, Luc Legar and Louis Jankowski, "The Relationship Between Aerobic Capacity and Physical Activity in Blind and Sighted Adolescents," *Journal of Visual Impairments and Blindness* 85 (1991): 382–84; Pam Stevenson, "The Pedagogy of Inclusive Youth Sport: Working towards Real Solutions," in *Disability and Youth Sport*, ed. Hayley Fitzgerald (London: Routledge, 2009); Kamil Yazicioglu et al., "Influence of Adapted Sports on Quality of Life and Life Satisfaction in Sport Participants and Non-Sport Participants with Physical Disabilities," *Disability and Health Journal* 5, no. 4 (2012): 249–53.

7   Sherrill and Williams, "Disability and Sport."

8   DePauw and Gavron, *Disability and Sport*.

9   Dada and Ukpata, "Sport Participation," 137.

10 DePauw and Gavron, *Disability and Sport*.

11 Pierre Barayagwiza, "Factors Related to Sport Preferences among Youth with Physical Disability in Rwanda" (PhD diss., University of the Western Cape, 2011); and Wladimir Andreff, "The Correlation Between Economic Underdevelopment and Sport," *European Sport Management Quarterly* 1, no. 4 (2001): 252–56.

12 *Sport and Development*, "Sport and Disability," *Sport and Development*, n.d., http://www.sportanddev.org/learnmore/sport_and_disability2/.

sporting events[13] are prevalent in developing countries. For instance, India has been criticized for having little involvement with disability cricket due to funding constraints.[14]

Developed countries, on the other hand, are said to have made considerable progress in enhancing the full potential of PWDs. They have done this through sports thanks to federal legislation and political pressure,[15] which is why their methods are regarded as best disability sport practice. This has necessitated the availability of sport participation opportunities "from the grassroots to elite levels for PWD to showcase their abilities in sport" in these countries.[16] Karen Losch argued that what makes disability sport successful in developed countries is that it is regarded as a low-cost means of fostering greater inclusion and well-being for PWDs.[17] This is particularly true in Australia where "sport has been identified as a low-cost and effective means to foster positive health and well-being, social inclusion. and community building for people with disability."[18]

In the British context, Elling and Claringbould noted that the end of the twentieth century witnessed an emerging discourse that promoted diversity, inclusion, and cohesion through the participation of PWDs in football[19] as a way of tackling social exclusion of this population.[20] Such policy documents as the *Disability Football Strategy 2010–2012* called for professional football clubs in Britain to "create opportunities . . . for anyone with a disability to get involved in football—whether as a player, referee, administrator, coach,

---

13   Sport and Development, "Sport and Disability."
14   "Disability Chief Calls on ICC to Raise Its Game," *This Ability*, October 4, 2016, https://www.thenews.com.pk/print/154695-Disability-chief-calls-on-ICC-to-raise-its-game.
15   DePauw and Gavron, *Disability and Sport*.
16   Barayagwiza, "Sport Preferences," 2; "Disability Sport Project," Australian Sports Commission (ASC), n.d., http://www.ausport.gov.au/participating/disability/get_involved/sports_ability.
17   Karen Losch, "A Case of Wheelchair Tennis," *ThinkSport: A Journal of Sport and Recreation* 2, no. 4 (March 2015): 71–78.
18   ASC, "Disability Sport Project."
19   Agnes Elling and Inge Claringbould, "Mechanism of Inclusion and Exclusion in the Dutch Sports Landscape: Who Can and Wants to Belong?" *Sociology of Sport Journal* 22, no. 4 (2005): 498–515.
20   Kris Southby, "Learning-Disability, Football Fandom and Social Exclusion" (PhD diss., Durham University, 2012), 35.

or spectator."[21] Likewise, in Canada, the increased benefits of physical activity and participation in sport for PWDs has seen the country implementing a number of projects promoting sport participation for this population as a way of curbing increasing health-care costs.[22] However, it should be noted that although developed countries are often referred to as supportive of disability sport initiatives, some of these countries have not completely broken down the barriers to sport participation in that they have not correctly implemented the extant disability policies.[23] Recent statistics on disability sports in the United States indicate that sports participation among PWDs is significantly lower across all age groups.[24]

In recent years there have been calls for governments to promote and meaningfully integrate sport for PWDs into society, but disability sports' full potential as a powerful way of redressing the historical exclusion of PWDs is only beginning to be realized.[25]

Benefits of Sport Participation for PWDs

Apart from participation in sports and exercise as an important right, proponents have noted that sports activity has numerous benefits for PWDs that are also applicable to nondisabled persons. For Richard Bailey and colleagues, disability sport participation has long-term health benefits such as improving the efficient functioning of the body.[26] Research has shown that involvement

---

21 "English Football's Ongoing Work to Tackle All Forms of Discrimination," *The FA*, n.d., http://www.thefa.com/football-rules-governance/inclusion-and-anti-discrimination/ policies-and-plans.

22 Penny Parnes and Goli Hashemi, "Sport as a Means to Foster Inclusion, Health and Well-Being of People with Disabilities," *Literature Reviews on Sport for Development and Peace* 124 (2007): 135.

23 Goli Hashemi, "Promoting Health and Social Participation: An Analysis of Disability Related Policies in the North West Province of Cameroon" (PhD diss., University of London, 2006).

24 Dada and Ukpata, "Sport Participation," 137.

25 Dada and Ukpata, "Sport Participation," 136; and Global Partnerships on Children with Disabilities, *Thematic Paper: Disability Inclusive Physical Activity and Sport in the Post-2015 Development Agenda and Sustainable Development Goals* (New York: UNICEF, 2015).

26 Richard Bailey et al., "The Educational Benefits Claimed for Physic Sport: An Academic Review," *Research Papers in Education* 24, no. 1 (2009): 3; and Parnes and Hashemi, "Sport as a Means," 133.

in adaptive sports can significantly improve participants' health.[27] For example, sport has been found in various studies to promote mental well-being;[28] reduce the risk of chronic illnesses;[29] lower levels of anxiety and decrease stress;[30] improve general mood and depressive and anxiety disorders in select psychiatric patients;[31] lower the prevalence of obesity;[32] reduce dependency on pain and depression medication;[33] and improve blood circulation, muscle strength, balance, and coordination.[34]

Apart from health benefits, Parnes and Hashemi argued that sports among PWDs "may also bring numerous benefits to a community both at a social and an individual level."[35] Both of these aspects are important in facilitat-

---

27 Ashley Bohnert, "Wheelchair Basketball Athletes: Motives for Participation" (master's thesis, East Carolina University, 2016), 2.
28 Kenneth Fox, "The Complexities of Self-Esteem Promotion in Physical Education and Sport," in *Sports and Physical Activity-Moving towards Excellence*, ed. T. Williams, L. Almond, and A. Sparks (London: E & FN Spon, 1992); and Denise Jones, "The Recreational Experience in South Africa: Critical Issues in Defining the Term," *International Council for Health, Physical Education, Recreation, Sport and Dance Journal* 37, no. 2 (1995): 1–24.
29 John Durstine et al., "Physical Activity for the Chronically Ill and Disabled," *Sports Medicine* 30, no. 3 (2000): 207–19; and Gregory Heath and Peter Fentem, "Physical Activity Among Persons with Disabilities—Public Health Perspective," *Exercise and Sport Science Review* 25 (1997): 195–234.
30 Jeffrey Martin, "Psychosocial Aspects of Youth Disability Sport," *Adapted Physical Activity Quarterly* 23, no. 1 (2006): 65-77; Kristen Lars, Goran Patriksson, and Bengt Fridlund, "Parents' Conceptions of the Influence of Participation in a Sport's Programme on Their Children and Adolescents with Physical Disabilities," *European Physical Education Review* 8, no. 2 (2003): 139–156.
31 Tim Meyer and Andreas Broocks, "Therapeutic Impact of Exercise on Psychiatric Diseases—Guidelines for Exercise Testing and Prescription," *Sports Medicine* 30, no. 4 (2000): 268–279.
32 Peter Bukhala, "A Survey of the Current Status of Physical Activity Level of Students with Disabilities at Kenyatta University, Kenya," *African Journal of Applied Human Sciences* 1, no. 1 (2009): 31–35; James Rimmer, Jennefer Rowland, and Kiyoshi Yamaki, "Obesity and Secondary Conditions in Adolescents with Disabilities: Addressing the Needs of an Underserved Population," *Journal of Adolescent Health* 41 (2007): 224–229.
33 Dada and Ukpata, "Sport Participation," 136.
34 Rohwer, "Benefits of Sport."
35 Parnes and Hashemi, "Sport as a Means," 133.

ing social inclusion or integrating PWDs into mainstream society.[36] At an individual level, PWDs who engage in sports have greater peer relations and improved social interactions.[37] According to the World Health Organization, participation in sport gives PWDs opportunities to make new friends and maintain social networks.[38]

Kumar argues that nondisabled people tend to focus on a person's disability rather than on an individual's abilities or skills.[39] This form of discrimination keeps nondisabled persons from appreciating and experiencing the full potential of PWDs, further perpetuating the negative attitudes.[40] It could be argued that sports have the potential to break down these negative attitudes by changing the community's perceptions of PWDs' capabilities. In light of this, proponents argue that sports have the capacity to "[move PWDs'] disability into the background."[41] This will positively result in nondisabled people learning to see that PWDs can do supposedly impossible things.[42]

---

36 Dada and Ukpata, "Sport Participation," 136.
37 Elaine Blinde and Lisa McClung, "Enhancing the Physical and Social Self Through Recreational Activity: Accounts of Individuals with Physical Disabilities," *Adapted Physical Activity Quarterly* 14 (1997): 327–344; Deborah Shapiro and Jeffrey Martin, "Athletic Identity, Affect, and Peer Relations in Youth Athletes with Physical Disabilities," *Disability and Health Journal* 3, no. 2 (2010): 79–85; and Karen DePauw, "Current International Trends in Research in Adapted Physical Activity," in *Sports and Physical Activity-Moving towards Excellence*, ed. T. Williams, L. Almond, and A. Sparks (London: E & FN Spon, 1992).
38 World Health Organization, *Review of Best Practice in Interventions to Promote Physical Activity in Developing Countries* (Geneva: WHO, 2005), https://www.who.int/dietphysicalactivity/bestpracticePA2008.pdf?ua=1.
39 Anant Kumar, "Making the Disabled, Differently-Abled Access Higher Education and Employment," in *Enabling Access for Persons with Disabilities to Higher Education and Workplace: Role of ICT and Assistive Technologies* (Cincinnati: Never-the-Less, n.d.), 65.
40 Kumar, "Differently-Abled," 65.
41 Dada and Ukpata, "Sport Participation," 138–139; Losch, "Wheelchair Tennis," 73; Claudine Sherill, *Young with Disability in Physical Education/Physical Activity/Sport In and Out of Schools: Technical Report for the World Health Organization* (Geneva: World Health Organization, 2004), https://www.icsspe.org/sites/default/files/YOUNGPEOPLE.pdf.
42 Dada and Ukpata, "Sport Participation," 138–139.

In addition to that, Fuluchi argued that sport works to improve the inclusion and well-being of persons with disabilities in two ways.[43] First, sport changes how communities think and feel about persons with disabilities, reducing stigma and discrimination associated with disability. Secondly, sport changes how persons with disabilities think and feel about themselves, thus empowering them and helping them recognize their potential.[44] Sport not only improves the economic development of those with disabilities and helps to make them marketable but also helps reduce the isolation PWDs often feel, so that they are able to integrate more fully into community life.

The growing body of evidence that confirms the social and health benefits of sports participation has also been documented in the higher education context, where it has been argued that students with disabilities (SWDs) enjoy sports for the same reasons as their nondisabled peers. The benefits of SWDs in particular participating in sports were noted in Blinde and Taub's study of twenty-eight male university students with physical and sensory disabilities at a Midwestern American university.[45] These students noted that sport participation increased their integration into university life[46] among other benefits. Other authors have noted that sport participation helps maintain self-discipline,[47] which can positively increase the SWD's academic achievement.[48] This has been confirmed in one study that showed that learners with disabilities who participate in sports activities perform better academically.[49] Likewise, a high percentage (92 percent) of SWDs at Kenyatta University who were sampled in Bukhala's study also confirmed that participation in sport was a very important component in helping them cope with

---

43   K. Fuluchi, "My Hope for an Inclusive Society Sports," in *United Nations Convention on the Rights of Persons with Disabilities* (New York: United Nations, 2006), http://www.un.org/wcm/webdav/site/sport.

44   Dada and Ukpata, "Sport Participation," 138.

45   Elaine Blinde and Diane Taub, "Personal Empowerment Through Sport and Physical Fitness Activity: Perspectives from Male College Students with Physic Sensory Disabilities," *Journal of Sport Behaviour* 22, no. 2 (1999): 181–202.

46   Blinde and Taub, "Personal Empowerment."

47   Bailey et al., "Educational Benefits," 3.

48   International Council of Sport Science and Physical Education (ICSSPE), "World Summit on Physical Education," *Berlin: International Council of Sport Science and Physical Education*, 2001.

49   Mwangi Wanderi, Andanje Mwisukha, and Peter Bukhala, "Enhancing the Full Potential of Persons with Disabilities Through Sports in the 21st Century with Reference to Kenya," *Disability Studies Quarterly* 29, no. 4 (2009).

their academic lives.[50] Dada and Ukpata's survey of sixty purposively selected SWDs from three Nigerian universities found that sports participation aided in integrating these students more fully into the university by reducing their social isolation.[51]

South African Historical Background

Nelson Mandela's vision for South Africa was a society that is "accessible and open to everyone." He believed that disabled children are "entitled to an exciting and brilliant future." He found it moral and just to take away barriers from disabled people, such as a poor education or lack of money, so that they could live prosperous lives.[52]

As a signatory of the CRPD, the South African government has enacted various policies to address the sporting and recreational needs of SWDs in higher education institutions (HEIs) in an effort to increase the social inclusion of SWDs. These measures are included in legislation such as the 1997 *White Paper on the Integrated National Disability Strategy*; the 2011 *White Paper on Sport and Recreation*; the 2012 *Green Paper for Post-School Education Training*; the 2014 *Draft Social Inclusion Policy Framework for Public Higher Education and Training Institutions*; the 2015 *White Paper on the Rights of Persons with Disabilities*, and the 2015 *Guidelines for the Creation of Equitable Opportunities for People with Disabilities in South African Higher Education*. All these policies oblige universities to provide conducive environments for the equal participation of SWDs in SARAs. Article 6 of the *South African Disability Human Rights Charter*, moreover, stipulates that disabled people should be able to engage in recreational activities and sports and that accessible facilities and financial aid will be provided for these initiatives. Despite this supportive policy, however, research indicates that SWDs have few sports participation opportunities on South African campuses.[53]

---

50 Bukhala, "A Survey of the Current Status," 31.
51 Dada and Ukpata, "Sport Participation," 138.
52 President Nelson Mandela, speech given at the opening of the First Annual South African Junior Wheelchair Sports Camp, Johannesburg, South Africa, December 4, 1995, https://www.sahistory.org.za/archive/speech-president-nelson-mandela-opening-first-annual-south-african-junior-wheelchair-sports.
53 Shernal Wright, "Accessibility of Recreational Sports for Students with Disabilities at the University of the Western Cape (master's thesis, University of the Western Cape, 2007); Matsobane Laka, "The University of the Western

In particular, Mantsha's study of SWDs at the University of Venda found that this institution's failure to prioritize disability sport stemmed from a lack of appropriately educated staff members.[54] Similar challenges were also raised by the University of Venda SWDs who were sampled in Tugli and colleagues' study.[55] Wright's study of SWDs at the University of the Western Cape found that the inaccessibility of sports facilities has been pointed to as the major reason for SWDs' nonparticipation in sport.[56] The other major reason that South African universities fail to prioritize sport for SWDs is that most of these universities tend to focus more on the academic rather than social needs of SWDs.

This was confirmed by one study that included SWDs at the University of Venda, which found that extracurricular activities were considered a secondary matter by far for SWDs at this institution.[57] Likewise, Mgulwa and Young's study of sports administrators at the University of the Western Cape found that this institution was failing to support the participation of SWDs

---

Cape Campus Recreational Sport Service Delivery" (honors diss., University of the Western Cape, 2009); Charl Roux and Cora Burnett, "The Extent to Which Students with Disabilities Are Included in Elite Sports at Higher Education Institutions," *African Journal for Physical, Health Education, Recreation and Dance* 16, no. 4 (2010): 120–131; Foundation of Tertiary Institutions of the Northern Metropolis (FOTIM), *Disability in Higher Education: Project Report* (Johannesburg, South Africa: FOTIM, 2011), http://www.students.uct.ac.za/usr/disability/reports/annual_report_10_11.pdf; Augustine Tugli et al., "Perceptions of Students with Disabilities Concerning Access and Support in the Learning Environment of a Rural-Based University," *African Journal of Physical, Health Education, Recreation and Dance* 1, no. 2 (2013): 356–64; Nadia Mgulwa and Marié Young, "University Sports Administrators' Perceptions on Campus Recreation Services for Students with Physical Disabilities," *Journal of Community and Health Sciences* 9, no. 1 (2014): 9–20; Augustine Tugli, "Extra-Curricular Encounters and Needs in the Learning Environment: The Case of Students with Disabilities at University of Venda," *International Journal of Science Education* 10, no. 1 (2015): 97–102; Tshifhiwa Mantsha, "Educational Support of Students with Disabilities at Institutions of Higher Learning in South Africa: A Case Study of the University of Venda" (PhD diss., University of Venda, 2016).

54 Mantsha, "Educational Support," 56.
55 Tugli et al., "Perceptions of Students," 101.
56 Wright, "Accessibility of Recreational Sports."
57 Tugli et al., "Perceptions of Students," 101.

in SARAs at all levels, as most funds were allocated to academic development.[58] This support of academic inclusion at the expense of sport inclusion is a contradiction of the 2015 *Guidelines*, which enjoins HEIs to create equitable opportunities for SWDs in all areas of university life, including the social life of the university.[59] Against this background, it has been recommended that the Department of Higher Education and Training (DHET) support all HEIs with funding specifically allocated to promote extracurricular activities, including indoor games for all categories of disabilities.[60]

The Study

The purpose of the present study was to describe and assess the measures being taken by South African universities to promote the participation of SWDs in SARAs. In order to do so, a critical review of various international and national instruments aimed at promoting the social inclusion of SWDs was conducted. Secondly, twenty-eight qualitative interviews with disability unit staff members (DUSMs) were conducted in order to gain insight into the measures these units are taking to ensure that SWDs are provided with equal participation opportunities in SARAs. In order to critically analyze how SWDs are currently faring in extracurricular activities, particularly SARAs, the present study employs othering as a useful theoretical lens.

The theory of othering was coined within postcolonial theory[61] and is useful in providing an understanding of the ways in which power relationships between the PWDs and those without disabilities are structured.[62] Othering is defined as the exclusion and marginalization of particular groups from the mainstream due to projected differences.[63] It is often "different" physical features that make PWDs victims of the othering process by

---

58   Mgulwa and Young, "Sports Administrators' Perceptions," 18.
59   Colleen Howell, "Guidelines for the Creation of Equitable Opportunities for People with Disabilities in South African Higher Education," *Cape Higher Education Consortium*, 2015.
60   Tugli et al., "Perceptions of Students," 101.
61   Sune Jensen, "Othering, Identity Formation and Agency," *Qualitative Studies* 2, no. 2 (2011).
62   Joy Johnson et al., "Othering and Being Othered in the Context of Health Care Services," *Health Communication* 16, no. 2 (2004): 255–71.
63   Johnson et al., "Othering and Being Othered."

nondisabled people, who make rules and standard labels that render PWDs as "outsiders."[64] It follows from this that whether intentional or unintentional, othering practices serve to reinforce and reproduce positions of domination, where SWDs are forced into a subordinate role.[65]

Several studies have employed the theory of othering to critically examine issues of discrimination on the grounds of racism, sexism, and gender.[66] To date, there is no study that has applied the othering theory to issues of disability in higher education, yet SWDs in South African HEIs are facing what Wispelaere and Casassas referred to as "double-discrimination" barriers not only to access but also to success in HEIs.[67] The only available literature that has attempted to examine the othering practices in relation to the experiences of PWDs[68] has focused mainly on the othering of PWDs in mainstream news and entertainment media.[69] The othering theory has much in common with ableism, which is a discriminating philosophy and practice that considers the nondisabled to be superior to the disabled.[70] Ableism also emphasizes disability as a "physical, moral, emotional, mental, and spiritual deficit."[71] Within the mainstream education context, Bathseba Opini argued that the construction of SWDs as the "other" negatively results in them being pushed to the periphery to occupy a subordinated status, which subsequently

---

64   Bathseba Opini, "A Review of the Participation of Disabled Persons in the Labour Force: The Kenyan Context," *Disability and Society* 25, no. 3 (2010): 273; and Johnson et al., "Othering and Being Othered."

65   Mary Lee Roberts and Martin Schiavenato, "Othering in the Nursing Context: A Concept Analysis," *Nursing Open* 4 (2017): 174; Michelle Fine, "Working the Hyphens: Reinventing Self and Other in Qualitative Research," in *Handbook of Qualitative Research*, ed. Norman Denzin and Yvonna Lincoln (London: SAGE, 1994).

66   Jensen, "Identity Formation," 65.

67   Jurgen de Wispelaere and David Casassas, "A Life of One's Own: Republican Freedom and Disability," *Disability and Society* 29, no. 3 (2014): 413.

68   Susan Wendell, *The Rejected Body* (New York: Routledge, 1996).

69   Leonard Kriegel, "The Cripple in Literature," in *Images of the Disabled, Disabling Images*, ed. Tom Joe and Alan Gartner (Santa Barbara, CA: Praeger, 1987).

70   Sarah Amin, "A Case for the Inclusion of Disability in Democratic Governance," *Journal of International Service* 22, no. 2 (2013): 40.

71   Ema Loja et al., "Disability, Embodiment and Ableism: Stories of Resistance," *Disability and Society* 28, no. 2 (2013): 198.

deprives them of equal access to educational opportunities.[72] This theory can thus be useful in understanding the power structures and barriers confronting SWDs when they try to access SARAs.

Role of Encouraging SWDs to Participate in SARAs

Scholars writing within the context of psychology of encouragement have highlighted the positive impact of encouraging individuals involved in challenging situations.[73] This includes competitive sports, as they require substantial effort.[74] Encouraging SWDs to participate in sport therefore becomes critical, especially given the prevalence of negative attitudes that aim to summarily disqualify PWDs' engagement.[75] Research has called for South African HEIs to encourage their SWDs to participate in SARAs, which are beneficial to the students' holistic development.[76] Some of the participants in this study view providing encouragement as the most important tool in eliminating SARA barriers for SWDs. They feel it is imperative to motivate SWDs to overlook their physical limitations and rather focus on their abilities so they can excel in sport. As Nobuhle said: "At this university we encourage our students to participate in every activity. . . . Every student must be equal to everyone; they should be doing anything that they want without any obstacle. Being on a wheelchair does not mean that I am unable—I'm able."[77]

---

72 Opini, "Disabled Persons in the Labour Force," 273.
73 Deborah Azoulay, "Encouragement and Logical Consequences Versus Rewards and Punishment: A Re-Examination," *Journal of Individual Psychology* 55 (1999): 91–99; and Thomas Sweeney, *Adlerian Counseling and Psychotherapy: A Practitioner's Approach* (New York: Taylor and Francis, 2009).
74 Joel Wong, "The Psychology of Encouragement: Theory, Research, and Applications," *Counseling Psychologist* 43, no. 2 (2015): 184.
75 Marie Hardin, "Marketing the Acceptably Athletic Image: Wheelchair Athletes, Sport-Related Advertising and Capitalist Hegemony," *Disability Studies Quarterly* 23, no. 1 (2003): 108–25; and DePauw and Gavron, *Disability and Sport*.
76 Roux and Burnett, "Students with Disabilities Included in Elite Sports," 120.
77 Nobuhle, interview by author, 2017.

Disability is often equated with vulnerability,[78] and this creates unequal power relations between the nondisabled and PWDs, in which the latter are treated as alien based on their physical characteristics.[79] Such negative attitudes are also prevalent when it comes to PWDs participating in sport in primary schools, as some educators view sport as "nothing more than leisure." These educators, therefore, encourage more time spent on academics.[80] Musengi and Mudyahoto conducted a study of fifteen pupils with various disabilities from five selected public primary schools in Masvingo, Zimbabwe, in order to examine how these schools include pupils with various disabilities in physical education and sports in general.[81] Both authors found that the majority of pupils with disabilities were not accepted in sports activities by most nondisabled peers and teachers, who had low expectations of disabled students.[82] These teachers and nondisabled students viewed sports as "competitive events in which pupils with disabilities were unlikely to do well" and more likely to get hurt.[83] Some participants in the present study also used similar perceptions as grounds for discouraging SWDs from participating in sport.

> I think there are sporting events that [our students] could participate in. . . . But [their disabled] bodies don't deal with stress the same way that our bodies [do]. . . . They get tired easily, they get sick easily, and when they get sick, it takes them longer to recover than it does for the rest of us . . . I don't think [sports] should be something that should be forced for the student.[84] The involvement of students with disabilities is a challenge. The work pressure is a lot. They have to work that much harder than other students. . . . We know that the work pressure is really hectic. So student involvement is minimal because of academic pressure.[85]

---

78   Willie Bryan, "The Disability Rights Movement," in *Readings for Diversity and Social Justice,* ed. Maurianne Adams (Oxford: Psychology Press, 2000): 337.
79   Jenny Morris, *Pride against Prejudice* (London: Women's Press, 1991): 29.
80   Barbara Churcher, *Physical Education for Teaching* (London: George Allen and Unwin, 1980).
81   Martin Musengi and Tapiwa Mudyahoto, "Quality of Sports Participation by Pupils with Disabilities in Inclusive Education Settings in Masvingo Urban," *Electronic Journal for Inclusive Education* 2, no. 6 (2010): 1–17.
82   Musengi and Mudyahoto, "Quality of Sports Participation," 6.
83   Musengi and Mudyahoto, "Quality of Sports Participation," 14.
84   Sally, interview with the author as a participant in this study, 2017.
85   Nadine, interview with the author as a participant in this study, 2017.

These narratives show that difference in the form of an impairment is a foundational attribute to the othering process.[86] In reality, these participants' perceptions are based merely on uneducated assumptions, as they seem to have little or no knowledge about the benefits of participation in sport for all PWDs. For instance, Sally's assumptions about the frailty of physically disabled bodies as a barrier have been contested by SWDs surveyed in Bukhala's study.[87] That study found that physical discomfort, medical problems, and medication were the least mentioned (4 percent) hindrances to SWDs participation in sport.[88] Rather, participants pointed to "inaccessible facilities, lack of encouragement, lack of information, lack of equipment, inappropriate activities, and lack of skills" as the actual barriers.[89]

By contrast, participant Melissa believes that equal opportunities for sport participation should be provided to SWDs, as this has beneficial outcomes such as helping them to live a self-disciplined lifestyle, which will subsequently enhance their academic achievement and holistic social integration into the university community.

> It's not even about disabilities. I find that any student who really plays sport, whether for a social club or on national level, excels in academics as well. There is a sense of discipline that runs through your sport into your life, into your studies. They make better friends, they get their own support structure, they even contribute to the awareness of other people to see them as people playing like they do.[90]

However, not all agree that encouragement and motivation need to be emphasized. Although the participation of PWDs in sport is regarded as an important right in various international and South African policy documents, authors have contested that sport participation is not as fundamental within an education context.[91] Some argue that inclusion in sport should not be regarded the same way as inclusion in education, as inclusion in sport

---

86 Mary Canales, "Othering: Toward an Understanding of Difference," *Advances in Nursing Science* 22 (2000): 16–31.
87 Bukhala, "A Survey of the Current Status."
88 Bukhala, "A Survey of the Current Status," 33.
89 Bukhala, "A Survey of the Current Status, "33.
90 Melissa, interview with author as participant in this study, 2017.
91 Florian Kiuppis, "Inclusion in Sport: Disability and Participation," *Sport in Society* 21, no. 1 (2016): 4–21.

is often voluntary.[92] Therefore nonparticipation in sport should not necessarily be equated with social exclusion or a violation of rights, particularly because "not everyone, regardless of whether they have disabilities, wants to take part in sport."[93] Some of my participants subscribed to this narrative, believing that participation in sport is an individual choice and that the more one enjoys sport, the more that particular person will practice sport consistently.[94] Drawing on Katleko's soccer team initiative case, Amanda emphasizes the point that self-motivation alone is important if SWDs are to enjoy sport participation and that their encouragement should not come from their DUSMs.

> In terms of sport, there is this lovely initiative: Katleko's soccer team. Many years ago, . . . the Disability Awareness Movements (DAM) wanted to set up a soccer team in order to raise awareness and also bring sort of integration with disabled students outside and able-bodied students, so they thought of soccer as it is a big sport nationally. I think they are playing in first division or second division soccer at the university and that's combined with students with disabilities and able-bodied students. So, that's something that has been running for quite a while. Well it's not to win; they are doing very well, but initially they just thought of this, just to have a soccer team because they did not have many disabled members to form a team, so they included others. That's again a nice example of mainstreaming, where disabled and nondisabled students actually took the lead in getting friends that are able-bodied to come and join them, and they are really enjoying it.[95]

Furthermore, there is a growing body of literature indicating that enjoyment of sport is one of the reasons that PWDs continue participating in athletic activities[96]. Some participants agree with this notion, stating that

---

92   Kiuppis, "Inclusion in Sport," 5.
93   Ramón Spaaij, Jonathan Magee, and Ruth Jeanes, *Sport and Social Exclusion in Global Society* (Abingdon, UK: Routledge, 2014).
94   Susan Shaw, Douglas Kleiber, and Linda Caldwell, "Leisure and Identity Formation in Male and Female Adolescents: A Preliminary Examination," *Journal of Leisure Research* 27, no. 3 (1995): 245–263.
95   Amanda, interview with the author as a participant in this study, 2017.
96   Jerrold Greenberg, George Dintiman, and Barbee Myers, *Physical Fitness and Wellness: Changing the Way You Look, Feel, and Perform* (Washington, DC: Library of Congress Cataloging in Publication Data, 2004); Xiaolin Yang et al., "Factors Explaining the Physical Activity of Young Adults: The Importance of Early Socialisation," *Scandinavian Journal of Medicine & Science in Sports* 9, no. 2 (1999): 120–127; Sharon Huddleston, Jane Mertesdorf, and Kaori

PWDs who enjoy sport enough will therefore not need encouragement from anybody else in order to participate in sport. Rather, these participants believe that SWDs have the agency to independently make informed choices regarding their participation. They also believe that some SWDs choose to not participate in sport and focus on their academic work instead.

> At the moment, I believe that if the students themselves are proactive, then they will participate in sport. It depends on what the students themselves want. It is also important that they take control of their own inclusion: that is not my unit's responsibility.[97]

> It's a WITS thing. WITS sports have never been strong because the students are more academically focused. Which is a dangerous thing to say, but that's the history of this institution.[98]

However, great self-motivation and enjoyment are often not enough to break down barriers to sports participation. In the South African educational system, public special schools have been blamed for providing learners with a low standard of schooling,[99] as some of their teachers do not have the necessary training to accommodate such diverse learner capacities.[100] Despite this academic inclusion challenge, participant Puleng applauded special schools for creating an enabling environment for identifying and developing sport talent among learners with disabilities,[101] as this participant's university is failing in this regard.

> Prioritizing academic inclusion over social inclusion is what is happening at this university, but it's killing the students' talents in sport because they come here after high school. Special schools are good in cricket and good in athletics and

---

Araki, "Physical Activity Behaviour and Attitudes toward Involvement among Physical Education, Health and Leisure Services Pre-Professionals," *College Student Journal* 36, no. 2 (2002): 555–573.

97   Beverly, interview with the author as a participant in this study, 2017.
98   Amanda, interview.
99   Howell, "Guidelines"; Mbulaheni Maguvhe, "Teaching Science and Mathematics to Students with Visual Impairments: Reflections of a Visually Impaired Technician," *African Journal of Disability* 4, no. 1 (2015): 1–6.
100 Dana Donohue and Juan Bornman, "The Challenges of Realising Inclusive Education in South Africa," *South African Journal of Education* 34, no. 2 (2014): 4.
101 Barrie Houlihan and Pippa Chapman, "Talent Identification and Development in Sport," *Sport in Society* 20, no. 1 (2017): 107–125.

they come here and it's like zero! They want to get involved, but they don't know how because it's like they are expecting us to do something about it, but we are not doing anything about it. They will even go to [Further Education and Training (FET)] colleges to join the blind cricket club, yet we have this big Disability Unit. It's like their dreams die because there is no club for them here; there is no team for them; there is no support for them to continue their sporting.[102]

Puleng's narrative sheds light on how nondisabled students are privileged, as they are guaranteed opportunities to continue or start participating in sport at university. Most universities' sport facilities are designed with non-disabled students in mind, neglecting SWDs who need adapted sport facilities in order to take part in sport.

Role of Viewing SARAs as an Important Right

As shown above, the international and South African disability policy framework supports the participation of SWDs in SARAs as an important right that all HEIs ought to respect and promote. Participants who uphold this human rights policy framework are of the opinion that universities should prioritize sport participation for the disabled through a holistic approach to achieving inclusive education beyond the conventional academic inclusion approach. According to Lynch, in order for mainstream educational institutions to be truly inclusive, they need to integrate SWDs not only educationally but socially as well.[103]

> The other aspect, which is non-academic [and] where I think as universities we have a long way to go, is to do with sport and recreation for students with disabilities. It's an area that I think universities need to play an active role, because when you are talking about inclusion that means all your students should be free to participate fully and equally in any activity as registered students. So our view really is all embracing; that from the classroom, to your residences, to your education, to competitive sport that you need to actually ensure that all your students, particularly students with disabilities . . . have equal participation and opportunities like anybody else.[104]

---

102 Puleng, interview with the author as a participant in this study, 2017.
103 James Lynch, *Inclusion in Education: The Participation of Disabled Learners* (Paris: UNESCO, 2001).
104 Thembani, interview with the author as a participant in this study, 2017.

> I think disability support is not just about equipment without having a personal touch; it's really about wanting to see your students succeeding in everything they do. . . . I think sports is one aspect of social inclusion, how they interact with each other, who they date. I think we need to conceptualize all those aspects when we support our students.[105]

Although the CRPD states that the accessibility to information and communication is important in enabling PWDs to fully enjoy all human rights and fundamental freedoms,[106] lack of information regarding SARAs remains a major barrier preventing SWDs from participating in sport activities.[107] SWDs sampled in previous studies reported several cases where they felt they were not made sufficiently aware of social events on campus because they were not well advertised.[108] Likewise, SWDs at Kenyatta University also reported that they did not participate in any sport activities because the university's sports and games department advertised information in inaccessible formats, particularly to blind students.[109]

Seeing that accessibility to information is a central right of SWDs if they are to participate equally in SARAs, the following participants made concerted efforts to ensure that relevant information was made readily available to students with diverse disabilities.

> So for me one of the most important things is to disseminate the information. So our role in that is to make the information accessible to the students, we can print something in Braille if it's needed, or we can provide a sign language interpreting if it's needed also. So disseminating information and disseminating accessible information I think is a big role that we play in creating opportunities. So if you create the opportunities and you disseminate the information and you create the space where this can happen, the choice in the end all remains the student's. But we don't want students to say, 'Oh, but I didn't know.'[110]
>
> If they are interested in sport, we link them up with people in Sports Admin. Because they are part of the university, they need to be not only here in this Disability Unit; they need to be out there. So if the student is interested

---

105 Catherine, interview with the author as a participant in this study, 2017.
106 United Nations, *Conventions on the Rights of Persons with Disabilities*, 3.
107 FOTIM, *Disability in Higher Education*.
108 FOTIM, *Disability in Higher Education*.
109 Bukhala, "A Survey of the Current Status," 33.
110 Charmaine, interview with the author as a participant in this study, 2017.

in, for example, sport, I make an appointment, I send them over to the Sport Department and I say, 'This student is interested in this. Please see how you can accommodate.'[111]

If sports participation is seen as a right, infrastructure resources will also be used to increase participation opportunities. Campuses that offered wheelchair-adjusted transport also allowed DUSMs to meaningfully realize the rights of their SWDs to participate in sport. The adjusted transport ensured that it was easy to commute SWDs to universities with more accessible sport facilities.

We don't have a swimming pool here at University of Johannesburg. So Mandeville Sport Club has hoists to get the disabled guys into the pool and the coaches et cetera et cetera, then we provide transport for you there whether you are a national swimmer or not. If you want to do swimming you have the right to go and swim, so that's how we see it.[112]

Furthermore, participation as a right negates negative assumptions about SWDs' ability to play sport. Participants who are aware of how most nondisabled people assume that "people with disabilities do not want to or cannot participate in sporting activities"[113] have taken on the responsibility of breaking these attitudinal barriers. They make an effort to prove that disability does not prevent a person from participating in, and enjoying, sport.

The barriers are still there; people should learn more about disability. Because if, for example, a student with a disability says, 'Okay, I want to take part of athletics,' some people will say, 'How will that blind student take part in athletics?' They should remove that mentality. Even if you are a blind student and you want to be an athlete, you can . . . because . . . blindness is not going to prevent this person from being an athlete. Instead, you can assist this person like this. . . . If a blind person is running and is next to a person, he or she runs as long as there is nothing in front. Even basketball, the wheelchair users can play basketball as well.[114]

---

111   Beverly, interview.
112   Melissa, interview.
113   Rohwer, "Benefits of Sport."
114   Nombuhle, interview with the author as a participant in this study, 2017.

Role of Infrastructure and Sport Facilities

Article 9[115] of the CRPD emphasizes accessibility as a fundamental concept of disability rights.[116] South Africa, however, seems to be lagging behind in this regard. The *White Paper on Sport and Recreation,* for instance, states that since the implementation of democracy in 1994 the South African government has made minimal efforts to provide accessible public sporting facilities to widen sport participation opportunities for PWDs.[117] Given this, some authors have associated the inadequate resources and lack of adaptable facilities for all people, including PWDs, with social exclusion.[118] Similarly, in the present study, participants from smaller universities have raised concerns about the lack of adaptable accessible facilities as the main hindrance that is preventing SWDs from participating in sport.

> Unfortunately, . . . I'm not in a position to talk about the sports part, because we don't do sport. Because big universities have more infrastructure, it's easier for them to accommodate students with disabilities; for us it makes it more difficult. That's what they want to do here, play goal ball. But we don't have enough infrastructure for those people, and there is not enough money for them because we only get a small amount for the sports and that money has to be divided for all necessary sports that is being offered; anything from dancing to choir and whatever.[119]

---

115 "To enable persons with disabilities to live independently and participate fully in all aspects of life, States Parties shall take appropriate measures to ensure to persons with disabilities access, on an equal basis with others, to the physical environment . . . and to other facilities and services open or provided to the public, both in urban and in rural areas."

116 Equal Access Monitor, *Accessibility of Infrastructure* (Equal Access Monitor, 2016), http://globaldisability.org/wp-content/uploads/2016/02/His-EqualAccessMonitor-Feb2016-EN.pdf, 1.

117 South African Sports Confederation and Olympic Committee (SASCOC), "Transformation Charter for South African Sport," in *2011 National Sport and Recreation Indaba* (Midrand, South Africa: SASCOC, 2011), https://www.srsa.gov.za/sites/default/files/Nat-Sport-and-Recreation-Plan.pdf, 16.

118 Ruth Levitas et al., "The Multi-Dimensional Analysis of Social Exclusion" (research paper, University of Bristol, 2007).

119 Richard, interview with the author as a participant in this study, 2017.

> There are no recreational facilities on this campus. There is a bar and that's about it. So there isn't any other recreational facilities; we don't have that. We haven't got anywhere in terms of access to recreation.[120]

These findings on the lack of accessible sport facilities are congruent with those of previous South African studies[121] and those of studies of SWDs in other African countries, including Kenya[122] and Nigeria.[123] These studies also pointed to lack of accessible facilities as the major barrier to sport participation for many SWDs. In light of this, it could be argued that the inaccessibility to sport facilities in these campuses relegate SWDs to the peripheries of physical activity venues, forcing them to remain passive participants.[124]

Some DUSMs in universities with no sport facilities are taking the responsibility to forge collaborative initiatives with other neighboring universities with sport facilities on behalf of SWDs interested in taking part in sport. Jarome noted that his university has "collaborated with University of Johannesburg" because it has more sports facilities. Consequently, some SWDs go to the University of Johannesburg in order to participate in sports.[125] Additionally, Amanda said:

> In terms of social things . . . for many years we have actually worked with University of Johannesburg (UJ). UJ is actually more advanced in terms of their sport offerings to students with disabilities, and there I fully support the idea of where you actually collaborate. So with sport I fully agree with that because you do not have enough blind students at one institution to form a team, yet if you work with UJ, the two together can make a strong team. So that's where regional collaboration is more important. So we have already had quite a number of meetings with UJ already in connection with collaborating for sport, which we also see as part of sport inclusion . . . So our sport people will communicate with them and get to some kind of arrangement to form a team or something like that.[126]

---

120 Beverly, interview.
121 Wright, "Accessibility of Recreational Sports"; and FOTIM, *Disability in Higher Education.*
122 Bukhala, "A Survey of the Current Status," 33; and Wanderi, Mwisukha, and Bukhala, "Enhancing the Full Potential."
123 Dada and Ukpata, "Sport Participation," 138.
124 Wanderi, Mwisukha, and Bukhala, "Enhancing the Full Potential."
125 Jarome, interview with the author as a participant in this study, 2017.
126 Amanda, interview.

By contrast, the following narratives highlight how universities with adequate sport facilities and resources could be said to be good practices exemplars as far as the inclusion of SWDs in SARAs is concerned. This is because these universities have the ability to provide their SWDs with a wide range of sports activities, both at recreational and competitive levels. They can also provide bursaries tailored for high-performance sport participants.

> Remember, University of Johannesburg focuses on high performance and elite sport; not all my athletes are elite athletes. But if you are a good student, I will provide any support structure for you to go and play sport. I have five basketball players, but only one in the national squad; the others are just playing it for fun, but they all use the same transport, so as a student I will provide you that infrastructure. I have to because you are a student at the University of Johannesburg. You don't have to excel in sport, but if you do excel, we will obviously provide all the additional services like physiotherapy, sports science backup, [and] medical support, and that is part of your bursary structure. Students who just play for social activities don't get a sports bursary, but they are not pushed aside, they can still [participate]. We have two vehicles; both of them are wheelchair accessible because we found that public transport does not work for them to their various training facilities. If you are a wheelchair tennis player and you want to get from one campus to another tennis court, we will transport you there. My responsibility is to bring in athletes; I provide them with all support structures I can for them to excel in their sport.[127]
>
> From a recreational perspective, I'm just thinking of students who are staying in residence that are wheelchair users. We do have bus access that they can also go to Rosebank, to the shops, and that's important. As far as recreation goes, we try and make everything accessible for all people; like the swimming pool in the Education campus has a lift to lower a wheelchair user into the water for swimming purposes.[128]

Role of Funding and Sport Participation

The South African government's disability funding cuts have placed SWDs at a substantial educational disadvantage compared to their nondisabled peers.[129] The participants whose views are cited below indicate that funding

---

127 Melissa, interview.
128 Ryan, interview with the author as a participant in this study, 2017.
129 Desire Chiwandire and Louise Vincent, "Funding Mechanisms to Foster Funding Inclusion in Higher Education Institutions for Students with

cuts have negatively affected several universities' capacities to effectively support disability sport. A lack of funds also means a lack of professional human resources, such as adequate DUSMs who specifically focus on issues of disability sports, as well as lack of adequate professional or qualified personnel like coaches and trainers.

> I'm probably the most outspoken about this because I don't think my opinions are based on just on reading things. I have lived it; I have experienced it. I have seen the struggles of my student athletes every day. . . . My budget in the university for sport [and] for athletes with disabilities is the smallest of all budgets for sport. From national government, the university receives up until today nothing to develop sport or high-performance athletes or mass participation.[130]
>
> I know that there are some Disability Units who have enough staff members to provide extracurricular activities to involve students with disabilities in sport, but this Disability Unit concentrates only on academics.[131]
>
> On this campus, we don't have a Disabled Sports Division, for instance. All our students need to go outside to a private trainer to get training. . . . So it's a lot of hustle to identify a person that is qualified to train persons with disabilities—say for instance, blind cricket. We don't have it on campus.[132]

Discussion

The failure of most South African universities to provide an enabling environment for SWDs to take part in sport activities perpetuates a culture of social exclusion.[133] Social exclusion as defined by Magumbate and Nyoni is the "process by which individuals or entire communities of people are systematically blocked from rights, opportunities, and resources available

---

Disabilities: A Critical Appraisal," *African Journal of Disability* 8 (2019); and Sibonokuhle Ndlovu and Elizabeth Walton, "Preparation of Students with Disabilities to Graduate into Professions in the South African Context of Higher Learning: Obstacles and Opportunities," *African Journal of Disability* 5, no. 1 (2016): 1–8.

130 Melissa, interview.
131 Beverly, interview.
132 Debbie, interview with the author as a participant in this study, 2017.
133 Roberts and Schiavenato, "Othering in the Nursing Context," 174.

to others."[134] Applying this definition to the findings of the present study, it follows that social exclusion is both directly and indirectly reinforced by universities that are failing to fully support SWDs who want to take part in SARAs. Such universities are those where SWDs have no or minimal sport participation opportunities because of disabling barriers, including lack of necessary infrastructure such as adapted sport facilities.

Another barrier identified in the present study is the lack of encouragement on the part of some DUSMs, who believe that encouraging SWDs is unnecessary because SWDs themselves need to be self-motivated to participate in sport . This rationale is problematic, as it absolves these institutions or DUSMs of the responsibility for taking proactive measures to ensure that SWDs' right to participate in sport is advanced. This creates a situation where sport participation becomes a privilege offered only to SWDs who are really passionate about sport—probably those participating at a competitive level. This form of partial inclusion is unacceptable, as it excludes those who want to participate at a recreational level.

Amin argued that widespread perceptions of incapability lead to "ableist" biases against PWDs.[135] Some DUSMs in this study could be said to be perpetuating such "ableist" biases, as they actively discourage students with physical disabilities from making sport as high a priority as academics. It could be argued that by seeing students' disabilities as a personal deficit that needs fixing,[136] these DUSMs create a sense of "otherness" by equating disability with vulnerability. Hence, this vulnerability subsequently becomes a rationale for unjustifiably treating PWDs differently,[137] which leads to DUSMs denying SWDs opportunities to participate in sport merely on the grounds of disability.

It should be noted that some of the present study's findings are important in contributing new knowledge concerning issues of participation of SWDs in sport because previous literature has only indicated challenges faced by

---

134 Jacob Mugumbate and Chamunogwa Nyoni, "Disability in Zimbabwe under the New Constitution: Demands and Gains of People with Disabilities," *Southern Peace Review Journal* 1 (2013): 4.

135 Amin, "A Case for the Inclusion," 40.

136 Nicola Martin, "Disability Identity—Disability Pride," *Perspectives: Policy and Practice in Higher Education* 16, no. 1 (2012): 15.

137 Jan Fook, "The Lone Crusader: Constructing Enemies and Allies in the Workplace," in *Breakthroughs in Practice: Theorizing Critical Moments in Social Work*, ed. Jan Fook and Lindsey Napier (London: Whiting and Birch, 2000).

SWDs. On the contrary, some universities could be said to be exemplars of best practices on the participation of SWDs in sport, particularly those universities whose DUSMs are making concerted efforts to promote the participation of SWDs in sport. It could be argued that such universities are those that take sport seriously, not only as a matter of human rights[138] but also as a matter of social inclusion. In this context, social inclusion can be defined as the process of improving the terms of participation in society for people who are disadvantaged, including those with disabilities.[139] Central to achieving social inclusion is the need to first tackle social exclusion by removing barriers hindering the full participation of PWDs in mainstream society.[140]

These best practices are evident from participants who were reported to be taking inclusionary steps, such as encouraging SWDs to participate in sport through ensuring timely dissemination of sport information in accessible formats. This form of encouragement instills strength, courage, perseverance, confidence, inspiration, motivation, and hope to current SWDs who are hesitant to participate in sport.[141] Other DUSMs have attempted to achieve social inclusion through forging collaborations with neighboring universities that have adapted facilities in order to overcome the challenge of inaccessible facilities in their own universities. Sport can be seen as one of the important tools for maximizing higher education experiences of SWDs, as it creates opportunities for friendships to develop. For instance, Katleko's soccer team clearly proves that PWDs enjoy sports for the same reasons as nondisabled participants.[142] This is also evidenced by some participants' narratives on their SWDs who visit neighboring universities with accessible adapted sport facilities to play sport with other SWDs or nondisabled students.

---

138 Paulo David, *Human Rights in Youth Sport: A Critical Review of Children's Rights in Competitive Sport* (London: Routledge, 2004), 7.
139 United Nations, "Identifying Social Inclusion and Exclusion," in *Leaving No One Behind: Report on the World Social Situation* (New York: United Nations, 2016), https://www.un.org/development/desa/dspd/report-on-the-world-social-situation-rwss-social-policy-and-development-division/rwss2016.html.
140 United Nations, "Identifying Social Inclusion."
141 Wong, "Psychology of Encouragement," 184.
142 Stephen Page, Edmund O'Connor, and Kirk Peterson, "Leaving the Disability Ghetto: A Qualitative Study of Factors Underlying Achievement Motivation Among Athletes with Disabilities," *Journal of Sport and Social Issues* 25, no. 1 (2001): 40–55.

Some South African policy documents have highlighted the importance of raising awareness in the entire nondisabled university community.[143] In light of this call, some of the participants in the present study have actively attempted to educate their university's nondisabled community on issues of SWDs' participation in sport, and this process has the potential to reduce the tendency to seeing the disability instead of the person.[144]

Conclusion

Jameel has criticized HEIs that focus only on academic inclusion, saying that they are perpetuating social exclusion by preventing SWDs from reaching their full potential at university.[145] Recent literature on South African HEIs continues to point to academic-oriented barriers such as inaccessibility of educational buildings and negative attitudes of nondisabled peer students and lecturers as the major factors hindering the academic performance of SWDs.[146] This dominant one-sided approach that promotes academic aspects of inclusion over social aspects of inclusion (including sport participation) creates what Martin referred to as "a sense of othering"[147] on the part of SWDs. Therefore, I propose that while supporting SWDs academically is important, it should not be the universities' only priority. A holistic, well-rounded education constitutes not just a means of achieving learning outcomes but also includes creating a welcoming space for social interaction.[148] This sense of othering can be equated to social exclusion, particularly in

---

143 Department of Government Printing Works, *Ministerial Committee Report: Draft Policy Framework for Disability in the Post-School Education and Training System* (Pretoria: Department of Government Printing Works, 2016), 39.

144 Dada and Ukpata, "Sport Participation," 139.

145 Syed Jameel, "Disability in the Context of Higher Education: Issues and Concerns in India," *Electronic Journal for Inclusive Education* 2, no. 7 (2011): 15.

146 Oliver Mutanga, "Students with Disabilities' Experience in South African Higher Education: A Synthesis of Literature," *South African Journal of Higher Education* 31, no. 1 (2017): 135–154.

147 Martin, "Disability Identity," 17.

148 Jean-Francois Trani et al., "Disabilities Through the Capability Approach Lens: Implications for Public Policies," *European Journal of Disability Research* 5 (2011): 143–157.

those South African universities that are failing to create equitable opportunities for SWDs to participate on par with their nondisabled peers in sport.

By contrast, the study also showed that universities that provide equitable opportunities for SWDs to participate in sport promote social inclusion, ensuring that SWDs reach their full potential at universities. Given this conducive environment, it is likely that SWDs in these universities will have high participation in a wide range of sport activities, and this will positively result in personal development in the form of "bringing out individual talents and abilities."[149] In light of these findings, I emphasize the need for the government to provide funding to universities to hire trained personnel, including coaches, to adapt presently inaccessible facilities and equipment and in general to honor their obligation to ensure that disability does not impose a barrier to those SWDs who wish to participate in SARAs both at recreational and competitive levels. I also propose that universities revise their policies so they are compliant with Article 30.5(b) of the CRPD and to address not only the academic but also the social needs of SWDs. One of the important ways in which South African HEIs can promote inclusive education is to promote the participation of SWDs in sport because doing so has significant social and health benefits. Universities should equally prioritize the participation of SWDs in SARAs as a holistic way of creating an enabling environment in which SWDs can flourish.

In the Kenyan context, Wanderi and colleagues have commended Kenyatta University as an exemplar of best practices in promoting and supporting the inclusion of SWDs in sport.[150] This is because Kenyatta University has a wide range of sports programs, adapted sport facilities, and human resources (such as professional coaches and volunteers) to serve SWDs with diverse disabilities who want to participate in sports at both recreational and competitive levels.[151] Given that these findings have shown that barriers to participation in sports do not emanate from the SWDs but rather the environment they live in,[152] I recommend that South African universities collaborate with such universities as Kenyatta University in order to share ideas about best practices.

---

149 Eli Bitzer and Ruth Albertyn, "Alternative Approaches to Postgraduate Supervision: A Planning Tool to Facilitate Supervisory Processes," *South African Journal Higher Education* 25, no. 5 (2011): 883.
150 Wanderi, Mwisukha, and Bukhala, "Enhancing the Full Potential."
151 Wanderi, Mwisukha, and Bukhala, "Enhancing the Full Potential."
152 Bukhala, "A Survey of the Current Status," 32.

Chapter Eighteen

Rehabilitation and the Realization of Disability Rights

Serges Djoyou Kamga

Introduction

In many countries in Africa and elsewhere, disabilities have long been associated with a curse or punishment from God, witchcraft[1], or illness. Consequently, the assumption is that a person with a disability needs medical attention. In this context, rehabilitation entails a range of medical responses often provided in medical facilities. Rehabilitation is associated with the notion of habilitation, which from a medical perspective seeks to provide appropriate therapies to patients. This understanding of rehabilitation and habilitation that has informed the early responses to disability were indeed characterized by the medical and welfare or charity models. The latter suggests that persons with disabilities often held in institutions need welfare assistance or charity to survive.

However, over the past decade or so, there has been a paradigm shift with the advent of the CRPD adopted in 2006 (A/RES/61/106). The convention calls for a human rights approach to disability, as well as adherence to a social

---

1 H. Jackson, "Approaches to Rehabilitation of People with Disabilities: A Review," *Journal of Social Development in Africa* 3, no. 1 (1988): 42.

model of disability. In this context, legislation and social policy should take into account the environmental barriers to the enjoyment of human rights by persons with disabilities. The CRPD in Article 26 provides for the right to habilitation and rehabilitation. It stipulates that "States Parties shall take effective and appropriate measures . . . to enable persons with disabilities to attain and maintain maximum independence, full physical, mental, social and vocational ability, and full inclusion and participation in all aspects of life." The States Parties shall do this through "habilitation and rehabilitation services" that are "based on multidisciplinary assessment of individual needs and strengths," "support participation and inclusion," "promote . . . training for professionals . . . working in [these] services," and "promote the availability [and] knowledge of assistive devices and technologies."[2]

Even so, persons with disabilities remain excluded and marginalized in our societies. According to Rosenthal and Kanter, "One of the most egregious forms of discrimination is the involuntary segregation of people in institutions."[3] Sometimes policies and programs intended to protect human rights may, paradoxically, violate these same rights. The aim of this chapter is to reflect on what needs to be done practically to ensure that rehabilitation policies and programs do not encroach upon disability rights but rather foster their enjoyment. Therefore, the chapter explores ways and avenues to give effect to Article 26 of the CRPD. It argues that the implementation of community-based rehabilitation and its extension to community-based inclusive development will ensure the full inclusion of persons with disabilities who enjoy their human rights. To this end, it unpacks the paradigm shift under the CRPD and its implication for rehabilitation, before focusing on moving forward, from a community-based rehabilitation perspective, toward the fulfillment of disability rights.

---

2   United Nations, "Article 26," *United Nations*, 2006, https://www.un.org/development/desa/disabilities/convention-on-the-rights-of-persons-with-disabilities/article-26-habilitation-and-rehabilitation.html.

3   Eric Rosenthal and Arlene Kanter, "The Right to Community Integration for People with Disabilities Under United States and International Law," *Disability Rights Education & Defense Fund*, n.d., https://dredf.org/news/publications/disability-rights-law-and-policy/the-right-to-community-integration-for-people-with-disabilities-under-united-states-and-international-law/#sdfootnote1sym.

Understanding the Paradigm Shift under the CRPD

Using a historical perspective, this section examines international disability discourse before the adoption of the CRPD—when the focus was on the medical model—and its transformation into the social and human rights models after the advent of this global instrument.

Pre-CRPD: The Medical Model

In the nineteenth and twentieth centuries, a disability was considered an inability due to ill health. A person with disabilities was therefore to be removed from the community in order to get treatment. In that context, the problem was to be solved by a therapist, psychologist, or any other medical practitioner trained to address the sickness. This was the manifestation of the medical model of disability.[4] The latter considers disability "a personal tragedy"[5] to be dealt with by medical practitioners concerned with functional limitations of the "patient."[6]

Associated with the medical model, moreover, was the charity or welfare model. This model was based on the idea that persons with disabilities who were sick and could not work would receive handouts or help from charity organizations and philanthropists. They had no rights and could only expect pity and compassion from good people, hence the term "charity model."[7] According to Duyan, "The Charity Model sees people with disabilities as victims of their impairment."[8] Nondisabled people should help persons with disabilities in whatever ways they can "because they are different." During

---

4 World Health Organization, *Towards Community-Based Inclusive Development* (Geneva: WHO, 2010), https://apps.who.int/bitstream/handle/10665/44405/9789241548052_introductory_eng.pdf;jsessionid=6D54E451E94C8A6FE0B9D858EBDDAD96?sequence=9.

5 G. Burton, I. Sayrafi, and S. Abu Srour, "Inclusion or Transformation? An Early Assessment of an Empowerment Project for Disabled People in Occupied," *Disability & Society* 28, no. 6 (2018): 812–825.

6 S. Burgstahler and T. Doe, "Disability-Related Simulations: If, When, and How to Use Them in Professional Development," *Review of Disability Studies: An International Journal* 1, no. 2 (2014): 4–17.

7 M. Retief and R. Letšosa, "Models of Disability: A Brief Overview," *HTS Teologiese Studies/Theological Studies* 74, no. 1 (2018): 1–86.

8 V. Duyan, "The Community Effects of Disabled Sports," *NATO Security Through Science Series E: Human and Societal Dynamics* 31 (2007): 71.

the operationalization of medical and charity models, no attention was paid to aspects of the environment that could have been further disabling for persons with disabilities.

Implication for Rehabilitation

Given the medical aspects associated with disability, rehabilitation was also provided using a medical model. In this context, rehabilitation was "[treatment(s)] designed to facilitate the process of recovery from injury, illness, or disease to as normal a condition as possible."[9] The aim of rehabilitation was to "restore" whatever was "lost due to injury, illness, or disease."[10] Rehabilitation and habilitation took place in medical facilities away from the community. The following excerpt from the United Nations' 1982 World Program of Action for the Disabled (Res 37/52) shows the scope of what was then encompassed by the concept of rehabilitation:

- Early detection, diagnosis, and intervention;
- Medical care and treatment;
- Social, psychological and other types of counselling and assistance;
- Training in self-care activities, including mobility, communication and daily living skills, with special provisions as needed;
- Provision of technical and mobility aids and other devices;
- Specialized education services;
- Vocational rehabilitation services (including vocational guidance), vocational training, placement in open or sheltered employment; and
- Follow-up.[11]

In this context, disability was a disease and nothing else. As such, it needed an adequate health-care system. Jackson explained that considering disability to be an individual problem, apart from the "physical environment," means that real social "problems [remain] hidden from the public eye."

---

9   "Rehabilitation," *The Free Definition*, n.d., https://medical-dictionary.thefreedictionary.com/rehabilitation.

10 Traumatic Brain Injury Info, "What Is the Definition of Rehabilitation?," *TBI Info*, n.d., http://www.repar.veille.qc.ca/info-tcc/What-is-the-definition-of.

11 United Nations, "World Programme of Action Concerning Disabled Persons," *United Nations*, 1982, https://www.un.org/development/desa/disabilities/resources/world-programme-of-action-concerning-disabled-persons.html#objectives.

Consequently, those in power feel less of a responsibility to care for those with disabilities. Disabled people are instead blamed for being victims.[12]

In this model, rehabilitation is generally synonymous with institutionalization. Yet the latter keeps persons with disabilities away from their families, creates "dependency, boredom and under-achievement, low self-esteem, stigmatization and loneliness,"[13] which effectively foster the social exclusion of persons with disabilities. Furthermore, isolating persons with disabilities in institutions promotes "cultural fear and beliefs about disability" and as such hinders the acceptance of persons with disabilities in the community.[14]

From the Medical Model to the Social Model

In recent decades, attention has moved from the medical features of disability to focus on social and environmental barriers faced by persons with disabilities. The marginalization and social exclusion of—and discrimination against—persons with disabilities were taken into consideration in the discourse on disablement. The WHO observes: "Disability was redefined as a societal problem rather than an individual problem and solutions became focused on removing barriers and social change, not just medical cure."[15] This development unequivocally echoed Hahn's view that disability originates from the "failure of a structured social environment to adjust to the needs and aspirations of citizens with disabilities."[16] In the same vein, it could be argued that under the social model features, disability is an externally imposed hindrance[17] that can be summed up as a form of persecution of individuals with disabilities.

In this context, rehabilitation factored in the environment in which persons with disabilities operated and how environmental barriers could be removed to foster social integration. This approach was echoed by the WHO, which adopted a resolution asserting its commitment to promoting

---

12 Jackson, "Approaches," 39–40.
13 Jackson, "Approaches," 41.
14 Jackson, "Approaches," 42.
15 WHO, *Community-Based*.
16 H. Hahn, "Public Support for Rehabilitation in Programs: The Analysis of US Disability Policy," *Disability, Handicap & Society* 1, no. 2 (1986): 128.
17 M. Nario-Redmond, J. G. Noel, and E. Fern, "Redefining Disability, Re-imagining the Self: Disability Identification Predicts Self-Esteem and Strategic Responses to Stigma," *Self and Identity* 12, no. 5 (2013): 469.

comprehensive rehabilitation programs and services, noting the importance of "full physical, informational, and economic accessibility in all spheres of life . . . in order to ensure full participation and equality of persons with disabilities."[18] This resolution clearly takes into consideration "accessibility in all spheres of life." It looks beyond medical issues and toward social integration/reintegration. This resolution was an appropriate remedy to disability as described by Hunt on behalf of Union of the Physically Impaired against Segregation. In his view, there is a difference between disability and impairment.

> [W]e define impairment as lacking part of or all of a limb, or having a defective limb, organ or mechanism of the body; and disability as the disadvantage or restriction of activity caused by a contemporary social organisation which takes no or little account of people who have physical impairments and thus excludes them from participation in the mainstream of social activities. Physical disability is therefore a particular form of social oppression.[19]

However, the push for a social model is not universally accepted. According to Hughes and Patterson, the social model of disability needs to do more to "problematize the body."[20] While the authors recognize that the social model has played an important role in "establishing a radical politics of disability, [it unfortunately] presupposes an untenable separation between body, culture, impairment and disability"; the authors thus call for a more "embodied, rather than a disembodied, notion of disability."[21]

This suggests that reducing disability to environmental barriers is not fully representative of disablement, which also encompasses problems with the body itself. Reducing disability to societal factors is a failure to recognize that "the physical and emotional pain and suffering experienced by disabled people due to their impairments has any impact upon their practical daily

---

18   United Nations, "Article 26."

19   Union of the Physically Impaired against Segregation, *Fundamental Principles of Disability, Union of the Physically Impaired against Segregation* (London: UPIAS, 1976), 3–4.

20   B. Hughes and K. Paterson, "The Social Model of Disability and the Disappearing Body: Towards a Sociology of Impairment," *Disability & Society* 12, no. 3 (1997): 326.

21   Hughes and Paterson, "Social Model," 326.

living."[22] From this standpoint, the call is to ensure that proponents of the social model acknowledge the subjective difficulties that may come about from impairments.[23] Prior to Lang, Crow had explained the weakness of social model theory: "For many disabled people personal struggles relating to impairment will remain even when disabling barriers no longer exist."[24]

Nevertheless, in spite of this controversy, it could be argued that even though struggles such as coping with physical pain are real and should be factored into the definition of disability, the social model is a valid framework that attempts to break down societal barriers that compound challenges faced by persons with disabilities. This is not to dismiss physical impairments but rather to open doors for people with disabilities even while recognizing and accounting for the difficulties arising from the pain they may experience.

While rehabilitation and habilitation cannot ignore the medical aspects of disability, medical features cannot be the sole focus. Relying exclusively on a medical model fosters the exclusion of marginalized individuals who do not enjoy independent living and the right to live in the community. In addition, reducing habilitation and rehabilitation to the medical model can feed into money-making schemes for some medical practitioners. Albrecht and Levy write:

> As demand for rehabilitation services increased and insurance benefits expanded, there was an incentive for physicians to enter the rehabilitation field. Under the aegis of designing comprehensive medical rehabilitation programs, hospitals, and physicians began to incorporate rehabilitation services into the medical model. Definitions of disabling conditions and appropriate treatment were expanded to include medical interventions and physical control. [25]

---

22 Raymond Lang, "The Development and Critique of the Social Model of Disability." Working Paper, Leonard Cheshire Disability and Inclusive Development Centre, University College, London (2007), 20, https://www.ucl.ac.uk/epidemiology-health-care/sites/iehc/files/wp-3.pdf.

23 Lang, "Development and Critique," 20–22.

24 L. Crow, "Including All Our Lives: Renewing the Social Model of Disability," in *Encounters with Strangers: Feminism and Disability*, ed. J. Morris (London: Women's Press, 1996), 9 and 209.

25 G. Albrecht and J. Levy, "Constructing Disabilities as Social Problems," in *Cross National Rehabilitation Policies: A Sociological Perspective*, ed. G. Albrecht (London: SAGE, 1981), 22.

So, the social model that calls for rehabilitation apart from institutions also seeks to protect persons with disabilities from predatory physicians. Mindful of this, the drafters of the CRPD ensured that disability issues were crafted within a human rights perspective with its positive implications on the right to rehabilitation and habilitation.[26]

After the CRPD: Moving beyond Disability as a Health and Welfare Construct

The CRPD epitomizes the human rights approach to disability. The significance of this shift cannot be overemphasized. Under its General Principles (Article 3), the CRPD provides for respect for inherent dignity, individual autonomy (including the freedom to make one's own choices), respecting the freedom of choice and the independence of persons with disabilities, accessibility, nondiscrimination, equal opportunity, and gender equality among other rights. These principles are important components of the right to rehabilitation and rehabilitation. Indeed, "the CRPD marks a shift from viewing persons with disabilities primarily as recipients of charity, medical treatment, special services and social protection towards recognizing them as . . . active members of society."[27]

This recognition is important for the enjoyment of the right to rehabilitation and habilitation. The latter in this context is a bridge for the insertion of persons with disabilities in the community to live independently and enjoy all the same rights as those who do not have a disability. Michailakis writes: "A human rights approach implies legal reasoning. . . . [It] implies, thus, among other things, the creation of a legislation which shall give persons with disabilities and their organizations the lever to ensure that there is effective advocacy for their rights."[28]

This is to say that the human rights discourse is an important factor in shielding persons with disabilities against social exclusion. From this perspective, rehabilitation and habilitation should reflect community-based

---

26 Lang, "Development and Critique," 2.
27 Christian Blind Mission, "A Human Rights-Based Approach to Disability in Development," *ReliefWeb*, August 2, 2013, https://reliefweb.int/report/world/human-rights-based-approach-disability-development.
28 D. Michailikis, "When Opportunity Is the Thing to Be Equalised," *Disability & Society* 12, no. 1 (1997): 19–20.

development principles. This approach affirming the positive identity of persons with disabilities is empowering as it recognizes the role of persons with disabilities in development. Swain and French explain in the following terms:

> The affirmative model directly challenges presumptions of personal tragedy and the determination of identity through the value-laden presumptions of nondisabled people . . . Embracing an affirmative model, disabled individuals assert a positive identity, not only in being disabled, but also in being impaired. In affirming a positive identity, disabled people are actively repudiating the dominant view of normality.[29]

This is to underline the significant place of the human rights model, which is instrumental in fostering the acceptance of difference and the recognition of disability as a variance of human diversity. The implementation of human rights models to disability encompasses community-based rehabilitation and community-based inclusive development.

Community-Based Rehabilitation

Originally, in line with the 1978 Declaration of Alma-Ata[30] that was crafted in the medical model approach to disability, community-based rehabilitation (CBR) was adopted to supplement this model. Its aim was to ensure physical accessibility of health care and rehabilitation services to persons with disabilities by bringing these centers closer to their community.[31]

Subsequently, in 1989, the WHO developed a more comprehensive CBR program targeting all stakeholders including persons with disabilities and their families and other members of the community who could play a role in fostering the inclusion of persons with disabilities.[32] The CBR was not simply focusing on persons with disabilities but on various sectors seeking their full rehabilitation and social inclusion. This development was given a major boost when the WHO and other UN agencies, as well as other global

---

29   J. Swain and S. French, "Towards an Affirmation Model of Disability," *Disability & Society* 15, no. 4 (2000): 578.

30   World Health Organization, *Declaration of Alma Ata: International Conference on Primary Health Care, Alma-Ata, USSR, 6–12 September 1978* (Geneva: United Nations, 1978), https://www.who.int/publications/almaata_declaration_en.pdf?ua=1.

31   A. Alwan, "Preface," in WHO, *Community-Based*, 1.

32   WHO, *Community-Based*, 23.

and national stakeholders, decided to ensure that CBR reduces poverty associated with disabilities. The CBR was owned by the community, which developed and fostered multisectorial collaboration with a massive participation of persons with disabilities.[33] This positive development that epitomizes the full inclusion of persons with disabilities led to the definition of CBR by the WHO as

> a strategy within general community development for the rehabilitation, poverty reduction, equalization of opportunities and social inclusion of all people with disabilities and promotes the implementation of CBR [programs] ... through the combined efforts of people with disabilities themselves, their families, organizations and communities, and the relevant governmental and non-governmental health, education, vocational, social and other services.[34]

In other words, CBR not only captures the need to address disabilities from a medical standpoint but also emphasizes the need to ensure that rehabilitation secures the dignity of persons with disabilities by fighting poverty, empowering them, and ensuring their right to autonomy and full independence. This is indeed in line with the CRPD, which compels states to ensure that rehabilitation capacitates persons with disabilities and enhances their ability to enjoy all their rights on an equal basis with others. This should be operationalized with the full and meaningful participation those beneficiaries of the rehabilitation services. In short, from a human rights perspective, rehabilitation and habitation should take place within communities where families are involved and not in isolated institutions. Rehabilitation is synonymous with noninstitutionalization. This view adopted by the CRPD was the position of the courts/commissions in numerous jurisdictions, namely in the United States, in the Inter-American, European, and African human rights systems.

Community-Based Rehabilitation and Human Rights in the US Courts

In *Olmstead v. L.C. ex rel. Zimring*, ("*Olmstead*"), based on the nondiscrimination provisions of the Americans with Disabilities Act of 1990, the United States Supreme Court was of the view that the denial of services to persons

---

33   WHO, *Community-Based*, 23–24.
34   WHO, *Community-Based*, 24.

with disabilities in the most integrated services amounted to discrimination.[35] In this vein, the court held that persons with mental disabilities have a right to live in the community, whenever suitable, and to obtain treatment there and not in institutions.[36] This decision was important for highlighting that confining persons with mental disabilities in institutions for treatment was discriminatory because those without mental disabilities received treatment within the community.[37] Echoing the court, Rosenthal and Kanter wrote:

> [T]his unnecessary confinement diminishes the individual's ability to have a social life and family relations, to receive an education, or to become economically independent through employment. Thus, undue institutionalization is discriminatory not only because it treats people with and without disabilities differently in terms of their access to mental health treatment, but also because it perpetuates negative stereotypes of people with mental disabilities as "incapable or unworthy of participating in community life," and deprives them of "everyday life activities" such as "family relations, social contacts, work options, economic independence, educational advancement, and cultural enrichment."[38]

Community-Based Rehabilitation and Human Rights in the Inter-American Human Rights System

In March 1999, the Inter-American Commission of Human Rights also guarded against keeping mental health in isolation. This was in the case of *Victor Rosario Congo v. Ecuador*. In this case, the Ecuadorian Mr. Congo, a mental health patient, died in pretrial detention after having been beaten by a guard, placed in solitary confinement, and denied appropriate medical and psychiatric care. The commission found that the degeneration of Mr. Congo's mental condition was caused by the fact that he was held in isolation, in contravention with Article 5 of the American Convention that prohibits inhuman and degrading treatment.[39] Based on this finding, the

---

35 Olmstead v. L.C. ex rel. Zimring 527 U.S. 581 (Supreme Court of the United States 1999).
36 Olmstead v. L.C.
37 Olmstead v. L.C., 601.
38 Rosenthal and Kanter, "Community Integration."
39 Victor Rosario Congo v. Ecuador 11.427 (Inter-American Commission on Human Rights 1999).

400   CHAPTER EIGHTEEN

Inter-American Commission of Human Rights was unequivocal about warning against institutionalization or isolation of mental health patients.

Community-Based Rehabilitation and Human Rights in the European Human Rights System

In July 2001, in the case of *Price v. United Kingdom*,[40] the European Court on Human Rights also underlined the need to avoid isolating persons with a mental disability, as this amounts to inhuman and degrading treatment of people with mental disabilities. This case was triggered by the detention of a mentally disabled woman for seven days in a jail where she was compelled to sleep in a wheelchair and left without an accessible bathroom. The court found this unacceptable and called for "extra vigilance to ensure that governments protect against inhuman and degrading treatment of people with mental disabilities, particularly those detained in institutions."[41] This decision clearly suggests the need to move from institutionalization to community-based rehabilitation in order to protect persons with disabilities against torture and degrading treatment.

Community-Based Rehabilitation and Human Rights in the African Human Rights System

In the African rights system, in 2003 the African Commission on Human Peoples' Rights in the case of *Purohit v. Gambia* also held that keeping a person with mental disabilities in an institution was discrimination under Article 2 of the African Charter, which prohibits discrimination. The applicants submitted the complaint on behalf of mental health patients detained under the Lunatics Detention Act (LDA) of The Gambia, which enabled the government to keep persons with mental disabilities in institutions. They also claimed that under the LDA there was no definition of "lunatic" or safeguards for patients under the act, and there was no requirement to acquire consent to treatment or to review treatment. Legal aid was not available to the patients under the act, and the patients were not allowed to vote.

The *Purohit* decision underlines that persons with disabilities have the right to participate in the community and enjoy life to the fullest, just as any other person would. The commission found the violations of specific rights:

---

40   Judgment in the Case of Price v. United Kingdom 512 (European Court of Human Rights 2001).

41   Rosenthal and Kanter, "Community Integration."

namely, the right to human dignity, to have one's cause heard, and to vote. It expressly held that persons with mental disabilities share and would like to realize the "same hopes, dreams, and goals" as other persons.[42]

In sum, the jurisprudence in America, Europe, and Africa (to list but a few jurisdictions) clearly emphasizes the need to foster community-based rehabilitation. In other words it is imperative to ensure that rehabilitation and habilitation take place away from prisons or so-called institutions. The latter disempowers persons with disabilities, hence the need to ensure their rehabilitation and habilitation within their communities with their meaningful involvement. This approach consecrates the human rights model of disability, which is vital to set persons with disabilities free from disablement.

The benefits of a well-developed community-based rehabilitation strategy cannot be overemphasized. It addresses the challenges of impairment as it raises awareness of disability in families and communities—and as such addresses the stigma attached to disability. Community-based rehabilitation is therefore vital to demystify disability and foster inclusion.[43] In highlighting the importance of community-based rehabilitation, Morris wrote:

> Our disability frightens people. They don't want to think that this is something that might happen to them. So we become separated from common humanity, treated as fundamentally different and alien. Having put up clear barriers between us and them, non-disabled people further hide their fear and discomfort by turning us into objects of pity, comforting themselves by their own kindness and generosity.[44]

Put differently, community-based rehabilitation will alleviate the fear about disability, for disability will be understood as a common element of human diversity.

Community-Based Inclusive Development

Community-based inclusive development (which refers to community-based rehabilitation) and habilitation for an inclusive society is a multisectoral strategy to ensure the full inclusion of persons with disabilities in the

---

42 Purohit and Moore v. The Gambia 241/2001 (African Commission on Human and Peoples' Rights 2003), https://www.escr-net.org/sites/default/files/caselaw/purohit_v_moore_judgment.pdf.
43 Jackson, "Approaches," 45.
44 J. Morris, *Pride against Prejudice* (London: Women's Press, 1991), 192.

communities.[45] This strategy seeks to ensure that no one is left behind in development initiatives. To this end, community-based inclusive development ensures that

> rehabilitation and habilitation [programs] often focus on three specific priorities: (a) promoting community-based, inclusive development that assists in mainstreaming disability in key development initiatives and, in particular, poverty reduction; (b) supporting stakeholders to meet the basic needs and enhance the quality of life of persons with disabilities and their families by improving access to the health, education, livelihood, and social sectors; and (c) encouraging stakeholders to facilitate the empowerment of persons with disabilities and their families by promoting their inclusion and participation in development and decision-making processes.[46]

In other words, community-based rehabilitation and habilitation for an inclusive society capacitates persons with disabilities and turns them into development actors by removing barriers that hinder their full participation. An initiative for community inclusivity contains fundamentals of self-consciousness and empowerment, which is likely to foster participation and access to strategy positions that are essential in effecting change.

Community-based inclusive development is a more progressive version of CBR. It fosters a multisectoral strategy to address the far-reaching needs of persons with disabilities: the ultimate aim being to address their marginalization and enhance their quality of life. It entails addressing health concerns and the livelihood of persons with disabilities. From this perspective, while undergoing habilitation and rehabilitation, persons with disabilities should be involved in development projects and other projects in their community. To this end, they should receive adequate assistive technology devices commensurate with their disabilities. These tools enable persons with disabilities to be involved in the design of projects and to enjoy the benefits of projects as well. These aspects of inclusive development should be factored in rehabilitation and habilitation of persons with disabilities as to ensure that no one is left behind.

In the African context, this will be in line with the African Disability Protocol, which compels state parties to

---

45 Convention on the Rights of Persons with Disabilities, 6th session (CRPD/csp/2013/4).
46 CRPD/csp/2013/4.

take effective and appropriate measures, including peer support, to enable persons with disabilities to attain and maintain maximum independence; full physical, mental, social, and vocational ability; and full inclusion and participation in all aspects of life, including by:

a) Organizing, strengthening, and extending comprehensive habilitation and rehabilitation services and [programs], particularly in the areas of health, employment, education and social services;
b) Promoting the development of initial and continuing training for professionals and staff working in habilitation and rehabilitation services;
c) Promoting the availability, knowledge, and use of appropriate, suitable and affordable assistive devices and technologies;
d) Supporting the design, development, production, distribution, and servicing of assistive devices and equipment for persons with disabilities, adapted to local conditions;
e) Developing, adopting, and implementing standards, including regulations on accessibility and universal design, suitable to local conditions.[47]

In this context, rehabilitation and habilitation serve as a roadmap for persons with disabilities to fulfill their rights in an inclusive society. Therefore, habilitation and rehabilitation should not only take care of health concerns of persons with disabilities but should also secure the total inclusion of persons with disabilities from a multisectoral perspective. This means that under community-based inclusive development, persons with disabilities should be equipped to fully participate in the social, cultural, economic, civil, and political life of their communities. This suggests that "imprisoning" persons with disabilities in institutions is illegal and punishable.

Besides engaging policymakers on the implementation of community-based inclusive development, it is important to also involve traditional leaders who generally have huge followings in many African communities. This approach of relying on traditional institutions to advance human rights embodies what Zwart calls the "receptor approach" to human rights.[48] This model ensures that the human rights discourse is presented to local communities through their leaders and languages and that it takes into account their local realities. This method would lead to the appropriation of resulting policies by local communities, and this will foster the inclusion of persons with

---

47 United Nations, "Article 26."
48 Tom Zwart, "Using Local Culture to Further the Implementation of International Human Rights: The Receptor Approach," *Human Rights Quarterly* 34 (2012).

disabilities in their settings. In this perspective, rehabilitation and habilitation will rely on the bottom-up approach, which would be instrumental to address the marginalization exclusion of persons with disabilities. This strategy would be fundamental in equally protecting families and caregivers of persons with disabilities, ensuring the establishment of an inclusive society where the right to equality is a reality.

Community-based inclusive development should be a bridge to highlight both the rights and place of people with disabilities in society. It should also serve to mainstream disability rights into all development endeavors. In this context, rehabilitation has nothing to do with institutionalization; it focuses on "accommodation" within family and communities, as well as "education, vocational training, and employment that are . . . critical for the successful integration of people with disabilities."[49]

Conclusion

The aim of this chapter was to examine the extent to which the rehabilitation of persons with disabilities leads to the realization of disability rights. It was found that historically persons with disabilities suffered exclusion and marginalization. They were considered ill, and all remedies were to be found in the medical sector—which is why the medical model was prevalent before the adoption of the CRPD. Although the social model considered barriers to inclusion, this model was not universally accepted, as numerous disability advocates called for the need to embed the body and physical disability, per se, in the disability discourse.

In this chapter, the CRPD was the agreed-upon human rights model of disability. To this end, it was found that community-based rehabilitation under the CRPD prohibits the institutionalization of persons with disabilities and calls for the habilitation and rehabilitation in their communities. It also highlights the need to rely on community-based inclusive development, which is a multisectoral strategy to ensure the full inclusion and independence of persons with disabilities in society. Ultimately, the chapter found that habilitation and rehabilitation within institutions hinder disability rights, while community-based rehabilitation and especially community-based inclusive development are essential for ensuring that disabled persons enjoy the same human rights as nondisabled persons.

---

49   Jackson, "Approaches," 41.

Conclusion

A Research Agenda for African Disability Studies

Anna Lee Carothers and Toyin Falola

We will now summarize the current status of those with disabilities in Africa, with Kenya as a starting point, in order to determine how disability studies in Africa should progress. Kenya in particular is worth examining first because it is considered one of the more progressive African countries when it comes to disability recognition and disability rights. Yet, even so, there is notable room for progress.[1] In 2009 the Ministry of Education, Science, and Technology in Kenya reported that among Kenyan students with disabilities, 90 percent either did not go to school or did not receive minimal accommodations for their needs.[2] The year 2009 was the last time the Ministry of Education, Science, and Technology released this report,[3] which means that about a decade's worth of the most updated information on Kenyan children with disabilities is missing. It is vital to uncover the most recent statistics in order to understand any improvements that have been made and to calculate what further improvements are still needed. The dearth of information on disabled children in Kenya reflects a greater problem. Research on disability

---

1   Ashley Lime, "Disability in Africa: 'I'm No Longer Ashamed of My Disabled Daughter,'" *BBC*, October 7, 2018, https://www.bbc.com/news/world-africa-45220690.
2   Republic of Kenya: Ministry of Education, Science and Technology, *Kenya National Special Needs Education Survey Report* (London: VSO International Oversees, 2009), https://www.vsointernational.org/sites/default/files/SNE%20Report_Full%20-2.pdf.
3   Lime, "Disability in Africa."

affecting both children and adults in low-income countries is scarce,[4] which means that research on disability affecting those of all ages across the African continent overall is scarce.

This fact is startling, considering how prevalent disability is in the world and specifically in Africa. In 2011, the World Report on Disability reported that the number of people with disabilities in the world rises as the world population ages.[5] According to the United Nations, in Africa alone there are about eighty million people who have some sort of disability, and this number is likely to increase over time.[6] This makes it all the more essential to gather relevant statistics on disabled individuals, young and old, across the African continent so that the lives of future generations can be sustained and enhanced. It is incumbent upon individuals involved in the disability studies field to spread their influence and knowledge to Africa so that disabled Africans and their stories are no longer ignored.

Yet in spite of the troubling statistics already mentioned, Kenya manages to set itself apart from many of its African neighbors; by comparison, it is indeed still one of the better places for Africans with disabilities to live. In Kenya, disabled individuals do not pay taxes, and sign language is the third most popular national language. Furthermore, David ole Sankok, the former National Council for Persons with Disability chairman, was able to convince President Uhuru Kenyatta that exams for disabled individuals be adapted to their specific needs after he encouraged the president to try to write his name while holding a pen in his mouth. As recently as August 2018, the president said that he would appoint those with disabilities to senior positions.[7] Certainly these facts are encouraging, although it is arguable whether other African countries can turn to Kenya as an example for implementation of disability rights. (Kenya is certainly far from an idyllic place for those with disabilities.)

As far as the rest of the African continent is concerned, it is apparent that the situation for disabled Africans is worrying. For example, according to

---

4   Arne H. Eide and Mitch E. Loeb, *Data and Statistics on Disability in Developing Countries* (London: Disability Knowledge and Research Programme, 2005).
5   World Health Organization and World Bank, *World Report on Disability* (Geneva: World Health Organization, 2011).
6   Kelsey Parrotte, "Why is Disability in Africa Increasing?" *The Borgen Project*, July 6, 2015, https://borgenproject.org/disability-africa-increasing/.
7   Lime, "Disability in Africa."

a report from the African Child Policy Forum, African children with disabilities at the turn of the twenty-first century were virtually "invisible" to society—even to their families. They were also more prone to be the victims of violence. Children with speech impairments were five times more likely to be physically abused or neglected and three times more likely to be sexually abused. Also, children with disabilities age five or younger had a mortality rate of 80 percent in some African countries.[8]

Across Africa, particularly in the poorest regions, only about 1 to 3 percent of children with disabilities receive an education because of the lack of accessible facilities and skilled teachers. Additionally, stigma against disability and the shame that comes with having a disability may further inhibit disabled children's educational attainment. In Africa, it is not uncommon for parents of children with disabilities to believe that they have been punished by God for their sins. Indeed, according to Damon Hill, the Patron of Disability Africa, African children with disabilities face conditions that are "unimaginably hard."[9]

Even if African countries have made some progress in recognizing the need to implement disability policies for not only children but also adults, the actual realization of these policies has been disappointing. In fact, the Convention on the Rights of Persons with Disabilities (CRPD) has failed to improve the lives of those with disabilities in the Global South generally.[10] There is a reason for this, academics have argued. Take Uganda as a case study, for instance. Uganda is another of the more "progressive" African nations when it comes to disability and has been inspired by US disability policies.[11] However, its attempt to replicate American policies has resulted in notable problems: for example, there has been "knowledge transfer" from a former colonialist entity (the Global North) to a former colonized entity (the Global South). When knowledge transfer of disability policy from the Global North to the Global South occurs, there is a "danger of replicating inherently

---

8 "Changing Attitudes to Child Disability in Africa," *Lancet* 384 (2014): 2000.
9 Parrotte, "Why is Disability in Africa Increasing?"
10 Shaun Grech, "Disability, Poverty and Development: Critical Reflections on the Majority World Debate," *Disability & Society* 24, no. 6 (2009): 771–784; and Helen Meekosha and Karen Soldatic, "Human Rights and the Global South: The Case of Disability," *Third World Quarterly* 32, no. 8 (2011): 1383–1397.
11 Patrick Ojok and Robert Gould, "A Comparison of Disability Rights in Employment: Exploring the Potential of the UNCRPD in Uganda and the United States," *Disability and the Global South* 6, no. 2 (2019): 1700.

unequal power relations . . . that links the 'problem' of disability to the need for industrialization and advanced development."[12]

The dangers of implementing policies from the Global North in the Global South are tremendous and should be acknowledged. Yet it is understandable why the Global South continues to try to repeat the successes in the Global North: those with disabilities in the Global South are undoubtedly in need of better care. Many Africans with physical disabilities who cannot afford wheelchairs or crutches may be forced to create their own stabilizers. Moreover, those with disabilities may struggle financially to support themselves as well as their families. Consequently, those with disabilities sometimes turn to begging.[13]

According to Goal 8 of the United Nations Development Program's Sustainable Development Goals, the nations of the world should implement nondiscriminatory policies in the workplace and in employment opportunities.[14] Inclusion in the workplace and in employment opportunities means that employers should not alienate current or potential employees for having disabilities. Even so, those with psychiatric disabilities are far less likely to be employed across the globe, much like those with physical disabilities. Certainly, it is just as important to consider mental disabilities as physical disabilities. The Organization for Economic Co-operation and Development (OECD) reported in 2010 that 30 percent to 45 percent of disability claims are due to mental health diagnoses and problems.[15] The phenomenon of discriminating against those with psychiatric disabilities is especially apparent in low- or middle-income countries (which includes countries on the African continent).[16] Part of this, of course, is due to the

---

12 Ojok and Gould, "Comparison of Disability Rights"; and Meekosha and Soldatic, "Human Rights and the Global South," cited in Ojok and Gould, "Comparison of Disability Rights," 1700.
13 Parrotte, "Why is Disability in Africa Increasing?"
14 United Nations Development Programme, "Goal 8: Decent Work and Economic Growth," *United Nations Development Programme*, 2020, https://www.undp.org/content/undp/en/home/sustainable-development-goals/goal-8-decent-work-and-economic-growth.html.
15 Organization for Economic Co-Operation and Development, *Mental Health, Disability and Work* (Paris: OECD, 2010).
16 Natalie Drew et al., "Human Rights Violations of People with Mental and Psychosocial Disabilities: An Unresolved Global Crisis," *Lancet* 378 (2011): 1664-1675; and Jody Heymann, Michael Ashley Stein, and Gonzalo Moreno, *Disability and Equity at Work* (Oxford: Oxford University Press, 2013).

struggles that inherently come with a mental health diagnosis. However, the diagnosis itself is only part of the problem.

Much of the problem also stems from mental health stigma that is prevalent globally but is especially pronounced in low- or middle-income countries.[17] This stigma does not have to persist, however, and there is much that can be done in these low- and middle-income countries for employees with mental health conditions to meet their best potential. Some research has indicated that if those with mental health conditions are given the treatment they need, they are more likely to remain in their jobs.[18] Indeed, without treatment, those with mental health conditions are more likely to suffer occupationally and socially.[19] Of course, one also cannot discount the research that indicates that those with mental health conditions who have found personal ways of handling their state and the related stigma also have succeeded in the workplace.[20] This means that employers and the government could potentially offer ways for those with mental health conditions to express their concerns and find ways to cope.

Bipolar disorder, depression, schizophrenia, and schizoaffective disorders are the main contributors to mental health–related disability.[21] However, in many African countries, it is almost impossible to be recognized for an

---

17 Abebaw Fekadu and Graham Thornicroft, "Global Mental Health: Perspectives from Ethiopia," *Global Health Action* 7, no. 1 (2014): 25447.

18 William Boyce et al., "Occupation, Poverty and Mental Health Improvement in Ghana," *ALTER-European Journal of Disability Research* 3, no. 3 (2009): 233–244.

19 Mirella Ruggeri et al., "Definition and Prevalence of Severe and Persistent Mental Illness," *British Journal of Psychiatry* 177, no. 2 (2000): 149–155.

20 Lana Van Niekerk, "Identity Construction and Participation in Work: Learning from the Experiences of Persons with Psychiatric Disability," *Scandinavian Journal of Occupational Therapy* 23, no. 2 (2016): 107–114; Lana Van Niekerk, "Participation in Work: A Source of Wellness for People with Psychiatric Disability," *Work* 32, no. 4 (2009): 455–465; and Lana Van Niekerk et al., "Time Utilisation Trends of Supported Employment Services by Persons with Mental Disability in South Africa," *Work* 52, no. 4 (2015): 825–833.

21 Michael Linden, "Definition and Assessment of Disability in Mental Disorders Under the Perspective of the International Classification of Functioning Disability and Health (ICF)," *Behavioral Sciences & The Law* 35 (2017): 124–134.

official mental health condition.[22] This lack of recognition has ethical repercussions, since denying individuals the proper resources needed for mental health treatment, as well as an occupation, denies these same individuals autonomy and stability. In addition, there are economic repercussions for the refusal to recognize those with mental health conditions in the workplace. Displacing those with mental health conditions from the workplace can cost the economy.[23] According to a study for the International Labour Organisation, excluding disabled individuals from the workplace can actually cause an economic loss of about 3.7 percent on average.[24]

However, it is important to emphasize how economic arguments for the inclusion of employees with disabilities is second to any ethical argument. First and foremost, we must acknowledge that people with disabilities are human beings. To exclude them for being disabled is to condemn them for something they cannot control. This is morally unjust and would suggest that human beings do in fact come only with price tags and not individuality, respect, and dignity.

Unfortunately, in spite of prevalent mental health stigma and the existence of mental health conditions in Africa, there are currently very few studies investigating employment issues for those with mental health conditions in Africa.[25] Lack of recognition of these issues practically assures the continued prevalence of misinformation on mental illness—for instance, the unprovable belief that supernatural beings,[26] rather than medical phenomena, cause

---

22 Matlhodi T. Mokoka, Solomon T. Rataemane, and Monika Dos Santos, "Disability Claims on Psychiatric Grounds in the South African Context: A Review," *South African Journal of Psychiatry* 18, no. 2 (2012): 34–41.

23 Gary R. Bond et al., "Does Competitive Employment Improve Nonvocational Outcomes for People with Severe Mental Illness?," *Journal of Consulting and Clinical Psychology* 69, no. 3 (2001): 489–501; Heymann, Stein, and Moreno, *Disability and Equity at Work*; and Karsten I. Paul and Klaus Moser, "Unemployment Impairs Mental Health: Meta-Analyses," *Journal of Vocational Behavior* 74, no. 3 (2009): 264–282.

24 Sebastian Buckup, *The Price of Exclusion: The Economic Consequences of Excluding People with Disabilities from the World of Work* (Geneva: International Labour Office, 2009).

25 I. D. Ebuenyi et al., "Barriers to and Facilitators of Employment for People with Psychiatric Disabilities in Africa: A Scoping Review," *Global Health Action* 11, no. 1 (2018): 8.

26 Ugo Ikwuka, Niall Galbraith, and Lovemore Nyatanga. "Causal Attribution of Mental Illness in South-Eastern Nigeria," *International Journal of Social Psychiatry* 60, no. 3 (2014): 274–279.

mental illnesses. One reason for the lack of research on this topic is because there is a disturbing lack of political interest in care for those with mental health conditions in Africa,[27] despite the ethical and economic ramifications for not helping these individuals. Consequently, it has been suggested that African governments institute initiatives that break stigmas related to mental illness, as well as programs that support workers with mental health conditions.[28]

Stigma related to disability of any kind needs to be addressed if Africa is to see a better future. As previously mentioned, many in Africa believe that supernatural reasons bring about mental disability. Just as many Africans also believe that supernatural reasons bring about physical disability. According to *The Lancet*, Africans typically cite "punishment from God, witchcraft, the fault of the mother, [and] reincarnation" as main causes for disability,[29] which justifies the ostracization of those with disabilities. But of course, none of this is backed up by scientific research. According to scientific research, disabled individuals in Africa came to their state as a result of valid issues that Africa should address, like poverty, lack of access to health care, and war.[30] Additionally, Africans with disabilities are more likely to be unemployed, uneducated, and generally excluded from social privileges like transportation and social networks.[31] All of these facts demonstrate how vital it is to understand how disability is not merely a medical or biological phenomenon but also a social and political phenomenon.

However, there is a caveat here. We are not saying that all cultural beliefs must be eradicated when treating disability. According to the social model of disability, the notion of "disability" is in fact a cultural construct as well as a biological phenomenon. In other words, even if a certain disability has

---

27 Benedetto Saraceno et al., "Barriers to Improvement of Mental Health Services in Low-Income and Middle-Income Countries," *Lancet* 370, no. 9593 (2007): 1164–1174.

28 Heymann, Stein, and Moreno, *Disability and Equity at Work*; H. Herzig and B. Thole, "Employers' Attitudes towards Employment of People with Mental Illnesses in Mzuzu, Malawi," *East African Medical Journal* 75, no. 7 (1998): 428–431; and Adenekan O. Oyefeso, "Attitudes towards the Work Behaviour of Ex-Mental Patients in Nigeria," *International Journal of Social Psychiatry* 40, no. 1 (1994): 27–34.

29 "Changing Attitudes," 2000.

30 "Changing Attitudes," 2000.

31 Martha Banda-Chalwe, Jennifer C. Nitz, and Desleigh De Jonge, "Impact of Inaccessible Spaces on Community Participation of People with Mobility Limitations in Zambia," *African Journal on Disability* 3, no. 1 (2014).

biological components that express themselves universally across time and place, this same disability will be interpreted differently by various cultures. Therefore, disability is given new meaning in every context. As a result, medical professionals may feel it is necessary to speak in a way that resonates with the patients and their loved ones by acknowledging their cultural beliefs. However, they will also explain how disability can have biological facets and notable social ramifications.[32] This sort of intervention is indeed effective, for it meets patients and their loved ones where they are spiritually and mentally while also utilizing research-based methods to guide treatment.

Nevertheless, there are certain beliefs found in the form of stigma that should be the main cause for concern. Beliefs in the form of stigma are pernicious because they lower the chances of treatment efforts. Stigma also allows able-bodied Africans to generalize all disabled people as being forever incapacitated[33] or forever financially dependent,[34] thereby making it unnecessary to give them ordinary citizenship rights. However, these stereotypes often prove false. Indeed, destigmatizing disability by showing the successes of those with disabilities is an essential way to obtain not only social justice but also more economic stability.[35] Of course, this is not to undermine or ignore those who have disabilities and who do primarily rely on caregivers. This population absolutely exists, especially as people age. Therefore, while the following few pages will discuss the counternarratives to disability, it is important to keep in mind how the dominant narrative of disabled individuals needing care should be just as thoughtfully considered. This dominant narrative will be addressed after the counternarrative.

---

32   Neeraja Ravindran and Barbara J. Myers, "Cultural Influences of Health, Illness, and Disability: A Review and Focus on Autism," *Journal of Child and Family Studies* 21 (2012): 311–319.

33   Edson Munsaka and Helen Charnley, "'We Do Not Have Chiefs Who are Disabled': Disability, Development and Culture in a Continuing Complex Emergency," *Disability & Society* 28, no. 6 (2013): 756–769; Leslie Swartz and Maria Marchetti-Mercer, "Disabling Africa: The Power of Depiction and the Benefits of Discomfort," *Disability & Society* 33, no. 3 (2018): 482–486.

34   Shimelis Tsegaye Tesemma, "Economic Discourses of Disability in Africa: An Overview of Lay and Legislative Narratives," *African Disability Rights Yearbook* 2 (2014): 145.

35   Tom Shakespeare et al., "Success in Africa: People with Disabilities Share Their Stories," *African Journal of Disability* 8, no. 0, a522 (2019), https://www.ncbi.nlm.nih.gov/ pmc/articles/PMC6489159/.

The Department for International Development/Economic and Social Research Council funded a project to ascertain why some disabled (physically and sensorially disabled) Africans in Uganda, Sierra Leone, Zambia, and Kenya lead successful lives and others do not, and which factors could allow disabled people in Africa to be successful. Success was defined as "[enjoying] economic prosperity on an equal basis with others," based upon the word choice of the CRPD.[36] Consequently, the researchers in this project looked for Africans with disabilities who were self-employed or employed in governmental or nongovernmental organizations. They then conducted in-depth interviews with these participants so that they could tell their own stories and dispel stereotypes surrounding disabilities.[37]

The researchers found that most of their participants were able to support themselves as well as their families. Furthermore, only one-tenth to one-third had incomplete educations, usually due to barriers like lack of money or living in rural areas without secondary schools. The rest of the participants were considered to be well educated through either accommodating or mainstream schools. Those who attended school at the university level had their fees paid for by the government. Notably, however, those who did not complete their education still succeeded financially because they attended vocational schools or completed apprenticeships in particular trades. Additionally, some of the participants who completed their education attributed their success to making their own walking sticks or switching schools if there was too much bullying or too little accommodation. All the participants displayed creativity and determination in order to overcome obstacles in their education or preprofessional lives.[38]

Also, all of the participants found that remaining positive and resilient were essential components to their success. One participant said: "If I start pitying myself I will fail, and nobody is caring about me and nobody is willing to help me, so I have to cope with whatever comes ahead of me."[39] To the researchers, this statement was significant in that it showed how those with disabilities in developing countries may not have access to sufficient health care and may as a result need to be self-reliant. Undoubtedly, the ability to be resilient and determined in times of difficulty was essential for the participants in this study, but the researchers also emphasized how attitude may not

---

36   Shakespeare et al., "Success in Africa."
37   Shakespeare et al., "Success in Africa."
38   Shakespeare et al., "Success in Africa."
39   Shakespeare et al., "Success in Africa."

always be enough. Indeed, it is necessary for future studies to observe what factors made certain Africans with disabilities successful so that African governments, activists, and scholars can take the appropriate measures to make all disabled Africans feel that they are valuable members of society.[40]

But while these counternarratives are inspiring, policymakers must also respectfully acknowledge the more dependent individuals with disabilities. Currently, these individuals—for instance, those with severe cognitive disabilities—are especially neglected by African governments.[41] Arguably, this is in part because these individuals do not offer immediate economic benefit, whereas individuals who can cope with their disabilities can still participate in the workforce. However, it is imperative to stress once again how the reasons for instituting rights for Africans with disabilities are not purely economic. There are ethical reasons as well, for offering aid to those with severe disabilities (and their caregivers) will allow for easier integration into society and the respect they deserve[42]

Indeed, the news for disability rights in Africa is not all positive, but there are numerous successes to be noted. The improvements made in Africa thus far touch on stigma, as well as other very real factors that affect people with disabilities in Africa every day. For instance, the South African Human Rights Commission in South Africa seeks to uphold constitutional democracy and the dignity of all South Africans. It was created under the Human Rights Commission Act 54 of 1994 and supported by the Constitution of the Republic of South Africa Act 200 of 1993. It focuses on seven key areas that relate to human life and dignity in South Africa. One of those seven key areas is disability. Approximately 7.5 percent of South Africans have a disability, and more than half of South Africans above the age of eighty-five are disabled. As in other regions of Africa, South African disabled individuals often are homeless and unemployed, as well as unable to secure adequate health care and education.[43] The commission has sought to address this problem by advocating for the rights of the disabled, as well as educating

---

40   Shakespeare et al., "Success in Africa."
41   Judith Anne McKenzie, "An Exploration of an Ethics of Care in Relation to People with Intellectual Disability and Their Family Caregivers in the Cape Town Metropole in South Africa," *ALTER* 10 (2016): 67–78.
42   McKenzie, "Exploration," 75.
43   South African Human Rights Commission, "Disability," *South African Human Rights Commission*, 2016, https://www.sahrc.org.za/index.php/focus-areas/disability-older-persons/disability.

others and training others on how to respect and treat those with disabilities.[44] The commission is required to be active in all of these things, in accordance with Promotion of Access to Information Act (2000). Furthermore, the Legal Services Unit (LSU) in South Africa has successfully protected human rights[45] by executing the goals and initiatives of the South African Human Rights Commission.[46]

Also of note, according to Section 184 of the Constitution of the Republic of South Africa, Act 108 of 1996, these are the responsibilities of the South African Human Rights Commission:

1. [It must] promote respect for human rights and a culture of human rights; promote the protection, development and attainment of human rights; and monitor and assess the observance of human rights in the Republic.
2. The Commission has the powers, as regulated by the national legislation, necessary to perform its functions, including the power (a) to investigate and report on the observance of human rights; (b) to take steps and secure appropriate redress where human rights have been violated; (c) to carry out research; and (d) to educate.
3. Each year, the Commission must require relevant organs of state to provide the Commission with information on the measures that they have taken towards the realization of the rights of the Bill of Rights concerning housing, health care, food, water, social security, education and the environment."
4. The Commission has the additional powers and functions prescribed by national legislation.[47]

On February 10, 2014, history was made when the first African Leaders Forum on Disability was held. At this event, African representatives from civil society, the government, and the development sector convened to discuss the stigma surrounding mental illness and how Africa as a continent will

---

44 South African Human Rights Commission, "Programmes," *South African Human Rights Commission*, 2016, https://www.sahrc.org/za/index.php/what-we-do/programmes.
45 South African Human Rights Commission, "Overview," *South African Human Rights Commission*, 2016, https:// www.sahrc.org.za/index.php/about-us/about-the-sahrc.
46 South African Government, "Constitution of the Republic of South Africa Act 200 of 1993," *South African Government*, 2019, https://www.gov.za/documents/constitution/constitution-republic-south-africa-act-200-1993.
47 South African Human Rights Commission, "Overview," https://www.justice.gov.za/legislation/constitution/SAConstitution-web-eng-09.pdf.

promote the rights of those with disabilities. The president of Malawi, Joyce Banda, hosted the forum and underscored the need to eradicate social stigma surrounding disability.[48]

According to the World Health Organization, Africa is the global region most impacted by HIV and AIDS. Young African women are the most susceptible to the infections. Happily, however, in 2017, there was a 30 percent decrease in HIV diagnoses in the east and south compared to 2010. In West Africa and Central Africa, the HIV diagnosis rate was down 8 percent, compared to 2010. Additionally, compared to 2010, there were 42 percent fewer AIDS deaths in the east and south and 24 percent fewer AIDS deaths in West Africa and Central Africa.[49]

Also noteworthy was that in 2015 the World Health Organization recommended a policy called Treat All. The policy seeks to eliminate the limitation of antiretroviral therapy (ART) to those with HIV and to provide preventative ART for those more likely to be exposed to HIV. These recommendations build upon preexposure prophylaxis (PrEP), a policy that provides counseling for those with HIV, HIV testing, sanitary injection tools, and condoms. PrEP and Treat All together aim to treat those with HIV/AIDS around the world (and especially in Africa) and end the HIV/AIDS epidemic by 2030.[50] It is especially critical for those with disabilities to be a primary focus for HIV/AIDS interventions, for research indicates that those with disabilities are at a higher risk of having acquired HIV.[51] In the past, vulnerable populations (including those with disabilities) have been excluded from campaigns that aim to prevent HIV, in part because it is wrongly assumed that those with disabilities are asexual or hypersexual in socially inappropriate ways. People with disabilities have also usually been unable to access the

---

48 UNICEF, "African Leaders Commit to the Rights of People with Disabilities," UNICEF (website), February 10, 2014, https://www.unicef.org/media/media_71902.html.

49 WHO, "HIV/AIDS," World Health Organization: Regional Office for Africa (website), 2018, https://www.afro.who.int/health-topics/hivaids.

50 WHO, "HIV/AIDS."

51 Poul Rohleder, Leslie Swartz, and John Philander, "Disability and HIV/AIDS: A Key Development Issue," in *Disability & International Development: Towards Inclusive Global Health*, ed. M. MacLachlan and L. Swartz (New York: Springer, 2009), 137–147.

resources needed for adequate treatment for their condition.⁵² This is a grave injustice from a human rights perspective.

Additionally, in January 2018, a new protocol to the African Charter on Human and People's Rights was adopted, and it is considered to be a monumental achievement for Africans with disabilities. It is meant to address how people with disabilities in Africa are disproportionately more likely to experience poverty and discrimination. It is also meant to purposefully include people with disabilities in social life and political decisions, particularly through budget making and the implementation of human rights agreements. In accordance with the standards from the United Nations Convention on the Rights of Persons with Disabilities, 53 African countries ratified the protocol.⁵³

On January 23, 2019, President Muhammadu Buhari of Nigeria signed the Discrimination against Persons with Disabilities (Prohibition) Act, 2018, into law. This is a true success for the twenty-five million Nigerians who, according to the World Health Organization in 2011, had a disability. In 2011 and 2015, the National Assembly approved and passed the Discrimination against Persons with Disabilities (Prohibition) Bill, 2009, but Goodluck Jonathan, who was the Nigerian president at the time, never signed the bill into law. The new bill for the cause had been passed by the House of Representatives in 2016 but apparently was not sent to the president until December 2018. The new law protects those with disabilities by forbidding discrimination based on their condition. It vows to create more accessible public spaces over the course of five years. It also establishes a National Commission for Persons with Disabilities, which will allow those with disabilities to acquire adequate education, health care, and schooling. At this point, it is up to the government to ensure that these stipulations in the law are enacted properly.⁵⁴

---

52 Rohleder, Swartz, and Philander, "Disability and HIV/AIDS"; Nora Groce, *HIV/AIDS and Disability: Capturing Hidden Voices* (Washington, DC: World Bank, 2004).

53 United Nations Human Rights Office of the High Commissioner, "African States Affirm the Rights of Persons with Disabilities in a New Landmark Protocol," *United Nations Human Rights Office of the High Commissioner* (website), February 15, 2018, https://www.ohchr.org/EN/NewsEvents/Pages/DisplayNews.aspx?NewsID=22661&LangID=E.

54 Anietie Ewang, "Nigeria Passes Disability Rights Law," *Human Rights Watch*, January 25, 2019, https://www.hrw.org/news/2019/01/25/nigeria-passes-disability-rights-law.

Worth noting, also, are African organizations that seek to help Africans with disabilities. For instance, Disability Africa is an organization that works with disabled youth in Zambia, the Gambia, Sierra Leone, and Kenya. The organization sends its representatives to various communities in these regions, and these communities then create situations where the able-bodied and disabled children can play together. These established activities are particularly impactful because they allow for disabled children to at long last interact meaningfully with their able-bodied peers. Furthermore, these activities provide perhaps the only form of accessible play for disabled children that will in turn eliminate the prejudices that able-bodied children may harbor. Along with activities, Disability Africa's representatives provide the older members of the community with parental support meetings, training sessions for volunteers who wish to help the disabled, and information on school inclusion programs that will better help prepare disabled children for more mainstream schools.[55] The representatives also offer the disabled children physiotherapy and help them find sufficient treatment. Through activities and helpful support, Disability Africa combines advocacy work and service delivery for its cause because, according to the organization's leaders, this is the only true way to accomplish enough for those with disabilities.[56]

But while there are certainly honorable nongovernmental organizations, both national and international, that seek to help those with disabilities, it is crucial to note how some of these entities may cater more to the desires of funders in the Global North rather than to the needs of the disabled people they ostensibly serve. For instance, programs that claim to be helping those in need in the Global South may place more power with the managers from the Global North, who then have the power to control funds in ways that may not best help those in need in the Global South. This, in turn, means that the programs may not be disability-inclusive, which denies disabled individuals the significant opportunity to speak up for change they want to see.[57] Consequently, those truly dedicated to the disability cause in

---

55 "What We Do," *Disability Africa*, n.d., https://www.disability-africa.org/what-we-do.

56 "Our Template," *Disability Africa*, n.d., https://www.disability-africa.org/our-template/.

57 Tsitsi Chataika and Judith A. McKenzie, "Global Institutions and Their Engagement with Disability Mainstreaming in the South: Development and (Dis)Connections," in *Disability in the Global South*, ed. S. Grech and K. Soldatic (Gewerbestrasse: Springer International, 2016), 423–436.

Africa need a nuanced and productive engagement with these organizations to ensure that their wealth is being used as effectively as possible for actual people with disabilities.

Based on our research, we propose the following points to be addressed for the future of disability studies as an academic discipline in Africa.

African and global academics in disability studies and disability rights activists should make a conscious effort to work with African disability rights organizations so that, together, the gap between academia and the common public can be closed. Indeed, vital information about Africans with disabilities can be spread to organizations that have the power and networking capabilities to perpetuate accurate and scientifically valid truths about disability. When academics and activists work with these disability rights organizations, they should especially emphasize two things: first, the importance of breaking stigma throughout African communities (particularly rural communities); second, the activation of African communitarian rhetoric—such as *ubuntu*, *ujaama*, *biaku ye* and their localized corollaries across the continent—to argue for the incorporation of people with disabilities fully into their communities.

Academics and activists should ensure that African disability rights organizations offer research-based resources for the visited communities. These resources should cover information about the proper medical and sociological reasons for disability, even if this also means acknowledging the harmful cultural beliefs about disability in various communities. These research-based resources should also cover coping tools for family members of those with disabilities, as well as for those with disabilities themselves.

Academics and activists should continue to work with disability rights organizations to strengthen grassroots movements that call upon governments to offer more public government-funded health care for those with disabilities. When there is more public support for those with disabilities, the political will for disability rights will increase. It will therefore be more likely that employment and poverty issues related to disabilities will decrease with governmental action. The key is for these organizations to cultivate progressively more effective grassroots movements.

It is important for academics and activists themselves to continue to work with African government officials on disability issues. Together, they should strive to create and promote laws that will hold employers accountable for implementing nondiscriminatory policies. They should also create laws that allow for more efficient health care for those with disabilities. For instance, there should be far greater prevalence of medication and stability tools (like crutches and wheelchairs) for those with disabilities. Additionally, there should be laws that allow for publicly funded counseling or counseling made available for workers with disabilities. In this way, individuals with disabilities can navigate society and the workplace and feel protected from harassment. Lastly, academics and activists should assist government officials in creating laws that establish more accessible transportation systems for those with disabilities—for instance, sidewalks, and ramps.

Academics and activists should also address stigma when coordinating with government officials. Governments should be encouraged to exercise their power to establish programs and campaigns that try to break stigmas surrounding disability. They can do this by spreading factual medical information about how disabilities come about and how they can be treated. They can also spread information about the lived realities that those with disabilities face—not just the negative realities but also the positive ones. When a powerful entity like the government presents information about how people with disabilities can live fruitful and productive lives, it is likely to change hearts and minds in a society. Their words, in combination with efforts from academics, activists, and organizations, can craft a memorable message.

Academics and activists should work with African governments to ensure that children with disabilities receive effective health care and schooling. If these children do not receive the assistance they need (with the appropriate accommodations in their education), they will fall behind the rest of their peers early in life. They will then not receive the same advantages that could make them productive and fulfilled adult citizens. Investing in children means an investment in the future.

Academics and activists should work with medical experts to spread knowledge of and access to HIV treatment, as well as safe sex education. In this way, HIV and AIDS rates in Africa will continue to drop and, hopefully, more Africans will practice safer sex. Academics and activists should also work to break the sexual stigma against those with disabilities. They should collaborate with medical experts to spread the knowledge that disabled individuals are more likely to contract HIV and are therefore especially in need of resources.

Academics and activists should continue to encourage the academy to fund research projects on those with disabilities in Africa. In this way, academics and activists can gather more information on what makes Africans with disabilities successful (or not). They can then effectively lead government officials and African disability rights organizations toward promoting the best behaviors, treatments, and interventions for those with disabilities.

It is highly unlikely that positive change can be made without an interest and earnest pursuit in studies on Africans with disabilities.

Academics must work in various circles and networks to provide more equity for those with disabilities. For example, they should collaborate with African government officials and encourage them to incorporate disability into their international cooperation agenda. They should partner with lawyers and litigators to advance protection of rights of persons with disabilities in court. They should interact regularly with businesses to discuss the importance of including those with disabilities in the workplace and also to facilitate practical solutions such as ensuring discounts on assistive devices for disabled people.

Academics need to ensure that while research on disability is being implemented, the dignity of those with disabilities is maintained. Those with disabilities should not be seen as lab rats or zoo animals to be observed. They should be seen and treated as human beings first and foremost. If these individuals are capable, they should be given the chance to exercise autonomy and express their wishes during the course of a study.

Academics should work with traditional leaders to ensure that custodians of African culture turn to their own cultures when including people with disabilities in their own communities. For instance, traditional leaders can encourage custodians to use *ubuntu* in order to recognize the disabled people in their work. Also, Anglophile academics and activists have the potential to work with Indigenous, Francophile, Lusophone, and Arabic language academics and activists in order to develop disability discourses across linguistic and cultural barriers.

Academics and activists should work with nongovernmental organizations and international non-governmental organizations to move toward interventions that are dictated more by the needs of people with disabilities than by the desires of donors in the Global North. Specifically, academics and activists should work with leaders and members of DPOs to incorporate more equitable acceptance, membership, and leadership from people with disabilities who are women, lower class, with less education, and/or part of the LGBTQ community.

Through pursuit of this research agenda, we believe that the progress made toward disability rights and disability studies in Africa will continue, and—more importantly—inequities surrounding those with disabilities will be minimized.

Selected Bibliography

References were chosen based on their importance to the contributors' works in this volume as well as their relevance to the subject of disability in Africa generally.

Barclay, Jennifer L. "Differently Abled: Africanisms, Disability, and Power in the Age of Transatlantic Slavery." In *Bioarchaeology of Impairment and Disability*, edited by Jennifer F. Byrnes and Jennifer L. Muller, 77–94. New York: Springer, 2017.

Berghs, Maria. *War and Embodied Memory: Becoming Disabled in Sierra Leone*. New York: Routledge, 2012.

Bukhala, Peter. "A Survey of the Current Status of Physical Activity Level of Students with Disabilities at Kenyatta University, Kenya." *African Journal of Applied Human Sciences* 1, no. 1 (2009): 31–35.

Chataika, Tsitsi. "Inclusion of Disabled Students in Higher Education in Zimbabwe." In *Cross-Cultural Perspectives on Policy and Practice-Decolonizing Community Contexts*, edited by Jennifer Lavia and Michele Moore. New York: Routledge, 2010.

Cole, Ernest. *Theorizing the Disfigured Body: Mutilation, Amputation, and Disability Culture in Post-Conflict Sierra Leone*. Trenton, NJ: Africa World, 2014.

Dada, Oluseyi, and Christiana Ukpata. "Sport Participation and Facilities as Predictors of Marketable Skill in Sport for Persons with Disability in Nigerian Universities." *European Journal of Special Education Research* 2, no. 5 (2017).

De Coster, Jori. "A Dialogue with Society: Disability, Theatre and Being Human in Kinshasa, DR Congo." In *Rethinking Disability: World Perspectives in Culture and Society*, edited by Patrick Devlieger, Beatriz Miranda-Galarza, Steven E. Brown, and Megan Strickfaden, 181–199. Antwerp-Apeldoorn: Grant, 2016.

Devlieger, Patrick. "Disability and Community Action in a Zimbabwean Community: Priorities Based on a Biocultural Approach." *Journal of the Steward Anthropological Society* 22 (1994): 41–57.

———. "The 'Why' of Disability: From an Existential to a Transmodern Perspective." In *Rethinking Disability: World Perspectives in Culture and Society*, edited by Patrick Devlieger, Beatriz Mairanda-Galarza, Steven E. Brown, and Megan Strickfaden, 389–397. Antwerp: Grant, 2016.

Eide, Arne H., and Benedicte Ingstad, ed. *Disability and Poverty: A Global Challenge*. Bristol: Bristol University Press, 2011.

Grech, Shaun, and Karen Soldatic. *Disability in the Global South: The Critical Handbook*. Cham, Switzerland: Springer, 2016.

Grischow, Jeff D. "Kwame Nkrumah, Disability and Rehabilitation in Ghana, 1957–1966." *The Journal of African History* (2011): 179–199.

Harknett, S. G. "Cultural Factors in the Definition of Disability: A Community Study in Nyankunde, Zaire." *African Journal of Special Needs Education* 1 (1996): 18–24.

Ingstad, Benedicte, and Susan Reynolds Whyte, ed. *Disability and Culture*. Berkeley: University of California Press, 1995.

———. *Disability in Local and Global Worlds*. Berkeley: University of California Press, 2007.

Kamga, Serges Djoyou. "Inclusion of Learners with Severe Intellectual Disabilities in Basic Education Under a Transformative Constitution: A Critical Analysis." *Comparative and International Law Journal of Southern Africa* 49, no. 1 (2016): 24–52.

Livingston, Julie. *Debility and the Moral Imagination in Botswana*. Bloomington: Indiana University Press, 2005.

McKenzie, Judith Anne. "An Exploration of an Ethics of Care in Relation to People with Intellectual Disability and Their Family Caregivers in the Cape Town Metropole in South Africa." *ALTER* 10 (2016): 67–78.

Mukuria, Gathogo, and Julie Korir. "Education for Children with Emotional and Behavioral Disorders in Kenya: Problems and Prospects." *Preventing School Failure* 50, no. 2 (2006): 49–54.

Naami, Augustina, and Reiko Hayashi. "Empowering Women with Disabilities in Northern Ghana." *Review of Disability Studies* 7, no. 2 (2007).

Nepveux, Denise, and Emily Smith Beitiks. "Producing African Disability Through Documentary Film: Emmanuel's Gift and Moja Moja." *Journal of Literary and Cultural Disability Studies* 4, no. 3 (2010): 237–254.

Quayson, Ato. *Aesthetic Nervousness: Disability and the Crisis of Representation*. New York: Columbia University Press, 2007.

Tungaraza, Frida D. "The Arduous March toward Inclusive Education in Tanzania: Head Teachers' and Teachers' Perspectives." *Africa Today* 61, no. 2 (2014): 109–123.

United Nations. *Convention on the Rights of Persons with Disabilities and Optional Protocol*. New York: United Nations, 2006. http://www.un.org/disabilities/documents/convention/convoptprot-e.pdf.

Watermeyer, Brian, Leslie Swartz, Theresa Lorenzo, Marguerite Schneider, and Mark Priestley, ed. *Disability and Social Change: A South African Agenda*. Cape Town: HSRC, 2006.

World Health Organization. *World Report on Disability*. Geneva: World Health Organization, 2011. https://www.who.int/publications/i/item/world-report-on-disability.

Contributors

ELIZABETH L. B. AGBETTOR is a development practitioner with over fifteen years' experience in the disability field. She is currently a PhD student at the University of Cape Town studying disability. Her research focus is livelihood development in the informal sector for women with visual impairments in Ghana. She works with the Ghana Blind Union as Programmes Manager for Inclusion. She championed the development of National Inclusive Education Policy launched in 2015 and the Marrakesh Treaty ratified in Ghana in 2017. She is currently a member of the national committee on the implementation of inclusive education in Ghana. She is the executive director of Action on Empowerment, a local organization that focuses on the development of girls.

SALOUA ALI BEN ZAHRA is associate professor of Arabic language, literature, and culture at Appalachian State University. She obtained her master's and doctoral degrees from the University of Minnesota. She is originally from Tunisia, where she studied English and Italian at the university of Tunis-Carthage and taught at various Tunisian universities. Her book *Arab Voices, Agencies and Abilities: Disability Portrayals in Muslim World Literature and Culture* was published by Lexington Books in 2017.

MARIA BERGHS is an anthropologist with a PhD in sociology and social policy. She is an Early Career Research Fellow at De Montfort University in the United Kingdom. She works in the field of medical anthropology and sociology, specializing in disability studies. Her research interests include disability, global health (sickle cell), humanitarianism, ethics, gender, and West Africa (Sierra Leone).

ANNA LEE CAROTHERS is pursuing her master's of education, with a concentration in social studies, at the University of Texas at Austin. She received her bachelor of arts in psychology and in Plan II Honors, with a minor in educational psychology, at the University of Texas at Austin. Her current research focuses on pedagogical topics like inclusion, cultural competence, counternarratives, and students' mental wellness in the classroom.

DESIRE CHIWANDIRE holds a PhD in Political and International Studies from Rhodes University, South Africa. His doctoral thesis focused on the social inclusion of students with disabilities at South African higher education institutions. He is currently a postdoctoral fellow at the Chair for Critical Studies in Higher Education

Transformation (criSHET), Nelson Mandela University. He also teaches undergraduate and postgraduate courses in Critical Disability Studies and Political Studies at Rhodes University. His research interests broadly focus on Disability Politics specifically the intersectionality of race, class, gender, and disability in South African educational and workplace environments.

ERNEST COLE is the John Dirk Werkman Professor of English and chair of the English Department at Hope College, Michigan, where he teaches postcolonial literature. He is the author of two monographs, *Theorizing the Disfigured Body* (2014) and *Space and Trauma in the Writings of Aminatta Forna* (2017); and two collected volumes, *Emerging Perspectives on Syl Cheney Coker* with Eustace Palmer (2014) and *Ousmane Sembene: Writer, Filmmaker, and Revolutionary Artist* with Oumar Cherif Diop (2017). He taught African literature at Fourah Bay College, Gambia College, and the University of the Gambia. He is presently associate editor of *African Literature Today*.

TOYIN FALOLA is the Jacob and Frances Sanger Mossiker Chair in the Humanities and a Distinguished Teaching Professor at the University of Texas at Austin. A celebrated scholar of global stature, Prof. Falola has published numerous books and essays in diverse areas. He has received various awards and honors, including the Jean Holloway Award for Teaching Excellence, the Texas Exes Teaching Award, and seven honorary doctorates. He is the series editor of Carolina Studies on Africa and the Black World, among several others.

FIKRU NEGASH GEBREKIDAN is professor of history at St. Thomas University in Fredericton, Canada. Subjects he regularly teaches include African history, world history, genocide, race and racism, slavery, historiography, and disability. He is the author of *Bond without Blood: A History of Ethiopian and New World Black Relations, 1896–1991* (Trenton, NJ: Africa World Press, 2005). He has authored over a half-dozen book chapters and journal articles, including "Disability Rights Activism in Kenya, 1959–1964: History from Below," *African Studies Review* 55, no. 3 (December 2012): 101–121.

KATHRYN LINN GEURTS is professor of anthropology in the Global Studies Department at Hamline University in St. Paul, Minnesota. She is the author of *Culture and the Senses: Bodily Ways of Knowing in an African Community* (University of California Press, 2002) as well as numerous articles on the disability rights movement in Accra, Ghana. She has been the recipient of Guggenheim and Rockefeller Foundation fellowships, a National Institute of Mental Health postdoctoral award, and a Fulbright-Hays grant.

NIC HAMEL is a doctoral candidate in performance as public practice at the University of Texas at Austin. His areas of research interest include disability activism, postcolonial theory, post-Marxism, queer aesthetics, and theater for social change. His dissertation focuses on issues of activist theater and performance strategies for people with intellectual disabilities in a variety of international contexts. More specifically, he examines questions of representation, agency, and structural support for contemporary disability-focused theater companies in Europe, Africa, and the United States.

SERGES DJOYOU KAMGA is a professor of human rights law at the Thabo Mbeki African School of Public and International Affairs, University of South Africa. His areas of interest include the right to development, the African renaissance, and disability rights. He publishes regularly in these areas.

THERESA LORENZO is professor of disability studies and occupational therapy and codirector of Inclusive Practices Africa research unit in the Department of Health and Rehabilitation Sciences, Faculty of Health Sciences, at University of Cape Town (UCT), South Africa. She worked for seven years at Tintswalo Hospital, Acornhoek, where she initiated community-based rehabilitation programs with communities in a rural health district. At UCT, she co-led the development of the first disability studies postgraduate programs in Africa, in collaboration with Disabled People South Africa and the Centre for Disability Studies at Leeds University, UK, which was launched in 2003. She is active in the African Network for Evidence of Action on Disability (AfriNEAD), the CBR Africa Network, and the Occupational Therapy Africa Regional Group (OTARG).

DENISE M. NEPVEUX is an assistant professor of occupational therapy at Utica College. As a 2002 Fulbright Scholar, Dr. Nepveux documented life stories of women in Ghana's disability movement. She continues to collaborate with Ghanaian activists and anthropologist Kathryn Geurts to study changing leadership styles, organizing strategies, gender relations, and transnational funding relationships in this movement. She has published research on sexual health knowledge, identity, and access to sexuality among LGBT youth self-advocates in Ontario and engages in elder organizing efforts in Syracuse, New York.

MARY NYANGWESO is professor and the J. Woolard and Helen Peel Distinguished Chair in Religious Studies at East Carolina University in North Carolina. Her specialization is religion and gender. Nyangweso received her master's in theology from Candler School of Theology, Emory University in Atlanta Georgia, and a PhD from Drew University in Madison, New Jersey. She is the author of *Female Genital Cutting: Mutilation or Cultural Right?* (Praeger, 2014), *Female Circumcision: The Interplay Between Religion, Gender and Culture in Kenya* (Orbis Maryknoll, NY:

2007) and co-author of *Religion, Gender-Based Violence, Immigration, and Human Rights* (Routledge, 2019). She is a trained sociologist, theologian, and human rights activist whose passion is social equality and empowerment of the marginalized.

Kolawole Olaiya joined the Anderson University English Department in the fall of 2015. His formal academic training includes a BA (Hon.) in dramatic arts from Obafemi Awolowo University Ile-Ife, Nigeria (1987); an MA in English (African literature) from the University of Maiduguri in Nigeria (1995); and a PhD in drama (with specialization in postcolonial drama) at the University of Toronto, (2007). Dr. Olaiya holds certificates in television production, directing, and scriptwriting form institutions in Nigeria, Ghana, France, and Germany. He has professional experience as an assistant director, producer, and director of theater and TV dramas in Nigeria and Canada. His research interests include Africa and African diaspora literatures, cultural studies, postcolonial studies, disability studies, film and television scriptwriting, and literary and film criticism.

Frances Emily Owusu-Ansah is a Catholic Sister of the Institute of the Daughters of the Most Holy Trinity (FST), and also a clinical psychologist and assistant professor at the Kwame Nkrumah University of Science and Technology (KNUST), Ghana. She is an international affiliate of the American Psychological Association (Division 12) and a member of the Ghana Psychological Council. Her passion and research have focused on adult psychotherapy, subjective well-being, disability issues, and indigenous knowledge. She served for years as the vice dean of students for the KNUST and is presently the founding head of the KNUST Counselling Center (KCC). She is the recipient of several awards, including Best Lecturer and the prestigious James Chair Professor of Psychology Award of St. Francis Xavier University, Nova Scotia, Canada.

Ozden Pinar-Irmak is a doctoral student at the University of Massachusetts at Boston in the Early Childhood Education and Care program. Her research areas include African immigrant families in early intervention services, early intervention and education programs for refugee children and their parents, and international inclusive education.

Emmanuel Sackey is a lecturer at the Center for Disability and Rehabilitation Studies, School of Public Health, Kwame Nkrumah University of Science and Technology, Kumasi, Ghana. He holds a PhD in development sociology from the University of Bayreuth, Germany. His research focuses on disability inclusive development, disability and political participation, social movements, civil society organizations and development, and related issues in disability studies and development sociology.

Angi Stone-MacDonald is an associate professor at the University of Massachusetts at Boston in the Early Education and Care in Inclusive Settings program and Associate Dean for Grants and Research in the College of Education and Human Development. She received her doctorate from Indiana University in special education and African studies. Her areas of research include early intervention, international special education for children with developmental disabilities, and teacher preparation for early intervention. Her current research agenda includes early intervention personnel preparation in the United States and inclusive early childhood education in Tanzania, Africa.

Ntombekhaya Tshabalala is founder director of Imijeloyophuhliso Foundation, South Africa. She is an intrepid social entrepreneur with twenty-five years' experience in the social and (partly) academic sectors, much of it working on promoting inclusive communities, social entrepreneurship, and building ecosystems for said communities. She is passionate about the use of photo-voice and cartoons as participatory action research tools to raise consciousness while mobilizing community groups into social action and inclusive and compassionate leadership. She envisions her major interest, that of contributing to disability and financial inclusion, achieved through the establishment of Financial Resource Centres, the community contact points where people collaboratively interrogate socioeconomic challenges and receive support and mentoring on sustainable ways of addressing financial challenges.

Index

Abeokuta, 108
ableism, 52, 67, 92, 179, 180, 270, 372
Aborigines, 100
abortion, 61
Accra, 22, 33, 119, 141, 149, 151, 153, 155, 293, 296, 319, 321, 326, 327, 344–46, 348, 351, 354, 359, 426
Adedeji, Joel, 197
Adelugba, Dapo, 197, 198, 199
Afghanistan, 165
African Charter, 25, 247, 261, 400, 417
African Child Policy Forum, 406
African Christians, 15
Africanism, 188
African Moralities, 80
African Muslims, 13
African ontologies, 79, 80, 84, 85, 87, 140, 149, 156
African Union, 256
African union policy documents, 256
Afrocentric, 8
Agbettor, Elizabeth Ladner Babi, viii, 45, 286
Aiken, Ama de-Graft, 143
albinism, 35, 36, 38, 103, 117, 121, 122, 129, 322
Aldersey, Heather, 28
Alger, Horatio, 96
Allina, Eric, 21
Alvarez, Francisco, 109
American Psychological Association, 55, 428
Amin, Idi, 116

Amkpa, Awam, 188
amputation, 30, 31, 45, 122, 137, 141, 161, 163–67, 169–72, 174–83, 204
Angola, 21, 30
Anlo, 10
Arab Spring, 41
Aristotle, 66
Ark of the Covenant, 110
Asch, Adrienne, 59
Asibey, Emmanuel Osei, 294
Australia, 54, 104, 364

Bailey, Richard, 365
Baka, 10, 97, 98, 99
Barclay, Jenifer L., 6–10, 423
Barth, Fredrik, 107
Bashuna, Ali Balla, 101
Baynton, Douglas, 65
BBC, 117, 121, 405
BDA (Busia Disabled Association), 156
Beier, Ulli, 194
Beijing, 320, 328
Bell, Chris, 53
Bemba, 106
Beng, 12
Benin, 36, 119, 121, 122, 250
Ben-Moshe, Liat, 57, 58
Berg, Alison, 144
Berger, Peter, 127
Berghs, Maria, vii, 23, 31, 44, 75–79, 105, 135, 141, 142, 425
Bérubé, Michael, 191
Bezzina, Lara, 41

Biafran, 201, 202
Biafran civil war, 201
bioethics, 53, 59, 87
blindness, 2, 12, 15, 45, 55, 102, 105–09, 112–14, 117, 120, 123, 128, 139, 154, 155, 158, 194, 195, 238, 252, 253, 262, 272, 291–96, 302, 304, 325, 336, 351, 378–80, 382, 384
Botswana, 2, 10, 22, 29, 30, 145, 147–49, 158, 194, 204, 424
Braidotti, Rosi, 139
Brégain, Gildas, 19, 20
Brisendon, Simon, 56
Britain. *See* United Kingdom
Brook, Peter, 107
Brotmacher, Leon, 101
Brueggemann, Brenda Jo, 50, 68
Buhari, Muhammadu, 417
Bukumunhe, Rosallie B., 14
Bulozi, 106
Burkina Faso, 41, 121
Burton, Richard, 101
Burundi, 36
Byrne, Peter, 213

Cameroon, 10, 36, 97, 98, 365
Campbell, Greg, 168, 175
Canada, 54, 311, 326, 365, 426, 428
Cape Verde, 40
Carothers, Anna Lee, v, vii, ix, 46, 47, 405, 425
CATCID (United Nations Convention against Torture and Other Cruel, Inhuman or Degrading Treatment or Punishment), 131
CBR (community-based rehabilitation), 42, 43, 45, 46, 288–90, 292, 305, 322, 397, 398, 402, 427
CDC (US Centers for Disease Control and Prevention), 47, 62

CEDAW (Convention on Discrimination against Women), 131, 320
Central Africa, 20, 416
Chad, 18
Chagga, 9, 119
Charlton, James, 144
Chataika, Tsitsi, 6, 11, 26, 40, 241, 418
Chiwandire, Desire, viii, 40, 46, 361, 384, 425
Christianity, 12–15, 44, 93, 94, 108–11, 128, 143, 264, 396
Clancy, Jim, 162
Clifford, James, 228
Coetzee, J. M., viii, 45, 228–38
Cole, Ernest, vii, 11, 30, 31, 45, 161, 162, 303, 423, 426
colonialism, 1, 3, 4, 7, 8, 15–22, 29, 81, 82, 91, 102, 105, 106, 109, 114, 139, 212, 229, 230, 231, 233–35, 258, 322
Conteh, Morlai Bizo, 171
Convention on the Rights of Persons with Disability, 321
Convention on the Rights of Person with Disabilities, 255, 256
Côte des Somalis, 20
Côte d'Ivoire, 9, 12
CPP (Convention's People's Party), 344
CRC (United Nations Convention on the Rights of the Child), 261
Crenshaw, Kimberlé, 126
CRPD (Convention on the Rights of People with Disabilities), 37, 38, 77, 86, 91, 133, 134, 242–45, 251, 256, 264, 289, 323, 324, 349, 355, 356, 358–60, 362, 369, 381, 388–91, 396, 398, 402, 404, 407, 413
cultural beliefs, 271
cyberculture, 67

DALY (Disability Adjusted Life Year), 78

Darwinian, 99
Davis, Lennard, 6, 29, 53, 54, 57, 58, 61, 72, 111
deafness, 3, 15, 40, 51, 70, 106, 108–10, 123, 139, 154, 155, 157, 158, 197, 245, 262, 272, 304, 326, 350, 351
De Coster, Jori, 34, 157, 158, 423
Denmark, 187
D'Errico, Nicole, 103
Devlieger, Patrick J., 9–12, 33, 34, 80, 81, 138, 139, 142, 157, 270, 423
DFID (Department for International Development), 258, 265
DHET (Department of Higher Education and Training), 371
Diamond, Jared, 97, 104
disability: African disability studies, 6, 24, 29, 30, 46, 80, 92, 93, 102, 105, 114; categorization, 50; children with disabilities, 12, 31, 32, 45, 83, 117, 118, 129, 133, 242, 243, 253, 256–66, 269, 272, 273, 276–79, 282–84, 304, 405–7, 420; disability community, 42, 54, 154, 192; disability rights, viii, 27, 33, 36, 42, 43, 49–51, 61, 115, 134, 246, 247, 249, 323, 358, 359, 373, 389, 390, 407, 408, 412, 417, 426; disability rights activists, 51, 53, 419; disability studies scholars, 1, 4, 52, 53, 62, 66; disabled soldiers, 139; ethics and disability, 87; feminist disability scholars, 63, 64; invisible disabilities, 57; mentally disabled, 226; studies, 2, 50, 52, 62, 64
Disability Discrimination Act, 56
disabilization, 241
Donnelly, Jack, 131, 132
Down syndrome, 61
DPOs (isabled people's organizations), 31, 32, 33, 41–44, 46, 135, 138, 149, 305, 319, 320, 322–29, 336, 338–41, 345–48, 353, 354, 358, 360, 421
DRC (Democratic Republic of the Congo), 144
Duala, 20
Dube, Andrew, 134
Duret, Eric, 178
DUSMs (disability unit staff members), 361, 371, 376, 380, 382, 384–86

East Africa, viii, 9, 12, 17, 20, 92, 101, 119, 255, 257, 259, 267, 268, 271, 274, 284, 285
Eastern Cape, 34, 305
Ebola, 78, 79
ECD (Early Childhood Development), 304
ECOMOG (Economic Ceasefire Monitoring Group), 167
Edemikpong, Ntiense Ben, 37
Egypt, 8, 9, 13, 41, 313
Eisland, Nancy, 127
Ekiti, 215
Engel, George L., 125
Erevelles, Nirmala, 5, 63, 71
Eritrea, 40
Esdros, Mamher, 112
Ethiopia, ii, 27, 93, 94, 101, 109, 110, 112, 118, 409
Ethiopian Orthodoxy, 111
eugenics, 61, 93
Eurocentric knowledge, 95
Euthanasia, 59
Evans-Pritchard, E. E., 140

Falola, Toyin, ii, iii, iv, vii, ix, 1, 8, 46, 47, 199, 405, 426
Fanon, Frantz, 4, 5
Feinstein, Sheryl, 103
feminist disability studies, 63, 64
FET (Further Education and Training), 378

FGM (female genital mutilation), 36, 37
Finkelstein, Victor, 3, 93, 94
Foundation for Human Rights Initiative, 264
France, 20, 40, 428
Franco-French, 19
French East Africa, 20
French National Assembly, 18
French West Africa, 19, 20

GAB (Ghana Association of the Blind), 154, 302
Gaddafi, Muammar, 41
Gambia, 112, 161, 162, 400, 401, 418, 426
Garland-Thomson, Rosemarie, 4, 49, 50, 62–66, 68–71
Gates, Henry Louis, 187
Gberie, Lansana, 167, 168, 170, 171
GBU (Ghana Blind Union), 291, 292, 294–96, 300, 302, 305, 346
Gebrekidan, Fikru Negash, vii, 33, 44, 91, 426
Geertz, Clifford, 100
gender-based violence, 129
gender policy, 321, 323, 324, 327
Gerimma, Aba, 109
Geurts, Kathryn Linn, vii, 22, 44, 426
GFD (Ghana Disability Federation), 322, 323, 324, 327
GFDO (Ghana Federation of Disability Organizations), 343, 344, 346, 347, 356
Ghana, viii, 10, 28, 33, 36–38, 45, 46, 119, 141, 142, 149–51, 153–55, 210, 212, 213, 257, 258, 290–92, 300, 302, 306–10, 319–26, 328, 340, 341, 343–50, 35–56, 358, 359, 409, 424–28
globalization, ii, 5, 71, 77, 141

global North, 3, 4, 11, 25, 29, 31, 42, 43, 78–81, 84, 87, 114, 141, 144, 187, 208, 321, 407, 408, 418, 421
global South, 2, 5, 22, 24, 25, 28–30, 35, 36, 40, 71, 75–78, 80, 91, 92, 114, 139, 145, 151, 205, 206, 224, 319, 321, 358, 407, 408, 418, 423
GNAD (Ghana National Association of the Deaf), 343, 344, 346
Goodley, Dan, 5, 6, 24, 29
Grech, Shaun, 22, 24, 29, 35, 76, 91, 407
GSB (Ghana Society for the Blind), 302, 346
GSPD (Ghana Society of the Physically Disabled), 343, 346
Guinea-Bissau, 13, 42

Haang'andu, Privilege, 40
Hamel, Nic, iii, iv, vii, 1, 45–47, 185, 427
Harar, 101
Harare, 117
Harkins, Eugene, 175
Harris, Cornwallis, 109, 110
Heaton, Matthew, 8, 15, 16
HEIs (higher education institutions), 40, 369, 371–73, 378, 387, 388
Henderson, Carol, 183
Hill, Damon, 407
Hilton, Leon, 191
HIV/AIDS, 34–36, 38, 122, 140, 142, 143, 157, 213, 312, 314, 416, 417, 420
Hogan, Patrick Colm, 195
Hollywood, 164
homophobia, 52
Hubeer, 9, 146, 147

Ibadan, 108, 118, 197, 220
Igbo, 10, 119
Igwe, Ifeoma Agela, 117

Ik, 107
Ikuenobe, Polycarp, 25
Iliffe, John, 106, 108
IMF (International Monetary Fund), 77
Ingstad, Benedicte, 2, 9, 12, 24, 31, 33, 35, 80, 81, 92, 138, 144–46, 151, 156, 423
Intersectionality, 64, 65, 126
Inuit, 100
Iraq, 165
Islam, 12–14, 19, 26, 31, 93, 94, 108, 109, 112, 113, 128
Issa, 101
Ituri Forest, 99

Janzen, John, 144
Jeyifo, Biodun, 185
Jinja, 116
Ju/'hoansi, 98

Kafer, Alison, 63, 67, 126, 127
Kalahari, 3, 98, 100
Kamara, Isatu, 171, 172
Kamara, Mariatu, 175
Kamga, Serges Djoyou, viii, 25, 38, 45, 46, 241, 242, 247, 249, 389, 424, 427
Kano, 108, 109
Kano Chronicle, 109
Kassam, Aneesa, 101
Katrak, Ketu H., 199, 200
Kayogoro, 117
Kebede, Mesele Terecha, 110
Kelani, Tunde, 211, 221, 222, 225
Kenya, ii, 11, 12, 15, 17, 31, 33, 35–37, 100, 101, 103, 119, 252, 254, 256, 257, 260, 261, 267, 272, 273, 366, 368, 382, 405, 406, 413, 418, 423, 424, 426, 427
Khadiya, 152
Kinshasa, 33, 34, 157, 158, 423
Kleege, Georgina, 50, 68

Krio, 163
Kuba, 106
Kuchera, Masimba, 117

LDA (Lunatics Detention Act), 400
LGBTQ+, 64, 421
Liberia, 83
Libya, 20, 21, 41
Lindfors, Bernth, 185
Livingston, Julie, 10, 22, 29, 147, 194, 204
Lobatse, 145
Lobo, Jeronimo, 111, 112
London, 2, 3, 5, 6, 8–11, 15, 20, 21, 26, 29, 35, 39, 40, 49, 71, 77, 78, 85, 86, 97, 101, 104, 106, 110–12, 119, 127, 132, 134, 135, 151–53, 188, 192, 228, 241, 248, 269, 274, 275, 285, 303, 311, 313, 363, 365–67, 372, 374, 385, 386, 394, 395, 401, 405, 406
Lorenzo, Theresa, viii, 6, 23, 32, 45, 130, 286, 424, 427
LSU (Legal Services Unit), 415
Lushoto, 277, 278, 279, 280, 281, 285

Maasai, 101, 102, 103
Maasailand, 102, 103
Maasiland, 12
Madagascar, 14, 15, 20, 40
Mahone, Sloan, 17
Makanda, 117
Maksini, Wandera, 116
malaria, 16, 140
Malawi, 26, 27, 36, 252, 411, 416
Mali, 7, 9, 111, 114
Mandela, Nelson, 3, 369, 426
Manninen, Bertha Alvarez, 61, 62
Marxism, 94
Mazrui, Ali A., 7
Mbembe, Achille, 3, 7, 194, 206, 207
Mbuti, 99, 100, 107

McCartney, Barney, 202
McDonald, David A., 24
McKenzie, Judith, 11, 27, 35, 77
McRuer, Robert, 5, 48, 66, 67
MDGs (Millennium Development Goals), 287
Meekosha, Helen, 5, 25, 71, 78, 92, 407
mental illness, 210, 212, 213, 215, 226, 409, 410
Middle East, 106, 111, 267
Miles, Susie, 42
Millennium Development goals and Education for All, 261
Miller, Patricia, 362
Mitchell, David T., 4, 88, 179, 189–91, 243, 284
MOES (Ministry of Education and Sport), 263
Mogadishu, 152
Molefi, Rra, 149
Mollien, Gaspard, 112
Morocco, 11, 32, 40
Mozambique, ii, 21, 40
Msiri, 106
Murove, M. F., 134, 135
Mutilations, 167
Mutua, Makau, 25

NABCO (Nation Builders Corps), 291
Namigambo, Sabina, 120
National Federation for the Blind, 55
NCPD (National Council for Persons with Disabilities), 349–53, 355, 359, 360
NEC (National Electoral Commission), 351
Neef, Max, 289
Neille, Joanne, 26
neoliberalism, 30, 139
neolithic, 97, 104, 105
Nepveux, Denise, 8, 46, 153, 319, 325

NGO, 31, 33, 43, 142, 157, 281, 282
Ngue, Julie Nack, 18, 194
Nguni language, 250
Nigeria, ii, 7, 10, 13, 14, 17, 33, 36, 39, 92, 117–19, 122, 147, 158, 186, 195, 199, 210–13, 217, 220, 227, 251, 313, 382, 410, 411, 417, 428
Nile River, 116
Nkoranza, 142
Nkrumah, Kwame, 4, 322, 344, 424, 428
Nollywood, viii, 35, 45, 209–12, 215, 216, 219, 221, 224, 227
NORAD (Norwegian Agency for Development Cooperation), 347
North Africa, 19, 26, 41
Norway, 2
Nyangweso, Mary, vii, 37, 44, 115, 427

Obafemi, Olu, 198, 199
Obatala, 119, 120, 194–97, 221, 224
Oduduwa, 119
OECD (Organization for Economic Co-operation and Development), 408
Olaiya, Kolawole, viii, 35, 45, 209, 224, 428
Olanrewaju, Abiodun, 211, 216
Oliver, Michael, 48, 49, 52, 94, 127, 179
Olodumare, 119, 224
Ologbojo, Ologbin, 199
Olorun, 120
Ontario, 54, 427
Orisha, 119, 194
Oromo, ii, 101
Òrùka Ìjọsí, 216, 217
Oseni, Taibat, 122
Osofisan, Femi, 201
Owusu-Ansah, Frances, 28
Owusu-Ansah, Frances Emily, viii, 45, 306, 428

Paleolithic, 95, 96
Parker, George, 178
Parmeleu, 102
Penn, Claire, 26
Pilgrim, David, 126
Pinar Irmak, Ozden H., 45, 255
Pinker, Steven, 96, 97
Pokot, 100
postcolonialism, 188
postmodernism, 49, 139
Power, Marcus, 21
pre–Neolithic Age, 97
PRSPs (Poverty Reduction Strategy Papers), 77
Puar, Jasbir, 72, 194, 205
punitive amputation, 30, 163, 164, 166, 169, 175, 176, 178, 180–82
PWDs (persons with disabilities), 38, 77, 245, 246, 344, 345, 347, 348, 350, 351, 354–56, 358, 359, 362–68, 371–77, 379, 381, 385, 386

Quayson, Ato, 186–94, 196, 202, 203, 205, 206, 215, 219, 228, 230, 424
Qur'an, 12

racism, 15, 18, 19, 30, 52, 76, 81, 93, 126, 372, 426
Rainbow School, 277, 278, 280
Red Sea, 101
Renne, Elishe, 147
Rose, Martha, 104
Rosenberg, Harriet, 98
RUF (Revolutionary United Front), 161–64, 167–69, 171–74
Rutachwamagyo, Kaganz, 12, 103
Rwanda, 22, 27, 31, 264, 265, 272, 363

Sahel Africa, 110, 111
Sahlins, Marshall, 96, 113
Salamanca Statement, 255, 256, 261
Salamanca World Conference, 256
Sandahl, Carrie, 55, 67
Sanger, Margaret, ii, 64, 65, 426
Sankok, David ole, 406
SARAs (sport and recreational activities), 361, 362, 369–71, 373, 378, 379, 383, 385, 388
SASSA (South African Social Security Agency), 304
Saxton, Marsha, 61
Scalenghe, Sara, 13, 93, 112
SCGs (Savings and Credit Groups), 297–99
Schalk, Sami, 67
SDGs (Sustainable Development Goals), 76, 86, 88, 287
SDS (Society for Disability Studies), 52
Sen, Amartya, 32, 268, 269, 285
Senegal, 18, 112
Senghorian regime, 18
sexism, 52, 372
sexuality, 26, 35, 140, 210, 215, 266
Shakespeare, William, 4, 49, 53, 125, 187, 267, 412–14
Sharia law, 31
Shewan highlands, 110
Shona, 11, 135
SICGs (Savings, Investments, and Credit Groups), 301, 303
SIDA (Swedish International Development Cooperation Agency), 115, 134
Siebers, Tobin, 51, 179, 180
Sierra Leone, 17, 30, 31, 43, 45, 78, 81–84, 141, 142, 158, 162–69, 171–76, 178, 182, 183, 413, 418, 423, 425
Simwe Hounto, 121
Slattery, Dennis P., 177
smallpox, 16
Snyder, Sharon L., 4, 179, 189, 190, 191

Sobchack, Vivian, 5
Somali, 101, 151–53, 273
Somalia, 9, 146, 151, 152, 265, 266, 273
Somaliland, 16, 30, 266
Songye, 11, 12
South Africa, 3, 6, 23–27, 31, 34, 37–41, 45, 54, 76, 77, 88, 105, 130, 250, 251, 258, 272, 288, 297, 300, 305, 306, 312, 352, 366, 369, 370, 377, 381, 409, 414, 415, 424, 425, 427, 429
Soyinka, Wole, vii, 45, 185–88, 190, 192–203, 205–08, 221
SSCIID (Section for the Study of Chronic Illness, Impairment, and Disability), 52
Standard Rules on the Equalization of Opportunities for Persons with Disabilities, 133, 255, 345
stone age, 96
Stone-MacDonald, Angi, viii, 9, 45, 92, 255, 267, 271, 429
sub-Saharan Africa, 11, 121, 242, 253, 254, 258, 271, 276, 283
Swartz, Leslie, 23, 24, 31, 35, 77, 78, 80, 81, 412, 416, 417, 424
Swaziland, 40
SWDs (students with disabilities), 40, 361, 362, 368, 369–81, 382–88

Talle, Aud, 101, 151, 152
Tanzania, 9, 11, 28, 36, 45, 101, 103, 117, 120–22, 257, 259, 260, 267, 270, 271, 276–81, 283, 284, 286, 424, 429
Tietze, Ulrich, 30
Tonoukouin, Sena Mireille, 121
Torner, Josephat, 120
TRC (Truth and Reconciliation Committee), 166, 167, 172
Tshabalala, Ntombekhaya, viii, 45, 286, 288, 429
Tswana, 22, 148
Tunisia, 14, 32, 41, 425
Turnbull, Colin, 99, 107

ubuntu, 22–26, 40, 80, 85, 86, 93, 105–08, 113, 118, 126, 134, 135, 250, 251, 253, 419, 421
Uganda, 32, 33, 37, 42, 83, 107, 116, 118, 134, 155, 156, 158, 257, 262–64, 272, 284, 407, 413
UNDESA (United Nations Department for Economic and Social Affairs), 92
UNESCO, 244, 255, 256, 258, 265, 287, 344, 350, 378
United Kingdom, 4, 18, 48, 52, 54, 56, 61, 99, 109, 271, 364, 400, 425
United Nations Commission on Human Rights, 130
United Nations Decade of Disabled Persons, 145
United Nations Declaration of the Rights of Children, 131
United Nations Human Rights Office, 121, 417
United States of America, iv, 48, 50–54, 56, 61, 68, 88, 138, 273, 280, 307, 312, 320, 321, 324, 351, 355, 365, 390, 398, 399, 407, 427, 429
Universal Declaration of Human Rights, 130, 261
UN (United Nations), 76, 77, 86, 88, 133, 136, 171, 320, 345, 351, 355, 398
UPIAS (Union of the Physically Impaired against Segregation), 52, 394
USAID, 258, 323

Walcott, Derek, 186

War-Affected Amputee Association, 142
Washington, DC, 15, 34, 41, 51, 63, 96, 348, 376, 417
WB (World Bank), 77
West Africa, 19, 20, 22, 84, 93, 94, 113, 119, 168, 171, 198, 199, 222, 300, 416, 425
Western Cape, 34, 88, 249, 363, 369, 370
WFP (World Food Programme), 171
WHO (World Health Organisation), 75, 78, 115, 122, 123, 130, 287, 289, 290, 294, 302, 303, 367, 391, 393, 397, 398, 406, 416, 417, 424
WID (World Institute on Disability), 61
Willis, John Thabiti, 199
World Bank, 47, 50, 77, 258, 406, 417
World Declaration on Education for All, 255
World War I, 20
World War II, 17, 96, 105, 138, 261

Wright, Derek, 119, 128, 186, 187, 196, 369, 370, 382

Yanomamo, 100
yellow fever, 16
YLD (Years Living with Disability), 78
Yoruba, 45, 108, 119, 186, 187, 193–200, 210, 211, 212, 216, 218, 220–25
Yorubaland, 10

Zahra, Saloua Ali Ben, viii, 14, 19, 26, 45, 228, 425
Zaire. *See* Democratic Republic of Congo
Zambia, 39, 411, 413, 418
Zeila, 101
Zimbabwe, 11, 27, 28, 35, 36, 40, 117, 119, 241, 250, 258, 374, 385, 423
Zola, Irving, 54, 55